1997
YEAR BOOK OF
GERIATRICS AND GERONTOLOGY®

Statement of Purpose

The YEAR BOOK Service

The YEAR BOOK series was devised in 1901 by practicing health professionals who observed that the literature of medicine and related disciplines had become so voluminous that no one individual could read and place in perspective every potential advance in a major specialty. In the final decade of the 20th century, this recognition is more acutely true than it was in 1901.

More than merely a series of books, YEAR BOOK volumes are the tangible results of a unique service designed to accomplish the following:

- to *survey* a wide range of journals of proven value
- to *select* from those journals papers representing significant advances and statements of important clinical principles
- to provide *abstracts* of those articles that are readable, convenient summaries of their key points
- to provide *commentary* about those articles to place them in perspective

These publications grow out of a unique process that calls on the talents of outstanding authorities in clinical and fundamental disciplines, trained literature specialists, and professional writers, all supported by the resources of Mosby, the world's preeminent publisher for the health professions.

The Literature Base

Mosby and its editors survey more than 1,000 journals published worldwide, covering the full range of the health professions. On an annual basis, the publisher examines usage patterns and polls its expert authorities to add new journals to the literature base and to delete journals that are no longer useful as potential YEAR BOOK sources.

The Literature Survey

The publisher's team of literature specialists, all of whom are trained and experienced health professionals, examines every original, peer-reviewed article in each journal issue. More than 250,000 articles per year are scanned systematically, including title, text, illustrations, tables, and references. Each scan is compared, article by article, to the search strategies that the publisher has developed in consultation with the 270 outside experts who form the pool of YEAR BOOK editors. A given article may be reviewed by any number of editors, from one to a dozen or more, regardless of the discipline for which the paper was originally published. In turn, each editor who receives the article reviews it to determine whether or not the article should be included in the YEAR BOOK. This decision is based on the article's inherent quality, its probable usefulness to readers of that YEAR BOOK, and the editor's goal to represent a balanced picture of a given field in each volume of the YEAR BOOK. In addition, the editor indicates when to include figures and tables from the article to help the YEAR BOOK reader better understand the information.

Of the quarter million articles scanned each year, only 5% are selected for detailed analysis within the YEAR BOOK series, thereby assuring readers of the high value of every selection.

The Abstract

The publisher's abstracting staff is headed by a seasoned medical professional and includes individuals with training in the life sciences, medicine, and other areas, plus extensive experience in writing for the health professions and related industries. Each selected article is assigned to a specific writer on this abstracting staff. The abstracter, guided in many cases by notations supplied by the expert editor, writes a structured, condensed summary designed so that the reader can rapidly acquire the essential information contained in the article.

The Commentary

The YEAR BOOK editorial boards, sometimes assisted by guest commentators, write comments that place each article in perspective for the reader. This provides the reader with the equivalent of a personal consultation with a leading international authority—an opportunity to better understand the value of the article and to benefit from the authority's thought processes in assessing the article.

Additional Editorial Features

The editorial boards of each YEAR BOOK organize the abstracts and comments to provide a logical and satisfying sequence of information. To enhance the organization, editors also provide introductions to sections or individual chapters, comments linking a number of abstracts, citations to additional literature, and other features.

The published YEAR BOOK contains enhanced bibliographic citations for each selected article, including extended listings of multiple authors and identification of author affiliations. Each YEAR BOOK contains a Table of Contents specific to that year's volume. From year to year, the Table of Contents for a given YEAR BOOK will vary depending on developments within the field.

Every YEAR BOOK contains a list of the journals from which papers have been selected. This list represents a subset of the more than 1,000 journals surveyed by the publisher and occasionally reflects a particularly pertinent article from a journal that is not surveyed on a routine basis.

Finally, each volume contains a comprehensive subject index and an index to authors of each selected paper.

The 1997 Year Book Series

Year Book of Allergy, Asthma, and Clinical Immunology: Drs. Rosenwasser, Borish, Gelfand, Leung, Nelson, and Szefler

Year Book of Anesthesiology and Pain Management®: Drs. Tinker, Abram, Chestnut, Roizen, Rothenberg, and Wood

Year Book of Cardiology®: Drs. Schlant, Collins, Gersh, Graham, Kaplan, and Waldo

Year Book of Chiropractic®: Dr. Lawrence

Year Book of Critical Care Medicine®: Drs. Parrillo, Balk, Calvin, Franklin, and Shapiro

Year Book of Dentistry®: Drs. Meskin, Berry, Kennedy, Leinfelder, Roser, Summitt, and Zakariasen

Year Book of Dermatologic Surgery®: Drs Greenway, Papadopoulos, and Whitaker

Year Book of Dermatology®: Drs. Sober and Fitzpatrick

Year Book of Diagnostic Radiology®: Drs. Federle, Gross, Dalinka, Maynard, Rebner, Smirniotopolous, and Young

Year Book of Digestive Diseases®: Drs. Greenberger and Moody

Year Book of Drug Therapy®: Drs. Lasagna and Weintraub

Year Book of Emergency Medicine®: Drs. Wagner, Dronen, Davidson, King, Niemann, and Roberts

Year Book of Endocrinology®: Drs. Bagdade, Braverman, Horton, Kannan, Landsberg, Molitch, Morley, Nathan, Odell, Poehlman, Rogol, and Ryan

Year Book of Family Practice®: Drs. Berg, Bowman, Davidson, Dexter, and Scherger

Year Book of Geriatrics and Gerontology®: Drs. Beck, Burton, Ostwald, Rabins, Reuben, Roth, Shapiro, and Whitehouse

Year Book of Hand Surgery®: Drs. Amadio and Hentz

Year Book of Hematology®: Drs. Spivak, Bell, Ness, Quesenberry, Wiernik, and Blume

Year Book of Infectious Diseases®: Drs. Keusch, Barza, Bennish, Poutsiaka, Skolnik, and Snydman

Year Book of Medicine®: Drs. Klahr, Cline, Petty, Frishman, Greenberger, Malawista, Mandell, and O'Rourke

Year Book of Neonatal and Perinatal Medicine®: Drs. Fanaroff, Maisels, Stevenson

Year Book of Nephrology, Hypertension, and Mineral Metabolism: Drs. Schwab, Bennett, Emmett, Hostetter, Kumar, and Toto

Year Book of Neurology and Neurosurgery®: Drs. Bradley and Wilkins

Year Book of Nuclear Medicine®: Drs. Gottschalk, Blaufox, Neumann, Strauss, and Zubal

Year Book of Obstetrics, Gynecology, and Women's Health: Drs. Mishell, Herbst, and Kirschbaum

Year Book of Occupational and Environmental Medicine®: Drs. Emmett, Frank, Gochfeld, and Hessl

Year Book of Oncology®: Drs. Ozols, Cohen, Glatstein, Loehrer, Tallman, and Wiersma

Year Book of Ophthalmology®: Drs. Wilson, Augsburger, Cohen, Eagle, Flanagan, Grossman, Laibson, Maguire, Nelson, Penne, Rapuano, Sergott, Spaeth, Tipperman, and Ms. Salmon

Year Book of Orthopedics®: Drs. Sledge, Poss, Cofield, Dobyns, Griffin, Springfield, Swiontkowski, Wiesel, and Wilson

Year Book of Otolaryngology–Head and Neck Surgery®: Drs. Paparella and Holt

Year Book of Pathology and Laboratory Medicine: Drs. Mills, Bruns, Gaffey, and Stoler

Year Book of Pediatrics®: Dr. Stockman

Year Book of Plastic, Reconstructive, and Aesthetic Surgery®: Drs. Miller, Cohen, McKinney, Robson, Ruberg, Smith, and Whitaker

Year Book of Podiatric Medicine and Surgery®: Dr. Kominsky

Year Book of Psychiatry and Applied Mental Health®: Drs. Talbott, Ballenger, Breier, Frances, Meltzer, Schowalter, and Tasman

Year Book of Pulmonary Disease®: Dr. Petty

Year Book of Rheumatology®: Drs. Sergent, LeRoy, Meenan, Panush, and Reichlin

Year Book of Sports Medicine®: Drs. Shephard, Alexander, Drinkwater, Eichner, George, and Torg

Year Book of Surgery®: Drs. Copeland, Bland, Deitch, Eberlein, Howard, Luce, Seeger, Souba, and Sugarbaker

Year Book of Thoracic and Cardiovascular Surgery®: Drs. Ginsberg, Wechsler, and Williams

Year Book of Urology®: Drs. Andriole and Coplin

Year Book of Vascular Surgery®: Dr. Porter

1997

The Year Book of GERIATRICS AND GERONTOLOGY®

Editor

John R. Burton, M.D.

Professor of Medicine, The Johns Hopkins University School of Medicine; Director, Division of Geriatric Medicine, Johns Hopkins Bayview Medical Center; Clinical Director, Division of Geriatric Medicine and Gerontology, The Johns Hopkins University, Baltimore, Maryland

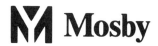 Mosby

St. Louis   Baltimore   Boston   Carlsbad   Chicago   Naples   New York   Philadelphia   Portland
London   Madrid   Mexico City   Singapore   Sydney   Tokyo   Toronto   Wiesbaden

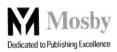

Mosby
Dedicated to Publishing Excellence

A Times Mirror
Company

Vice President and Publisher, Continuity Publishing: Kenneth H. Killion
Director, Editorial Development: Gretchen C. Murphy
Acquisitions Editor: Li Wen Huang
Developmental Editor, Continuity: Kelly Poirier
Associate Production Editor: Anna Wleklinski
Assistant Project Supervisor, Production: Sandra Rogers
Freelance Staff Supervisor: Barbara M. Kelly
Illustrations and Permissions Coordinator: Steven J. Ramay
Director, Editorial Services: Edith M. Podrazik, B.S.N., R.N.
Information Specialist: Kathleen Moss, R.N.
Information Specialist: Terri Santo, R.N.
Circulation Manager: Lynn D. Stevenson

1997 EDITION
Copyright © April 1997 by Mosby–Year Book, Inc.

Printed in the United States of America
Composition by Reed Technology and Information Services, Inc.
Printing/binding by Maple-Vail

Mosby–Year Book, Inc.
11830 Westline Industrial Drive
St. Louis, MO 63146

Customer Service:
customer.support@mosby.com
www.mosby.com/Mosby/CustomerSupport/index.html

Editorial Office:
Mosby–Year Book, Inc.
161 North Clark Street
Chicago, IL 60601
series.editorial@mosby.com

International Standard Serial Number: 0894-2757
International Standard Book Number: 0-8151-0640-8

Associate Editors

John C. Beck, M.D.
Professor of Medicine Emeritus, University of California, Los Angeles, California

Sharon K. Ostwald, Ph.D., R.N., C.S.
Theodore J. and Mary E. Trumble Professor; Director, Center on Aging, University of Texas–Houston School of Nursing, Houston, Texas

Peter V. Rabins, M.D., M.P.H.
Professor of Psychiatry, The Johns Hopkins University School of Medicine, Baltimore, Maryland

David B. Reuben, M.D.
Associate Professor of Medicine; Chief, Division of Geriatrics; Director, Multicampus Division of Geriatric Medicine and Gerontology, University of California, Los Angeles, California

Jesse Roth, M.D.
Raymond and Anna Lublin Professor of Medicine; Director, Division of Geriatric Medicine and Gerontology, The Johns Hopkins University School of Medicine, Baltimore, Maryland

Jay R. Shapiro, M.D.
Professor of Medicine, Division of Geriatric Medicine and Gerontology, The Johns Hopkins University School of Medicine; Program Director, General Clinical Research Center, Johns Hopkins Bayview Medical Center, Baltimore, Maryland

Peter J. Whitehouse, M.D., Ph.D.
Director, Alzheimer Center, University Hospitals of Cleveland; Professor of Neurology and Chief, Division of Behavioral and Geriatric Neurology, Case Western Reserve University, Cleveland, Ohio

Table of Contents

Journals Represented

Mosby and its editors survey more than 1,000 journals for its abstract and commentary publications. From these journals, the editors select the articles to be abstracted. Journals represented in this YEAR BOOK are listed below.

Acta Psychiatrica Scandinavica
Advances in Nursing Science
Age and Ageing
Aging: Clinical and Experimental Research
Alzheimer Disease and Associated Disorders
American Journal of Alzheimer's Disease
American Journal of Clinical Nutrition
American Journal of Epidemiology
American Journal of Gastroenterology
American Journal of Geriatric Psychiatry
American Journal of Medicine
American Journal of Ophthalmology
American Journal of Pathology
American Journal of Physiology
American Journal of Psychiatry
American Journal of Public Health
American Journal of Respiratory and Critical Care Medicine
American Journal of Surgery
Annals of Emergency Medicine
Annals of Epidemiology
Annals of Internal Medicine
Annals of Neurology
Applied Nursing Research
Archives of Family Medicine
Archives of General Psychiatry
Archives of Neurology
Archives of Ophthalmology
Archives of Otolaryngology–Head and Neck Surgery
Bone
British Journal of Psychiatry
British Journal of Urology
British Medical Journal
Canadian Medical Association Journal
Cancer Research
Cell
Circulation
Circulation Research
Clinical Cancer Research
Clinical Pharmacology and Therapeutics
Diabetes Care
Endocrinology
European Urology
Family Practice
Gerontologist
Hypertension
International Journal of Geriatric Psychiatry
International Journal of Nursing Studies

Journal of Affective Disorders
Journal of Clinical Endocrinology and Metabolism
Journal of Clinical Epidemiology
Journal of Clinical Immunology
Journal of Clinical Investigation
Journal of Experimental Medicine
Journal of General Internal Medicine
Journal of Gerontological Nursing
Journal of Gerontology
Journal of Immunology
Journal of Neurology
Journal of Neuropsychiatry and Clinical Neurosciences
Journal of Urology
Journal of the American College of Cardiology
Journal of the American Geriatrics Society
Journal of the American Medical Association
Journal of the National Cancer Institute
Laboratory Investigation
Lancet
Mechanisms of Ageing and Development
Medical Care
Medicine and Science in Sports and Exercise
Nature
Neurology
New England Journal of Medicine
Oncology Nursing Forum
Ophthalmology
Proceedings of the National Academy of Sciences
Prostate
Psychiatric Services
Psychological Assessment
Psychosomatic Medicine
Qualitative Health Research
Research in Nursing and Health
Scandinavian Journal of Urology and Nephrology
Schizophrenia Bulletin
Science
Stroke
Urologia Internationalis
Urology
Western Journal of Nursing Research

STANDARD ABBREVIATIONS

The following terms are abbreviated in this edition: acquired immunodeficiency syndrome (AIDS), cardiopulmonary resuscitation (CPR), central nervous system (CNS), cerebrospinal fluid (CSF), computed tomography (CT), deoxyribonucleic acid (DNA), electrocardiography (ECG), health maintenance organization (HMO), human immunodeficiency virus (HIV), intensive care unit (ICU), intramuscular (IM), intravenous (IV), magnetic resonance (MR) imaging (MRI), and ribonucleic acid (RNA).

NOTE

The YEAR BOOK OF GERIATRICS AND GERONTOLOGY® is a literature survey service providing abstracts of articles published in the professional literature. Every effort is made to assure the accuracy of the information presented in these pages. Neither the editors nor the publisher of the YEAR BOOK OF GERIATRICS AND GERONTOLO- GY® can be responsible for errors in the original materials. The editors' comments are their own opinions. Mention of specific products within this publication does not constitute endorsement.

To facilitate the use of the YEAR BOOK OF GERIATRICS AND GERONTOLOGY® as a reference tool, all illustrations and tables included in this publication are now identified as they appear in the original article. This change is meant to help the reader recognize that any illustration or table appearing in the YEAR BOOK OF GERIATRICS AND GERONTOLOGY® may be only one of many in the original article. For this reason, figure and table numbers will often appear to be out of sequence within the YEAR BOOK OF GERIATRICS AND GERONTOLOGY®.

Publisher's Preface

We are pleased to further expand our multidisciplinary approach to geriatric medicine by adding the new chapter "Geriatric Nursing" to this and subsequent editions of the YEAR BOOK OF GERIATRICS AND GERONTOLOGY. Please join us in welcoming Sharon K. Ostwald, Ph.D., R.N., C.S., director of the Center on Aging at the University of Texas–Houston, to our editorial board.

Introduction

The 1997 YEAR BOOK OF GERIATRICS AND GERONTOLOGY is the best ever. We have added a chapter, "Geriatric Nursing," and a new editor, Sharon K. Ostwald, Ph.D., R.N., C.S. We welcome most enthusiastically her contributions to the YEAR BOOK. I am sure you will find them valuable. Geriatric medicine, by its very nature, is multidisciplinary, and there is now emerging literature about geriatric nursing that is important to disseminate.

I also am pleased that all of last year's associate editors have remained and have contributed remarkably to making this edition extraordinary. John Beck, M.D., and David Reuben, M.D., have continued to be responsible for the chapter about clinical geriatrics. Peter Rabins, M.D., M.P.H., has developed the chapter about geriatric psychiatry. Peter Whitehouse, M.D., P.h.D., has developed the chapter about geriatric neurology. And Jesse Roth, M.D., and Jay Shapiro, M.D., jointly created the chapter about gerontologic research.

I would like to personally thank all of the associate editors for an outstanding job with the 1997 edition. They have labored altruistically and diligently over the months in the long process of selecting articles and writing editorial comments. Their timely effort has allowed us to get the manuscript to press on time and to make the book pertinent for readers.

From November 1995 through October 1996, literally thousands of articles are reviewed by the editors. Those that are selected are felt to be representative of important, useful, new knowledge in our field. As I review the 1997 edition, I believe that it contains an enormous amount of information and new ideas valuable for all health care professionals who are working with the elderly or who are interested in the science of aging. This year, the table of contents and the subject index have been well developed so that the reader can easily find subjects of interest that may be covered in different chapters.

I also would like to thank very much the administrative assistants of each of the editors, without whose tireless and dedicated help we simply could not create this YEAR BOOK. The handling of hundreds of articles by each editor and the reworking of comments is a tough job, and they have done it extremely well. These individuals are Kathy Barnes-Sanchez (Roth), Maritsa Lemasson (Shapiro), Kate Jakobsen (Rabins), Faith Reidenbach (Whitehouse), Stephanie Ngo (Reuben), and Dianne Kirven (Oswald).

I would also like to specially acknowledge the extraordinary commitment to this project of my administrative assistant, Sharon Kuta. Her work during the many months of preparation and in doing again and again the editorial comments has helped tremendously in strengthening the value of this book.

The associate editors and I also would like to thank the staff of Mosby–Year Book, Inc.—especially Kelly Poirier, who has again been the developmental editor for this edition. She and her staff do a tremendous job in keeping track of the articles and developing the abstracts so that they are cohesive and crisp.

We still have adhered to our principle of not abstracting review papers. For that reason, I would like to use this introduction to call your attention to an outstanding series of reviews that appeared in the July 5, 1996, issue of *Science*.[1] That entire issue is an extremely rich resource of reviews that cover all aspects of our field. Included are papers about demography and important issues related to funding of health care for the elderly; neurology and drugs that combat Alzheimer's disease; longevity genes; theories about aging, including information about oxidative stress; caloric restriction; replicative senescence; menopause; and the aging of multiple pace makers. The entire series is extremely well done and would be a valuable resource to anyone looking for a treasure to keep on file and refer to from time to time.

I am sure that you will find the 1997 YEAR BOOK OF GERIATRICS AND GERONTOLOGY a very worthwhile review. I certainly have found it so.

John R. Burton, M.D.

Reference

1. *Science* 273:42–74, 1996.

1 Clinical Geriatrics

Introduction

Among the major new research findings of the past year, perhaps the most important have been those related to trophic factors. Although many of these studies must still be regarded as preliminary, clinical trials of growth hormone and estrogen in older persons have been published. A case series indicates that testosterone injections to men who have low serum testosterone levels improved strength. Not all the news has been good, however. Growth hormone did not improve functional ability and was associated with frequent side effects. These articles are just the first of many that will explore the effects of these potent hormones and attempt to identify the appropriate therapeutic niche that they will fill.

Several important studies of osteoporosis also have been published, including a randomized clinical trial of alendronate, a bisphosphonate, which may be a major advance in the treatment of established osteoporosis. In contrast, data from another clinical trial dampen the enthusiasm for vitamin-D supplementation. The risk factors for osteoporotic fractures among men are beginning to be identified through an Australian cohort study.

The importance of risk factors for cardiac and cerebrovascular disease continues to be explored with contributions from both the Established Populations for Epidemiologic Studies of the Elderly and the Honolulu Heart Study. Moreover, studies attempting to ameliorate these risk factors with the use of exercise, weight loss, and estrogens have begun to clarify the efficacy and appropriate choice of these treatments.

Several health services research articles demonstrate the effectiveness of innovations in health care delivery, including a nurse practitioner–based in-home preventive services program, a geriatric multidisciplinary approach to preventing readmissions for congestive heart failure, and a strategy to improve compliance with recommendations from comprehensive geriatric assessment. Observational studies and randomized clinical trials also have contributed to our understanding of the management of specific diseases of major importance to older persons, including benign prostatic hyperplasia, diabetes mellitus, and pressure sores.

Some of these studies will immediately change the way we practice medicine. Others are just the next chapters in stories that continue to unfold. Such evolution of the discipline of clinical geriatrics is a large part of the joy of caring for our elderly patients.

David B. Reuben, M.D.

Successful and Healthy Aging

Successful Aging: Predictors and Associated Activities
Strawbridge WJ, Cohen RD, Shema SJ, et al (California Public Health Found, Berkeley; California Dept of Health Services, Berkeley)
Am J Epidemiol 144:135–141, 1996   1–1

Introduction.—A growing interest in preventing disease and promoting health in older individuals has led to an examination of "successful" aging. Although there is no agreed-upon standard for what constitutes successful aging, the definition adopted for this study assumes the ability to perform without difficulty all the basic physical activities expected of an adult. A group of men and women aged 65–95 years was followed up for 6 years to determine predictors of successful aging.

Methods.—Study participants were members of the Alameda County Study, a longitudinal investigation of factors related to health and mortality. In 1984, 508 cohort members aged 65 years or older completed questionnaires covering matters of health, sociodemographic variables, and behavioral and psychosocial factors. At 6-year follow-up, 356 of the 381 surviving members of the 1984 cohort responded to a second questionnaire. Those who were aging successfully could execute 13 basic activities without difficulty or assistance and 5 physical performance activities with no more than a little difficulty.

Results.—The group of survivors had a mean age of 71.9 years and included 209 women (59%) and 147 men (41%); 88% were white and 12% were black. Whereas nearly 60% were scored as aging successfully in 1984, that proportion decreased to 35% in 1990. Eighteen individuals showed improvement, moving from not aging successfully in 1984 to aging successfully in 1990. There was a strong relationship between baseline successful aging and follow-up successful aging. After adjusting for baseline status, sex, and age, positive predictors of successful aging in 1990 were income above the lowest quintile, 12 or more years of education, and white ethnicity. After adjusting for all variables, behavioral and psychosocial predictors were the absence of depression, having close personal contacts, and walking often for exercise (Table 2). The likelihood of successful aging was reduced by the presence of certain chronic medical conditions.

Conclusions.—Individuals who age successfully and are able to function independently have a good quality of life. Many do paid or volunteer work and participate regularly in activities they enjoy. Their physical health status is generally high, they are not too tired to do things they enjoy, and they report feeling pleasure and excitement more than depression.

TABLE 2.—Baseline Predictors of 1990 Successful Aging for 356 Alameda Study Cohort Members Aged 65–95 Years at Baseline Interviewed in 1984 and 1990

1984 Baseline predictor	OR*	95% CI*
Baseline successful aging and sociodemographic predictors		
Baseline successful aging	7.21	4.06–12.78
White ethnicity	2.12	0.93–4.86
Income above lowest quintile	2.01	0.99–4.11
Aged 65–74 years compared with older	1.82	1.02–3.27
≥12 years of education	1.67	0.98–2.84
Male sex	1.30	0.79–2.11
Married	0.82	0.45–1.51
Chronic conditions		
Diabetes	0.10	0.01–0.79
Asthma	0.27	0.05–1.36
Stroke	0.34	0.07–1.61
Chronic obstructive pulmonary disease	0.41	0.17–0.97
Arthritis	0.43	0.26–0.71
Hearing problems	0.48	0.25–0.89
Cancer	0.73	0.36–1.49
Behavioral and psychosocial predictors		
Not often depressed	1.82	1.05–3.16
Has five or more close personal contacts	1.76	1.02–3.02
Often walks for exercise	1.70	0.98–2.96
Moderate alcohol use	1.48	0.83–2.62
Does not currently smoke cigarettes	1.22	0.60–2.47

* Based upon logistic regression models. All models include age, sex, and baseline successful aging. Behavioral and psychosocial predictors also include adjustments for ethnicity, income, education, and number of chronic conditions.
Abbreviations: OR, odds ratio; CI, confidence interval.
(Courtesy of Strawbridge WJ, Cohen RD, Shema SJ, et al: Successful aging: Predictors and associated activities. *Am J Epidemiol* 144:135–141, 1996.)

▶ Why do some persons age successfully whereas others do not? The authors of this study used prospective Alameda County Study data to identify predictors of successful aging, as defined by functional status and physical performance measures, during the subsequent 6 years. The strongest predictor was successful aging at the baseline interview. Other predictors included white ethnicity, younger age (65–74 years compared with 75 years or older), the absence of specific chronic conditions (diabetes, arthritis, chronic obstructive pulmonary disease, or hearing problems), and specific behavioral or psychosocial factors ("not often depressed," 5 or more close personal contacts, and walking often for exercise). As expected, those who had aged successfully were more engaged in work and leisure activities, had fewer sick days and saw doctors less frequently, and had better mental health. Although some of these predictors are immutable, others (e.g., walking for exercise, increasing personal contacts) may be changed. Perhaps the more important question is whether better management of the chronic diseases associated with unsuccessful aging can make a difference.

D.B. Reuben, M.D.

Physical Activity and Immune Senescence in Men

Shinkai S, Kohno H, Kimura K, et al (Ehime Univ, Japan; Hiroshima Univ, Japan; Suzugamine Women's College, Hiroshima, Japan; et al)
Med Sci Sports Exerc 27:1516–1526, 1995   1–2

Objective.—Immune senescence is primarily a result of a decrease in distribution and function of T cells. Because exercise changes many immune parameters, a study was conducted to compare age-related changes of immune function between young and older sedentary men and older male runners.

Methods.—Counts of immunocompetent cells, natural killer (NK) cell activity, proliferative responses to mitogens PHA and PWM, allogenic mixed lymphocyte reaction, and interleukin (IL)-1β, IL-2, IFN-γ, and IL-4 cytokine production were determined from the venous blood of 17 older recreational runners (average age, 63.8 years), 10 age-matched sedentary controls (average age, 65.8 years), and 16 young sedentary controls (average age, 23.6 years). Elderly runners had jogged an average of 56 minutes 5 days a week for an average distance of 39 km for 17 years. Before each of 5 blood drawings, individuals did not exercise for the previous 36 hours and did not eat or drink anything but water in the previous 10 hours.

Results.—Both of the older groups had significantly lower CD3+ and CD8+ counts, a significantly higher percentage of CD16+, a higher CD4/CD8 ratio, and higher percentages of activated T cells and "memory" helper and cytotoxic T cells than did the younger group. There was no change in NK cell activity or other cytokine production in older individuals. Proliferative responses to PHA and PWM were significantly reduced in older individuals, although proliferative responses of the older runners and rates of IL-2, IFN-γ, and IL-4 production were significantly higher than were those of the older sedentary group. Production of IL-2 was somewhat decreased in the older groups. There were no significant differences between the 2 older groups in numbers of immunocompetent cells.

Conclusion.—Regular endurance exercise in older men appears to slow the development of immune senescence and the decline of cytokine production.

▶ During the past several years, numerous studies have indicated the benefit of exercise in reducing falls, improving osteoarthritis, and preventing disability. In this small cross-sectional study, researchers in Japan demonstrated that elderly runners have better immune function than age-matched sedentary controls. In particular, when compared with their sedentary peers, the elderly runners showed much higher responses to phytohemagglutinin and to pokeweed mitogen, although these responses were not as large as those occurring in younger controls. Cytokine production, particularly IL-2, was high in elderly runners, as high as young control group subjects. Running, however, did not attenuate the age-related changes of lymphocyte subsets.

Although cross-sectional studies of convenience samples do not permit a cause-and-effect relationship to be determined, such data support a potential beneficial role for exercise in maintaining immune function. It would be most helpful if some of the many clinical trials of exercise in older persons that are currently in progress would include preintervention and postintervention measures of immune function.

D.B. Reuben, M.D.

A Home-based Exercise Program for Nondisabled Older Adults
Jette AM, Harris BA, Sleeper L, et al (New England Research Insts, Watertown, Mass; Boston Univ; MGH Inst of Health Professions, Boston; et al)
J Am Geriatr Soc 44:644–649, 1996   1–3

Background.—The benefits of enhanced physical activity among the elderly have been reported. However, more research is needed on the feasibility and efficacy of enhanced physical activity among more representative elderly populations. To determine whether a program called Strong-for-Life would be beneficial, community-dwelling, nondisabled, elderly participants in the program were evaluated.

Methods.—One hundred two individuals, aged 66–87 years, were enrolled in the randomized, controlled trial. Program efficacy was defined by changes in isokinetic upper and lower extremity muscle strength, psychological well-being, and health status.

Findings.—Several significant short-term benefits were associated with 12–15 weeks of exercise, especially in men. The younger individuals had a 10% improvement in knee extensor stength, compared with control patients. The older men significantly differed from control patients in perceived anger, tension, and overall social functioning. In general, men significantly improved in perceived vigor. The program did not benefit women psychologically.

Conclusions.—The Strong-for-Life program produced the best results among individuals aged 66–73 years, especially men. The psychological and social benefits occurred mostly among older male participants.

▶ There are now many studies that show the positive benefits of enhancing levels of physical activity in older individuals. They have largely been done in a purely research mode and therefore have tested the efficacy of exercise rather than the feasibility and effectiveness of exercise in older individuals.

This article describes an in-home strength-training strategy designed specifically for older individuals. It reports on its effectiveness in a community-dwelling sample of individuals 65 years of age and older who had no disability and tested the hypothesis that the program would result in increased lower and upper extremity strength, enhance psychological well-being, and result in measurable improvements in overall health status.

This study showed positive short-term physiologic, psychological, and social benefits to the participants in the home-based strength-training program. Physiologic results, although modest, were clearest among those younger than age 73 years, whereas psychological and social benefits were seen predominantly in the older participants and particularly in men. One of the confounding problems in this study was that there were variable degrees of adherence.

J.C. Beck, M.D.

Reducing Frailty and Falls in Older Persons: An Investigation of Tai Chi and Computerized Balance Training
Wolf SL, and the Atlanta FICSIT Group (Emory Univ, Atlanta, Ga)
J Am Geriatr Soc 44:489–497, 1996   1–4

Introduction.—Identifying and using interventions that can decrease frailty and fall-related injuries in older adults is an important public health priority. Older Chinese adults have been practicing Tai Chi (TC) for more than 3 centuries. This ancient martial art is practiced in the United States

TABLE 5.—Adjusted Estimates From the Anderson-Gill Extension of the Cox Proportional Hazards Model

Variables	Risk Ratio	95% Confidence Interval	P
Time to one or more falls			
FICSIT fall definition			
Tai Chi indicator (0 or 1)	0.511	(0.361, 0.725)	0.017
Balance Training indicator (0 or 1)	0.976	(0.710, 1.341)	0.879
Fell last year	1.756	(1.336, 2.308)	0.0006
Fear of falling	1.160	(1.009, 1.335)	0.0004
Trouble falling asleep	0.606	(0.511, 0.717)	0.00006
Atlanta site specific fall definition			
Tai Chi indicator (0 or 1)	0.525	(0.321, 0.860)	0.010
Balance Training indicator (0 or 1)	1.136	(0.733, 1.760)	0.569
Fell last year	2.016	(1.378, 2.950)	0.0003
Fear of falling	1.417	(1.180, 1.700)	0.0002
Trouble falling asleep	0.611	(0.483, 1.770)	0.00003
Time to one or more injurious falls			
Tai Chi indicator (0 or 1)	0.812	(0.327, 2.020)	0.655
Balance Training indicator (0 or 1)	1.174	(0.490, 2.810)	0.719
Fell last year	3.104	(1.476, 6.530)	0.003
Fear of falling	1.456	(1.039, 2.040)	0.029
Trouble falling asleep	0.915	(0.598, 1.399)	0.680

Abbreviation: FICSIT, Frailty and Injuries: Cooperative Studies of Intervention Techniques.
(Courtesy of Wolf SL, and the Atlanta FICSIT Group: Reducing frailty and falls in older persons: An investigation of Tai Chi and computerized balance training. *J Am Geriatr Soc* 44(5):489–497, 1996.)

mostly by older Asian adults to enhance balance and body awareness. Its health claims have not been evaluated by Western scientific methods. Computerized balance training (BT) provides feedback about balance through the use of transducers imbedded in the floor of a moveable platform. Tai Chi, BT, and an exercise control group (ED) were compared to determine their effects on biomedical, functional, and psychological indicators of frailty (primary outcomes) and their influence on the occurrence of falls (secondary outcomes) in adults age 70 years or older.

Methods.—Two hundred older adults participated in this prospective, randomized, controlled clinical trial. Research subjects were evaluated at baseline and completion of a 15-week intervention by blinded data collectors for: psychosocial, demographic, functional, and biomedical outcomes and fall-related variables from the Frailty and Injuries: Co-operative Studies of Intervention Techniques (FICSIT) database. The occurrence of falls was monitored throughout. Research subjects were randomized to participate in either TC, BT, or ED. Patients in TC met weekly and were encouraged to practice TC at least 15 minutes twice daily. Participants in the ED group were encouraged not to change exercise levels and met weekly for discussions on health-related topics. Research subjects in the BT worked once a week on the platform with the goal of progressively increasing sway to the limits of postural stability.

Results.—Left-hand grip strength was more likely to decline by follow-up in the BT and ED groups, but not the TC group. Compared to baseline, the TC group showed reductions in systolic blood pressure before and after a 12-minute walk after TC participation. Participants in the BT and ED groups improved their walking distance in the 12-minute walk at follow-up, compared to baseline. Those in the TC group decreased the distance they walked by 0.02 miles. Compared with the ED group, TC participants had a reduced fear of falling and increased sense of being able to do all that they would like to do after the TC intervention. The significant risk factors for falling were: fall occurrence in the past year, fear of falling, and trouble falling asleep. The risk of falls was reduced by 47.5% in the TC group after participation in a 15-week TC program (Table 5).

Conclusions.—Participation in a 15-week TC program made a significant difference in the occurrence of falls in elderly adults. Several TC participants reported anecdotal incidents of near falls that they were able to avoid with their new body awareness. Approximately half of the TC group continued to meet as a group informally after the 15-week program.

▶ Several years ago, the National Institute on Aging funded several studies of interventions to improve frailty and/or reduce the effects of falls. The results of this initiative, FICSIT, are now beginning to be published. In 1994, Tinetti et al. published their findings on a multifactorial intervention to reduce the risk of falling.[1] Now, Wolf and colleagues report a comparison of 2 exercise approaches, TC (an ancient Chinese martial arts form) and computerized BT, to mitigate indicators of frailty and reduce the occurrence of falls. Tai Chi was performed by older persons in classes for 15 weeks, and participants were encouraged to practice at least 15 minutes, twice a day at home. The computerized BT was designed to train the older person to move his or her center of mass with no foot displacement to direct a cursor to various targets on a screen.

The findings of the study indicated that TC conferred a variety of health benefits compared with computerized balance training and an education-only control group. Among the most striking of these was a 48% reduction in the number of falls and a 49% gain in the time until 1 or more falls occurred. Although quite promising as a choice of exercise interventions, to be successful, TC programs will have to achieve long-term adherence. Secondary nonadherence has been the Achilles heel of many exercise programs, as participants have dropped out because of illness or simply because of loss of interest. Despite their potential benefit, these life-style changes are among the most difficult to sustain.

D.B. Reuben, M.D.

Reference

1. Tinetti ME, Baker DI, McAvay G, et al: A multifactorial intervention to reduce the risk of falling among elderly people living in the community. *N Engl J Med* 331:821–827, 1994.

▶ The FISCIT, a group of research projects funded by the National Institute on Aging, are identifying some excellent interventions that can reduce frailty and fall-related injuries in older people. Falls are a major cause of death and disability among the elderly; the annual incidence of hip fracture alone is approximately 250,000 persons with the cost of treatment approaching $7 billion. In this article, the effects of 2 exercise approaches are evaluated in community-dwelling persons 70 years of age and older. Tai Chi, an ancient martial arts form, was shown to have a favorable impact on frailty and to reduce the risk of multiple falls by 47.5%. Another article in this same issue of the *Journal of the American Geriatrics Society* reports a related FICSIT study in which TC was successfully used as a 6-month maintenance program after intensive balance and/or weight training in community dwellers older than age 75.[1] If proved effective, TC provides a low-technology, low-cost, low-impact form of exercise that may appeal to many elderly individuals in community and institutional settings.

S.K. Ostwald, Ph.D., R.N.

Reference

1. Wolfson L, Whipple MA, Derby C, et al: Balance and strength training in older adults: Intervention gains and Tai Chi maintenance. *J Am Geriatr Soc* 44:498–506, 1996.

State-Specific Changes in Physical Activity Among Persons Aged ≥65 Years: United States, 1987–1992

(Centers for Disease Control and Prevention)
JAMA 274:1500–1501, 1995   1–5

Background.—Although regular physical activity is known to provide important health benefits, most elderly Americans have sedentary lifestyles. State-specific trends in the prevalence of physical inactivity during leisure time among the elderly were analyzed for 1987–1992.

Methods.—Data from the Centers for Disease Control (CDC) Behavioral Risk Factor Surveillance System (BRFSS), a population-based telephone survey of the noninstitutionalized population, were used in the analysis. The survey included 83,858 people aged 65 years and older living in 49 states and the District of Columbia. Thirty-three reporting areas participated in the BRFSS each year between 1987 and 1992. In addition, a state-specific method and an aggregate method were used to project physical inactivity levels in 1997.

Findings.—The median prevalence of no reported leisure-time physical activity declined from 43.2% in 1987 to 38.5% in 1992 for the 33 reporting areas. Consistent reductions occurred in Maryland, New Mexico, New York, and the District of Columbia. The greatest overall decrease in inactivity during the 6-year period occurred in Rhode Island, which had a 21.5% decline. Massachusetts reported a 15% decline; Ohio, 14.1%; New Mexico, 12.7%; and Maryland, 10.1%. The greatest overall increases in prevalence of inactivity occurred in Montana, West Virginia, Maine, and Georgia. Based on the state-specific and aggregate methods of projection, the median prevalences of no lesisure-time activity for 1997 were 35.9% and 37.1%, respectively.

Conclusions.—In this report, data from the CDC's BRFSS were used to track state-specific trends in the prevalence of leisure-time inactivity among the elderly during a 6-year period. State-specific prevalences for 1997 were also projected.

▶ I selected this report from the CDC because it suggests that one of the national health objectives for the year 2000—the reduction of inactive older persons to 22% of the population—is not being met. With the use of 2 methods, it appears clear that the projected median prevalence of no leisure-time physical activity for 1997 will be either 35.9% or 37.1%—far from the year-2000 goal.

There are a number of limitations to this study, which include that (1) the data are self-reported without any validation; (2) it is possible that subjects may have been active for other reasons, such as their occupation or house work, which lead to misclassification; and (3) there may be variation related to age in the response to the survey questions addressing leisure-time physical activity.

J.C. Beck, M.D.

Survival After the Age of 80 in the United States, Sweden, France, England, and Japan

Manton KG, Vaupel JW (Sanford Inst of Public Policy, Duke Univ, Durham, NC; Odense Univ, Denmark)
N Engl J Med 333:1232–1235, 1995   1–6

Background.—Mortality among young Americans is greater than among residents of many European countries and Japan. These differences lessen in the 65- to 80-year-old age group. New data are now available for mortality comparisons among persons aged 80–100 years.

Methods.—Extinct-cohort methods were used to determine death rates among those born from 1880 through 1894 in the United States, Japan, Sweden, France, and England, including Wales. Only white Americans were included in the U.S. analysis. Extinct-cohort methods use continuously collected data from death certificates rather than census data, which are less reliable.

Findings.—Life expectancy at the age of 80 years and survival between 80 and 100 years of age in the United States significantly exceeded life expectancy in the other countries investigated. Cross-sectional data for 1987 were used to confirm this finding. In the United States, the mean life expectancy for an 80-year-old white woman is 9.1 years and for an 80-year-old white man, 7 years.

Conclusions.—Life expectancy for Americans between the ages of 80 and 100 years is higher than for the Swedish, French, English, or Japanese. The possible explanations for this include current American health policies and conditions as well as lingering cohort effects.

▶ This paper is an intriguing one because of the fascinating questions it raises about the possible outcomes of our present health care system. It is well known that the mortality rate of U.S. citizens is much higher than that of citizens of many other industrialized countries and this is particularly true before the age of 65. Between the ages 65 and 80, these differences gradually decline. This particular study addresses the mortality rates of people 80–100 years of age in this country and compares them to rates in 1 Asian and 3 European countries.

The results are described in the abstract, and I believe it is of interest to raise the possible causes for this dramatic difference in mortality rates of the oldest old. From a conceptual point of view, it might be related to current health policies and conditions or the long-term effects of earlier conditions. One might postulate that poor health insurance coverage is a major disadvantage to younger Americans, whereas older Americans, at least since the middle sixties, have had broad Medicare coverage. It is also possible that reduced survival of disadvantaged groups in this country decreases the heterogeneity of our older population. I know from personal experience that older Americans are much more demanding of high-quality health services than older persons in the other countries. Among the better educated in the United States there is also a much greater emphasis on altering behavior that might reduce risk factors for mortality at advanced ages. I also believe that most elderly in this country receive more effective medical care than in the countries with which this comparison was made.

In terms of some of these hypotheses, one might link the quality of medical and public health interventions in this country to the results that are described in this article, and in the present health care debate it would seem important to consider the mechanisms of success at older ages, as well as the problems that impact both younger and older Americans.

J.C. Beck, M.D.

Primary and Secondary Prevention

Ambient Air Pollution and Hospitalization for Congestive Heart Failure Among Elderly People in Seven Large US Cities
Morris RD, Naumova EN, Munasinghe RL (Med College of Wisconsin, Milwaukee)
Am J Public Health 85:1361–1365, 1995   1–7

Objective.—Although most studies of the health effects of air pollution have emphasized respiratory disease, there is evidence that air pollution may be even more harmful for patients with underlying cardiovascular disease. Several studies have demonstrated associations between high levels of air pollution and hospital admissions for cardiovascular disease. The link between air pollution and hospitalization for congestive heart failure was investigated.

Methods.—The analysis combined existing data on ambient levels of gaseous air pollution, weather conditions, and Medicare hospital admissions data from 1986 through 1989 for 7 U.S. cities: Chicago, Detroit, Houston, Los Angeles, Milwaukee, New York, and Philadelphia. The various data sources were used to generate daily values for hospitalization for congestive heart failure; maximum hourly temperature; and maximum hourly levels of carbon monoxide, nitrogen dioxide, sulfur dioxide, and ozone. The effects of single and multiple pollutants were evaluated in negative binomial regression analyses, with adjustment for temperature, seasonal conditions, and weekly cycles.

Results.—In both single pollutant and multipollutant models and for all 7 cities studied, there was a positive correlation between ambient carbon monoxide levels and hospital admissions for congestive heart failure. This relationship was unaffected by the season of the year, temperature variations, and other important gaseous pollutants. For each 10-ppm increase in carbon monoxide level, the relative risk of hospital admission for congestive heart failure increased by 1.10 to 1.37 (in New York City and Los Angeles, respectively). In Los Angeles, more than 11% of hospital admissions could be attributed to ambient carbon monoxide levels. In the other cities, the percentages ranged from 2% to 4.5% (Fig 1).

Conclusions.—As the ambient carbon monoxide level in the air of American cities increases, so does the number of hospital admissions for congestive heart failure in the elderly. This relationship is not related to the

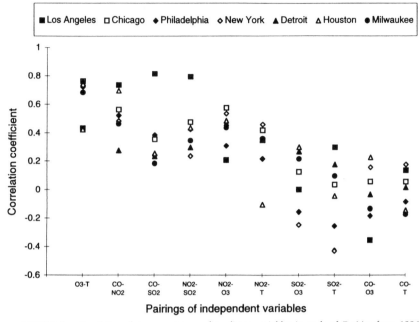

FIGURE 1.—Correlations between pairings of predictor variables in each of 7 cities from 1986 through 1989. *Abbreviations:* O3, ozone; CO, carbon monoxide; NO2, nitrogen dioxide; SO2, sulfur dioxide; T, temperature. (Courtesy of Morris RD, Naumova EN, Munasinghe RL: Ambient air pollution and hospitalization for congestive heart failure among elderly people in seven large US cities. *Am J Public Health* 85:1361–1365, 1995. Copyright American Public Health Association.)

effects of weather, seasonal factors, or other pollutants. Further study of the reasons for increased admission rates for congestive heart failure may produce useful strategies for public health intervention.

▶ Although environmental air pollution has been most consistently linked to respiratory illness, there has been some evidence that it has also been associated with morbidity and mortality caused by cardiovascular disease. To better explore this association, this study used Medicare Provider Analysis and Review files to measure hospital admissions for congestive heart failure and the Aerometric Information and Retrieval System collected by the Environmental Protection Agency for the same dates (1986–1989) in 7 U.S. cities.

The findings show a clear relationship with ambient levels of carbon monoxide in virtually all cities, with the strongest associations being in Los Angeles and New York. In Los Angeles, 11% of admissions for congestive heart failure among older persons could be attributed to ambient carbon monoxide. The relationships with other pollutants (nitrogen dioxide, sulfur dioxide, and ozone) were less consistent. This study reminds us of the importance of public health efforts to clean the environment as an adjunct to reducing the health consequences of congestive heart failure.

D.B. Reuben, M.D.

Prevention of Colorectal Cancer by Flexible Endoscopy and Polypectomy: A Case-Control Study of 32,702 Veterans
Müller AD, Sonnenberg A (Med College of Wisconsin, Milwaukee; Veterans Affairs Med Ctr, Albuquerque, NM)
Ann Intern Med 123:904–910, 1995
1–8

Background.—Colorectal endoscopy with flexible instruments has not been widely used for cancer prevention because of the lack of unequivocal evidence of its efficacy, its associated complications, and its expense. Before large numbers of individuals are regularly subjected to endoscopic procedures, these procedures must be shown to actually reduce the risk for cancer in the large intestine. The value of colonoscopy, flexible sigmoidoscopy, and polypectomy in protecting against the future development of colorectal cancer was investigated.

Methods.—A total of 8,722 patients with colon cancer and 7,629 with rectal cancer were compared with control groups matched for age, sex, and race and discharged at the same time. All patients and control subjects were U.S. military veterans. The number and type of endoscopic procedures of the large bowel performed between 1981 and the development of cancer were determined.

Findings.—Compared with control subjects, the patients were less likely to have had an endoscopic procedure of the large bowel before their diagnosis of cancer. The odds ratio for those with colon cancer was 0.51, and for those with rectal cancer, 0.55. The odds ratios were even lower for patients who had flexible sigmoidoscopy, colonoscopy, and polypectomy. When analyzed in separate 1-year periods, patients with cancer underwent significantly fewer procedures for up to 6 years before the onset of their cancer. Patients also had fewer inpatient and outpatient procedures than control subjects.

Conclusions.—In this study of U.S. military veterans, those who did not have colorectal cancer were approximately 50% more likely to have had endoscopic procedure than those who did have colorectal cancer. This is strong evidence of the efficacy of endoscopy as a tool for decreasing the risk of colorectal cancer. There are apparently no significant differences among the protective influences of various types of endoscopic procedures.

▶ This case-control study of a large population of older veterans tests the hypothesis that colonoscopy, flexible sigmoidoscopy, and polypectomy, when indicated, protect against the future development of colorectal cancer. The data show that veterans who did not have colorectal cancer at the time of the study were 50% more likely to have had an endoscopic procedure as compared with the matched controls. Furthermore, the benefit from an endoscopic procedure lasted for about 6 years. This study extends previous findings by showing that this beneficial effect is not limited to reducing mortality resulting from cancer but also aids in the prevention of cancer. The beneficial effect appears to apply to both the distal and proximal areas of the large bowel.

This study has several limitations, including the generic limitations of the case-control design. The investigators attempted to adjust for as many of these shortcomings as possible. In addition, the study was carried out in an exclusively veteran population, which consists primarily of men with low family incomes and increased exposures to risk factors such as alcohol consumption and smoking. Another limitation is that the data source—the Patient Treatment File of the Department of Veterans Affairs—records only the pertinent health care activity within the Veterans Affairs system. Because many veterans receive care outside the system, the Patient Treatment File cannot account for this. Furthermore, the Patient Treatment File only documents outpatient activity after 1990 so that a systematic error might have been introduced, but this would have applied to both the case-patients and the controls.

J.C. Beck, M.D.

HDL Cholesterol Predicts Coronary Heart Disease Mortality in Older Persons
Corti M-C, Guralnik JM, Salive ME, et al (Natl Inst on Aging, Bethesda, Md; Harvard Med School, Boston; Univ of Iowa, Iowa City; et al)
JAMA 274:539–544, 1995   1–9

Purpose.—Whether to offer aggressive treatment to older adults with an abnormal lipoprotein profile is an important clinical question. Total and high-density lipoprotein (HDL) cholesterol levels are known to be important risk factors for coronary heart disease (CHD) in middle age and early old age. However, the importance of these factors in old age is subject to debate. The relationship of total and HDL cholesterol to CHD mortality and events was studied among elderly individuals aged 71 years or older.

Methods.—The prospective cohort study included 2,527 women and 1,377 men from the collaborative, longitudinal Established Populations for Epidemiologic Studies of the Elderly (EPESE) study. Each of these subjects survived at least 1 year after an interview and measurement of their serum lipid levels. The main study outcomes were death from CHD and new CHD events in subjects with no CHD history or hospitalization. A low HDL cholesterol level was defined as less than 35 mg/dL, compared with a reference level of 60 mg/dL or more. Total cholesterol was considered high in subjects with a level of 240 mg/dL or more, compared with a reference range of 161–199 mg/dL.

Results.—Subjects with low HDL cholesterol had a 2.5 relative risk (RR) of death from CHD, after adjustment for the known CHD risk factors. Relative risk was 4.1 for subjects aged 71–80 years and 1.8 for those older than 80 years; the increased risk of CHD death was apparent in both men and women. Low HDL cholesterol also was associated with an increased risk of new CHD event (RR, 1.4).

For women, high total cholesterol carried a 1.8 RR for CHD mortality, but men had no associated increase in risk. In the overall study sample, each 1-unit increase in the ratio of total cholesterol to HDL cholesterol carried a 17% increase in the risk of CHD mortality.

Conclusions.—For individuals in their 70s and older, a low HDL cholesterol level carries a significant increase in risk of CHD mortality and new CHD events. In addition, a high total cholesterol level may increase the risk of CHD death for women. The results suggest the need for an individualized approach to lipid and lipoprotein screening and treatment for older adults.

▶ Because of the high prevalence of CHD in elderly persons, preventive strategies may be more cost-effective for this age group than for younger persons. Ideally, lessons learned from studies of younger populations, which have been more extensively analyzed, would be applicable to older persons with the same effect. Unfortunately, in the case of cholesterol (a strong and modifiable risk factor for CHD in middle-aged men), this lesson does not appear to be quite so certain. Two studies used data from the same cohort and yielded somewhat contradictory results. The New Haven, Conn, site of the Established Populations for Epidemiologic Studies of the Elderly (EPESE) found that increased total serum cholesterol, low HDL-C, and increased total serum cholesterol to HDL-C ratio were not associated with a significantly increased rate of all-cause mortality, CHD mortality, or hospitalization for myocardial infarction or unstable angina after adjustment for cardiovascular risk factors.[1] However, using data from all EPESE sites, low HDL-C (less than 35 mg/dL) was associated with a 2.5 increased risk of death during the 4.4-year (median) follow-up period. For women, but not men, total cholesterol also predicted mortality. The take-home message is not entirely clear with respect to screening for and treating older individuals with cholesterol abnormalities. For some subgroups (e.g., those who have documented CHD and those without functional disability), lipid measurement may be beneficial. However, better definition of these subgroups and evidence from clinical trials will be needed to guide appropriate therapy.

D.B. Reuben, M.D.

Reference

1. Krumholz HM, Seeman TE, Merrill SS, et al: Lack of association between cholesterol and coronary heart disease mortality and morbidity and all-cause mortality in persons older than 70 years. *JAMA* 272:1335–1340, 1994.

Total and High Density Lipoprotein Cholesterol as Risk Factors for Coronary Heart Disease in Elderly Men During 5 Years of Follow-up

Weijenberg MP, Feskens EJM, Kromhout D (Natl Inst of Public Health and Environmental Protection, Bilthoven, The Netherlands)

Am J Epidemiol 143:151–158, 1996   1–10

Background.—Although associations between serum total and high density lipoprotein cholesterol (HDL cholesterol) and risk of coronary heart disease are well established among middle-aged men, it is not clear whether these associations are applicable to elderly individuals. At present, studies investigating HDL cholesterol among elderly patients are few, but it has been suggested that low HDL cholesterol levels may be a more important predictor of coronary heart disease as age increases than elevated total cholesterol levels. Serum total cholesterol and HDL cholesterol as risk factors for the incidence of and mortality from coronary heart disease therefore were investigated among a group of elderly men.

Patients and Methods.—Eight hundred eighty-five men from the Dutch town of Zutphen were followed up during 5 years. Seven hundred ten of the participants were without a history of clinical coronary heart disease. The participant ages ranged between 64 and 84 years. After adjusting for age, body mass index, systolic blood pressure, and cigarette and alcohol use, associations between coronary heart disease and serum total and HDL cholesterol were determined.

Results.—No significant association between total cholesterol and the incidence of coronary heart disease was noted. For mortality, however, the relative risk, corresponding to a 1.00-mmol/L increase, was 1.40. No association between HDL cholesterol and disease-related mortality was identified, but the relative risk for the incidence of the disease, corresponding to a 0.26-mmol/L increase, was 0.80. The relative risk for coronary heart disease incidence, corresponding to a 0.05 increase, was 0.70 for the ratio of HDL cholesterol to total cholesterol.

Conclusions.—Among elderly men, both total and HDL cholesterol are important predictors of coronary heart disease; total cholesterol appears to be a more powerful risk factor for disease-related mortality, and HDL cholesterol is more strongly associated with the incidence of a first coronary heart disease event.

▶ I chose this article because it begins to clarify whether the association between serum total and HDL cholesterol levels and risk of coronary heart disease, so well established among middle-aged men, also applies to older individuals. This study is a prospective one among older individuals, the majority of whom were disease free at the onset of the study and who were followed up for a relatively short period. The results clearly show that, in elderly men followed up for 5 years, total cholesterol is an independent risk factor for mortality associated with coronary heart disease, whereas HDL cholesterol seems to be a stronger risk factor for the incidence of coronary heart disease. The study thus confirms observations made in the Framingham Study.[1] It further demonstrates that neither total nor HDL cholesterol in this age group appeared to be predictive for all-cause mortality. The finding that HDL cholesterol appears to be predictive of a first coronary disease event during a relatively short follow-up time stresses the short-term predictive importance of HDL cholesterol for coronary heart disease in older men.

J.C. Beck, M.D.

Reference

1. Castelli WP, Garrison RJ, Wilson PWF, et al: Incidence of coronary heart disease and lipoprotein cholesterol levels: The Framingham Study. *JAMA* 256:2835–2838, 1986.

Age-Related Changes in Stroke Risk in Men With Hypertension and Normal Blood Pressure

Curb JD, Abbott RD, MacLean CJ, et al (Univ of Hawaii, Manoa; Kuakini Med Ctr, Honolulu, Hawaii; Univ of Virginia, Charlottesville; et al)
Stroke 27:819–824, 1996   1–11

Introduction.—Stroke is a major cause of morbidity and mortality in older individuals, and hypertension has been identified as the single most powerful risk factor for stroke. Some studies, however, suggest that hypertension may be less important than other age-related factors in older age groups. To determine whether the relationship between hypertension

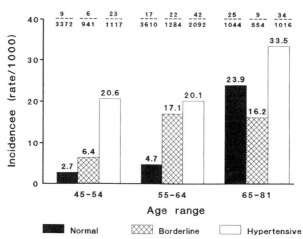

FIGURE 2.—Six-year incidence of stroke by hypertensive status and age group in Japanese-American men in Hawaii. Values at **top** are number of thromboembolic events/6-year person intervals at risk. (Courtesy of Curb JD, Abbott RD, MacLean CJ, et al: Age-related changes in stroke risk in men with hypertension and normal blood pressure. *Stroke* 27:819–824, 1996. Reproduced with permission. Copyright 1996, American Heart Association.)

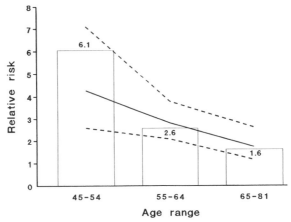

FIGURE 3.—Risk factor–adjusted 6-year relative risk of thromboembolic stroke for Japanese-American men in Hawaii with hypertension compared with those without hypertension by age, as well as a linear illustration of change in relative risk with age and 95% confidence limits (derived from the Cox model). (Courtesy of Curb JD, Abbott RD, MacLean CJ, et al: Age-related changes in stroke risk in men with hypertension and normal blood pressure. *Stroke* 27:819–824, 1996. Reproduced with permission. Copyright 1996, American Heart Association.)

and stroke changes with age, the 6-year incidence of stroke was examined in men enrolled in the Honolulu Heart Program.

Methods.—Participants in the Honolulu Heart Program were 8,006 men of Japanese ancestry who were born between 1900 and 1919 and living on the island of Oahu in 1965. Baseline screening data were collected from 1965 to 1968; updates on hypertension and other variables took place during two 6-year periods after baseline (1971–1974 and 1980–1982). Participants were followed for the first occurrence of a fatal or nonfatal stroke.

Results.—Across the period of follow-up, 2,267 incident cases of stroke were recorded: 187 thromboembolic, 63 hemorrhagic, and 17 of unknown type. There was an age-related increase in the prevalence of hypertension, from 20.6% among men aged 45–54 years to 38.9% for those aged 65 years and older. A significant increase in the incidence of thromboembolic stroke also accompanied increasing age, and the rate of increase was significantly steeper for normotensive men than for those classified as hypertensive at baseline (Fig 2). Compared with men without hypertension, those with hypertension showed a marked decline in the relative risk of thromboembolic stroke with increasing age (Fig 3). This decline resulted from the increasing incidence of stroke in normotensive men and was not attributed to a treatment effect among those on antihypertensive medication. Similar patterns, although with slightly weaker associations, were observed for hemorrhagic stroke.

Conclusions.—The age-associated increase in the incidence of stroke was most notable among men who were normotensive at the start of follow-up. This finding suggests that other factors associated with aging play an increasing role in the development of stroke as an individual ages.

► Several randomized clinical trials support the effectiveness of treating isolated systolic and systolic-diastolic hypertension in older persons. Nevertheless, many older persons with normal blood pressure and those who have normalized blood pressure as the result of antihypertensive therapy have strokes.

This report from the Honolulu Heart Program study provides a look at the age-related relative importance of hypertension as a risk factor for stroke. In this cohort, with increasing age, many more normotensive Japanese-American men had strokes; accordingly, there is an age-related decrease in the relative risk of incurring a stroke among those with hypertension compared with those without hypertension. Overall, the rate of stroke attributable to hypertension decreases from 50% among men aged 45–54 years to 18% among men aged 65–81 years. Hence, other factors must assume increasing importance with aging. These other factors are not well defined in this study. Although other factors (e.g., cholesterol, smoking, and atrial fibrillation) were predictive of thromboembolic events, the authors did not find age-related trends in their risk. They speculate that other factors such as changes in cerebral vessel wall integrity, physical inactivity, glucose intolerance, and coagulation factors may play a role.

D.B. Reuben, M.D.

A Randomized Controlled Trial of Stress Reduction for Hypertension in Older African Americans

Schneider RH, Staggers F, Alexander CN, et al (Maharishi Univ of Management, Fairfield, Iowa; West Oakland Health Ctr, Calif; Univ of Arkansas, Pine Bluff; et al)
Hypertension 26:820–827, 1995   1–12

Background.—Compared with white Americans, African Americans have a greater prevalence, incidence, and severity of hypertension. Hypertension also has an earlier onset, causes more target-organ damage, and is generally treated later and less adequately in African Americans. Stress reduction may be a useful treatment. The short-term efficacy and feasibility of 2 stress reduction approaches were compared.

Methods.—Two hundred thirteen African Americans were screened during an 18-month period for eligibility for the randomized, controlled, single-blind trial. One hundred twenty-seven persons aged 55–85 years were randomized. All had initial diastolic pressures of 90–109 mm Hg, systolic pressures of 189 mm Hg or less, and final baseline blood pressures of 179/104 mm Hg or less. Transcendental meditation (TM), progressive muscle relaxation (PMR), and a lifestyle modification education control program were compared.

Findings.—Transcendental meditation reduced systolic pressure by 10.7 mm Hg and diastolic pressure by 6.4 mm Hg, after adjustments for significant baseline differences. Progressive muscle relaxation reduced systolic and diastolic pressures by 4.7 and 3.3 mm Hg. The decreases asso-

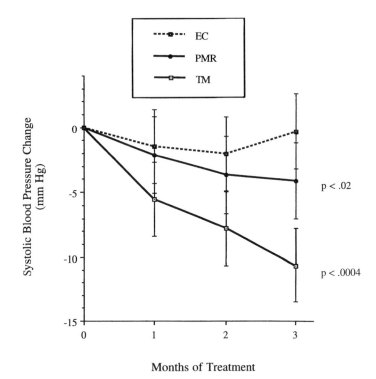

Months of Treatment

FIGURE 1.—Line graph shows mean changes in clinic systolic pressure over 3 months (follow-up minus baseline) with SEM. Probability values are for repeated-measures ANCOVA comparing each experimental group (TM and PMR) with control (EC). *Abbreviations: TM,* transcendental meditation (n = 36); *PMR,* progressive muscle relaxation (n =33); and EC, lifestyle modification education control (n = 35). (Courtesy of Schneider RH, Staggers F, Alexander CN, et al: A randomized controlled trial of stress reduction for hypertension in older African Americans. *Hypertension* 26:820–827, 1995. Reproduced with permission. Copyright 1995, American Heart Association.)

ciated with TM were significantly larger than those associated with PMR. Both groups had high levels of compliance (Fig 1).

Conclusions.—Stress reduction appears to be feasible and effective in the treatment of mild hypertension in elderly African Americans. Transcendental meditation is especially beneficial. Further research is needed to confirm these findings.

▶ The prevalence of hypertension among older African Americans is exceptionally high, and the resulting consequences are profound. Hence, any effective methods to lower blood pressure in this ethnic group are particularly welcome. This study tested 2 nonpharmacologic methods—TM and physical-based techniques for stress reduction (muscle relaxation exercises)—lowering blood pressure in older persons with mild hypertension who attended a primary care community health center.

During the course of 3 months, both methods lowered blood pressure (systolic more than diastolic) compared with a control group that received educational techniques for hypertension. Transcendental meditation was more effective. Although these results are encouraging, several points of caution should be noted. The sample size was small, and approximately half were already taking hypertensive medications. The elevation in blood pressure at baseline was very mild (mean blood pressure, 147/92 mm Hg). The follow-up was short, and the adherence rate was extremely high (97% of the TM group practiced "twice a day" or "almost twice every day." The research was also conducted by investigators from the Maharishi University of Management, who may have had a vested interest in the outcomes of the study. Nevertheless, if these results and benefits can be replicated in other settings, this nonpharmacologic treatment may be of substantial value in treating hypertension in this population.

D.B. Reuben, M.D.

Effects of Weight Loss vs Aerobic Exercise Training on Risk Factors for Coronary Disease in Healthy, Obese, Middle-Aged and Older Men: A Randomized Controlled Trial
Katzel LI, Bleecker ER, Colman EG, et al (Univ of Maryland, Baltimore; NIH, Baltimore, Md)
JAMA 274:1915–1921, 1995   1–13

Introduction.—In the aging population, weight loss and exercise to reduce obesity have the potential for important health benefits. Aerobic exercise and weight loss have both been recommended to reduce obesity and increase fitness. However, it remains unclear which of these interventions is more effective in reducing risk factors for coronary artery disease (CAD) in older individuals who are obese. Weight loss and aerobic exercise training were compared for their effect on CAD risk factors in obese middle-aged and older men.

Methods.—The randomized, controlled trial included 170 obese older men with a mean body mass index of 30 kg/m² and a mean age of 61 years. Each subject was assigned to 1 of 3 groups: a 9-month dietary intervention for weight reduction, a 9-month aerobic exercise training program, and a weight-maintenance control group. At the end of the interventions, the 3 groups were compared for changes in body composition, maximal aerobic capacity, blood pressure, lipoprotein concentrations, and glucose tolerance.

Results.—The interventions were completed by 44 of 73 in the dietary weight reduction group, 49 of 71 in the aerobic exercise group, and 18 of 26 in the weight maintenance group. The men in the weight loss group lost a mean of 9.5 lb, (10% mean weight reduction) with no change in maximal aerobic capacity. Those in the aerobic exercise group had a mean increase of 17% in maximal aerobic capacity with no change in weight. Weight loss was associated with a 2% decrease in fasting glucose concentration; an 18% decrease in insulin concentration; and decreases of 8% and 26% in glucose and insulin areas, respectively, during the oral glucose tolerance test (OGTT).

Aerobic exercise yielded no improvement in fasting glucose or insulin concentration, nor in glucose response during the OGTT, but it did produce a 17% decrease in insulin area on the OGTT. Analysis of variance showed that the decreases in fasting glucose and insulin levels and in glucose areas achieved in the weight loss group were significantly different from those in the aerobic exercise group. High-density lipoprotein cholesterol level increased by 13% and blood pressure decreased in the weight loss group but not in the aerobic exercise group. Multiple regression analysis suggested that the lipoprotein and glucose metabolism changes were related primarily to the reduction in obesity.

Conclusions.—For obese middle-aged and older men, weight loss is more effective than aerobic exercise in improving the CAD risk factor profile. Weight loss improves lipoprotein concentrations, glucose tolerance, postprandial insulin level, and blood pressure more than aerobic exercise without weight loss.

▶ Exercise is commonly regarded as a difficult-to-implement yet highly beneficial treatment for obese, middle-aged, and elderly persons. Exercise advocates tout benefits that are virtually protean in scope, ranging from increased longevity to reduced functional disability, and there are some data to support many of these claims. This randomized clinical trial casts doubt on the effectiveness of aerobic exercise for decreasing risk factors for CHD. In contrast, weight loss of 10% of body weight was much more effective in improving lipid profiles in middle-aged and elderly men. Unfortunately, the implementation and maintenance of such weight loss is just as difficult. The study is limited by a large (slightly more than one third) attrition rate, indicating the difficulty of implementing these therapies even among highly motivated volunteers. Moreover, the ability to maintain such weight loss beyond the study period is doubtful. Nevertheless, those highly motivated obese persons who can lose weight and maintain the weight loss may reap cardiovascular benefits.

D.B. Reuben, M.D.

Effects of Endurance Exercise and Hormone Replacement Therapy on Serum Lipids in Older Women
Binder EF, Birge SJ, Kohrt WM (Washington Univ, St Louis)
J Am Geriatr Soc 44:231–236, 1996   1–14

Background.—Hormone replacement therapy (HRT) generally reduces the rate of cardiovascular disease, an effect believed to be mediated partly by the favorable effects of estrogen on plasma lipoprotein concentrations. Physical activity also favorably affects serum lipids and lipoproteins. The effects of 11 months of exercise training and HRT, individually and combined, on serum lipids and lipoproteins were investigated.

Methods.—Seventy-one healthy postmenopausal women (age range, 60–72 years) were prospectively assigned to 1 of 4 groups: control, exer-

TABLE 2.—Effects of Exercise and/or Hormone Replacement Therapy (*HRT*) on Serum Lipids

| Variable | | Study Group | | | |
		Control (*n* = 17)	Exercise (*n* = 23)	HRT (*n* = 15)	Exercise + HRT (*n* = 16)
Total cholesterol (mg/dL)	Initial	205 ± 30	217 ± 34	216 ± 28	207 ± 24
	Final	206 ± 28	204 ± 31†	211 ± 27	194 ± 18*
HDL cholesterol (mg/dL)	Initial	54 ± 14	60 ± 17	52 ± 14	54 ± 12
	Final	53 ± 14	60 ± 17	63 ± 16†	63 ± 15†
LDL cholesterol (mg/dL)	Initial	121 ± 23	134 ± 31	140 ± 28	126 ± 26
	Final	126 ± 25	123 ± 27*	116 ± 28‡	101 ± 24†
Triglyceride (mg/dL)	Initial	134 ± 96	115 ± 63	107 ± 38	148 ± 71
	Final	136 ± 78	106 ± 53	152 ± 63†	151 ± 56

Different from initial: *$P < 0.05$, †$P < 0.01$, ‡$P < 0.001$.
Abbreviation: LDL, low-density lipoprotein.
(Courtesy of Binder EF, Birge SJ, Kohrt WM: Effects of endurance exercise and hormone replacement therapy on serum lipids in older women. *J Am Geriatr Soc* 44(3):231–236, 1996.)

cise alone, HRT alone, or exercise plus HRT. Women receiving HRT took conjugated estrogens, 0.625 mg/day, and trimonthly medroxyprogesterone acetate, 5 mg/day, for 13 days. Exercise included 2 months of low-intensity training followed by 9 months of rigorous exercise for 45 min/day for 3 or more days a week at 65% to 85% of maximal heart rate.

Findings.—After 11 months, total and low-density lipoprotein (LDL) cholesterol were reduced in the women in the exercise group. However, high-density lipoprotein (HDL) cholesterol and triglycerides were not affected. Women receiving HRT alone had reduced LDL cholesterol, increased HDL cholesterol, and unchanged total cholesterol. Women in the exercise plus HRT group had reduced total cholesterol and LDL cholesterol and increased HDL cholesterol. Exercise prevented the HRT-related triglyceride increase in this group (Table 2)

Conclusions.—In older postmenopausal women, exercise training and HRT seem to cause independent beneficial effects on serum lipids and lipoproteins. There are, however, disadvantages to each form of treatment. Exercise had no effect on HDL cholesterol, and HRT adversely affected triglycerides. Combining exercise and HRT seems to optimize lipid and lipoprotein response.

▶ Among postmenopausal women, the benefit of aerobic exercise on lipid profiles remains uncertain. Moreover, the effects of exercise compared with other pharmacologic methods of improving lipid profiles have not been well studied. This small, 2 × 2 factorial design, randomized clinical trial examined lipid profiles of women who exercised at least 3 times a week and those who received ERT. Exercise (with or without estrogen) improved total cholesterol, and estrogen (with or without exercise) improved HDL cholesterol. All intervention arms improved LDL cholesterol concentrations, and exercise, when combined with estrogen, ameliorated the estrogen-mediated increase in triglycerides. These findings seem to indicate that these 2 modalities tend to be complementary, although the analyses demonstrated no significant interaction effects. However, the sample size in each group was small and may have precluded the ability to fully explore such treatment interactions. Further studies will need to better define the roles of these 2 interventions in preventing heart disease in women.

D.B. Reuben, M.D.

Optimal Oral Anticoagulant Therapy in Patients With Nonrheumatic Atrial Fibrillation and Recent Cerebral Ischemia

Koudstaal PJ, for The European Atrial Fibrillation Trial Study Group (Univ Hosp Rotterdam Dijkzigt, The Netherlands)
N Engl J Med 333:5–10, 1995   1–15

Background.—Although oral anticoagulant therapy has been shown to effectively reduce the risk of stroke and systemic embolism in patients with nonrheumatic atrial fibrillation, the risk of major bleeding complications increases. The targeted therapeutic ranges of anticoagulant control have varied widely among studies, preventing a determination of the optimal intensity of oral anticoagulant therapy. Therefore, the international normalized ratio (INR)–specific incidence rates of ischemic and of major hemorrhagic events were calculated in patients with nonrheumatic atrial fibrillation.

Methods.—Data were collected on patients participating in a randomized trial of oral anticoagulant therapy for patients with atrial fibrillation who had recently had minor cerebral ischemic events. International normalized ratio–specific event rates were calculated by dividing the occurrence of ischemic or hemorrhagic events by the time the patient was treated at each range of anticoagulant intensity.

TABLE 2.—First Ischemic and Hemorrhagic Complications Among the Study Patients, According to the Internationalized Normal Ratio (*INR*) at the Time of the Event*

INR	PERSON-YR OF EXPOSURE	ISCHEMIC EVENTS		MAJOR BLEEDING		EITHER EVENT	
		NO.	NO./100 PERSON-YR	NO.	NO./100 PERSON-YR	NO.	NO./100 PERSON-YR
Unknown	72	4 (2)	7	2	3	7 (3)†	10
<2.0	40	7 (2)	18	0	0	7 (2)	18
2.0–2.9	186	3 (2)	2	2	1	6 (3)†	3
3.0–3.9	114	4 (2)	4	3 (1)	3	7 (3)	7
4.0–4.9	27	6 (1)	26	1	4	8 (2)†	30
≥5.0	10	1	10	5 (1)	50	6 (1)	60
All with known INR	377	21 (7)	6	11 (2)	3	34 (12)	9

* *Numbers in parentheses* are numbers of fatal events.
† Includes 1 patient with stroke of uncertain cause.
(Reprinted by permission of *The New England Journal of Medicine.* Koudstaal PJ, for The European Atrial Fibrillation Trial Study Group: Optimal oral anticoagulant therapy in patients with nonrheumatic atrial fibrillation and recent cerebral ischemia. *N Engl J Med* 333:5–10, 1995. Copyright 1995, Massachusetts Medical Society.)

Results.—Of the 4,883 INR values obtained for 214 patients over 377 patient-years, 56% were within the target therapeutic range of 2.5 to 3.9, 35% were below the target range, and 9% were above it. Thromboembolic and hemorrhagic events were least common when the INRs were between 2.0 and 3.9; hemorrhagic complications were most common when the INRs were 5 or higher; and thromboembolic risk was not reduced with an INR lower than 2.0 (Table 2).

Conclusion.—For the secondary prevention of thromoboembolic and hemorrhagic complications in patients with nonrheumatic atrial fibrillation who have sustained a recent minor cerebral ischemic event, the optimal therapeutic range for oral anticoagulants is an INR between 2.0 and 3.9, with a target of 3.0. International normalized ratios lower than 2.0 or higher than 5.0 should be avoided.

▶ Anticoagulation of most older patients with atrial fibrillation has strong support based on clinical trials and has been widely incorporated into clinical practice. However, most clinicians prescribe this treatment in older individuals with some apprehension because of the risk of hemorrhagic complications, especially among those who may be at risk for falls.

This secondary data analysis of the anticoagulation cohort (average age, 71 years) of the European Atrial Fibrillation Trial presents valuable information on the therapeutic window of anticoagulation and appropriate target for therapy.

This analysis found no treatment effect when the INR was below 2.0 and no substantial increase in major bleeding events unless the INR was 5.0 or greater. Of note, however, is that age older than 75 years was associated with a higher risk of major bleeding, independent of the level of anticoagulation. Accordingly, the authors recommend a target INR of 3.0 when for anticoagulating patients who have atrial fibrillation. Physicians caring for very old patients might aim for slightly lower INRs in this age group.

D.B. Reuben, M.D.

The Efficacy of Influenza Vaccine in Elderly Persons: A Meta-analysis and Review of the Literature

Gross PA, Hermogenes AW, Sacks HS, et al (Hackensack Med Ctr, New Jersey; New Jersey Med School, Newark; Mt Sinai Med Ctr, New York; et al)
Ann Intern Med 123:518–527, 1995   1–16

Background.—Influenza viruses in elderly persons can still be fatal or cause serious complications. Research on the efficacy of influenza vaccines in the elderly has yielded inconsistent findings. However, several studies have reported a decreased incidence of pneumonia and mortality with these vaccines. A meta-analysis of published studies on influenza vaccine efficacy in the elderly was performed.

Methods.—A MEDLINE search was conducted to identify cohort observational studies with mortality assessments. Other types of studies were also reviewed.

Findings.—In the 20 cohort studies included in the meta-analysis, the pooled estimates of vaccine efficacy were 56% for preventing respiratory illness, 53% for preventing pneumonia, 50% for preventing hospitalization, and 68% for preventing death. In 3 recent case-control studies, vaccine efficacy ranged from 32% to 45% for preventing hospitalization for pneumonia, from 31% to 65% for preventing hospital deaths from pneumonia and influenza, from 43% to 50% for preventing hospital deaths from all respiratory conditions, and from 27% to 30% for preventing deaths from all causes. The 1 randomized, double-blind, placebo-controlled trial reviewed demonstrated a 50% or greater reduction in influenza-related disease. The 2 recent cost-effectiveness studies reviewed confirmed that influenza vaccine effectively decreases influenza-related morbidity and mortality and results in important cost savings per year per vaccinated person.

Conclusions.—Many studies confirm that influenza vaccine decreases the risks for pneumonia, hospitalization, and death among the elderly during influenza epidemics when the vaccine strain used is similar to the epidemic strain. Thus immunization against influenza is an essential part of care for the elderly.

▶ This is a meta-analysis of 20 cohort studies, 3 case-control studies, and 1 randomized, double-blind, placebo-controlled study and is an excellent summary that all providers should be aware of. The meta-analysis conclusively demonstrates that morbidity and mortality are greatly reduced with influenza vaccination administered before the epidemic, provided the vaccine strain is either similar or identical to the epidemic strain. There are a number of limitations to this study, the first being that almost all of the studies in this meta-analysis were carried out in the institutional long-term care setting. Because of this, the persons in the studies were those with extensive underlying disease and one would anticipate that had a representative sample of elderly who were community based been included, the efficacy might have been still higher. It is important to realize that during the 1993–1994 season, approximately half of all elderly persons were receiving influenza vaccine annually. Although this represents a substantial change since the 1980s, it identifies a major unsolved problem involving both health providers and the public health system.

J.C. Beck, M.D.

General Clinical Care Of Older Persons

Do Too Many Cooks Spoil the Broth? Multiple Physician Involvement in Medical Management of Elderly Patients and Potentially Inappropriate Drug Combinations
Tamblyn RM, McLeod PJ, Abrahamowicz M, et al (McGill Univ, Montreal)
Can Med Assoc J 154:1177–1184, 1996   1–17

Introduction.—Problems can occur in prescribing medication for older patients who have a number of medical problems and are receiving care from several physicians. Without monitoring by a single pharmacy or primary care physician, a patient may be prescribed potentially inappropriate drug combinations (PIDCs) or 2 drugs from the same group. Factors that increase or decrease the risk of a PIDC were retrospectively examined in a cross-sectional study.

Methods.—Study participants were drawn from elderly Medicare registrants in 12 geographically defined health care regions in Quebec. Those eligible had visited at least 1 physician in 1990, were not living in a health care institution for the entire year, and had received at least 1 prescription for a cardiovascular drug, a psychotropic drug, or a nonsteroidal anti-inflammatory drug (NSAID). Data were obtained by reviewing physician and prescription claims. A PIDC was defined as a drug combination with established or probable evidence of a risk of adverse interaction and which could not normally be justified to achieve safe and effective treatment in an elderly patient.

Results.—A total of 51,587 patients, 82% of the sample of eligible participants, had been prescribed drugs from 1 or more of the 3 drug groups studied. These patients had a mean age of 74.7 years and received a median of 7 different drugs each. Most had a single primary care physician and had prescriptions filled at a single pharmacy, but two thirds had 2 or more prescribing physicians during the study period. Overall, 17.4% of patients had at least 1 PIDC during the year. Those receiving a psychotropic drug were most likely to have a PIDC, and the most common PIDC was concurrent prescription of 2 benzodiazepines. In all 3 drug groups (Fig 1), the number of prescribing physicians was the most important risk factor for a PIDC. Use of a single dispensing pharmacy lowered the risk of a PIDC in all drug groups, whereas the presence of a single primary care physician lowered the risk for cardiovascular and psychotropic PIDCs (Table 3).

Conclusions.—For elderly patients, the risk of a PIDC increases with the number of physicians involved in their care. Use of a single dispensing pharmacy and having a primary care physician can lower this risk.

▶ Among the arguments for identification of a primary care physician is the fragmentation of care provided when many physicians are involved. One particularly risky consequence of receiving care from many physicians is drug prescribing without adequate consideration of the medications that the

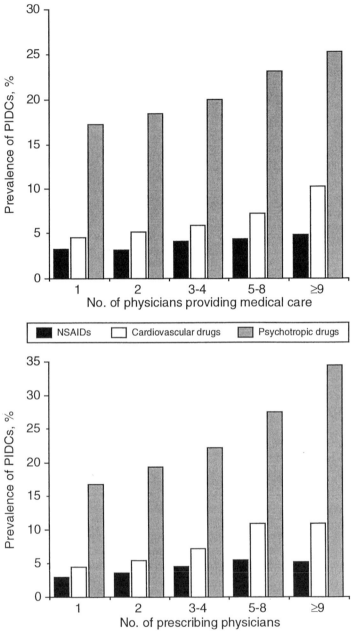

FIGURE 1.—Prevalence of potentially inappropriate drug combinations (PIDCs) by number of physicians providing medical care (**top**) and number of prescribing physicians (**bottom**), by type of drug combination. *Abbreviation: NSAIDs,* nonsteroidal anti-inflammatory drugs. (Courtesy of Tamblyn RM, McLeod PJ, Abrahamowicz M, et al: Do too many cooks spoil the broth? Multiple physician involvement in medical management of elderly patients and potentially inappropriate drug combinations. *Can Med Assoc J* 154:1177–1184, 1996.)

TABLE 3.—Proportion of Patients With a Single Primary Care Physician or a Single Dispensing Pharmacy Who Had a PIDC, by Type of Drug Combination

Variable	Type of Drug Combination: % of Patients With a PIDC		
	Cardiovascular	Psychotropic	NSAID
Single primary care physician			
Yes	5.1	18.3	3.8
No	7.1	22.1	4.0
Odds ratio	0.70*	0.79*	0.94
Single dispensing pharmacy			
Yes	5.0	18.7	3.5
No	7.2	22.4	4.6
Odds ratio	0.68*	0.79*	0.75*

* $P < 0.001$.

Abbreviation: PIDC, potentially inappropriate drug combination.

(Courtesy of Tamblyn RM, McLeod PJ, Abrahamowicz M, et al: Do too many cooks spoil the broth? Multiple physician involvement in medical management of elderly patients and potentially inappropriate drug combinations. *Can Med Assoc J* 154:1177–1184, 1996.)

patient is already receiving from another physician. Communication between providers may be inadequate. Moreover, patients may not accurately relate what medications they are taking and may use multiple pharmacies to fill their prescriptions.

In this study, researchers in Canada examined PIDCs as determined by expert reviewers and then examined the impact of having a single primary care physician to coordinate the care, as well as the impact of having a single pharmacy to monitor dispensing. Most of the PIDCs involved using multiple drugs of the same class or having the same physiologic effect (e.g., potassium-sparing diuretic with potassium supplement). Their results indicate that the greater the number of physicians providing medical care or prescribing medications, the higher the risk of PIDCs for cardiovascular drugs, psychotropic drugs, or NSAIDs. Having a single primary care physician reduced the odds of a cardiovascular or a psychotropic PIDC by 30% and 21%, respectively. Having a single dispensing pharmacy reduced the odds of a cardiovascular, a psychotropic, or an NSAID drug PIDC by 32%, 21%, and 25%, respectively. These findings indicate the need for better coordination of medical care and a network system among pharmacies to ensure that duplication and potential adverse drug interactions are brought to the attention of patients' physicians.

D.B. Reuben, M.D.

Fever in Geriatric Emergency Patients: Clinical Features Associated With Serious Illness

Marco CA, Schoenfeld CN, Hansen KN, et al (Johns Hopkins Bayview Med Ctr, Baltimore, Md; Johns Hopkins Hosp, Baltimore, Md)
Ann Emerg Med 26:18–24, 1995   1–18

Introduction.—Older patients, who account for an increasing percentage of emergency department (ED) admissions, often require more extensive evaluation and are more difficult to manage in several key clinical conditions, including fever. The importance of fever in geriatric patients seen in the ED was evaluated at a community hospital.

Methods.—At this urban, university-affiliated hospital, approximately 20% of visits are by adults aged 65 years or older. All patients in this age category who were seen with fever during the period from July 1991 through June 1992 were studied. Fever was defined as an oral temperature of 100.0°F or greater. Charts were reviewed for admitted patients, and those discharged were contacted for follow-up information at least 1 month after the ED visit. A number of clinical features were analyzed for the significance of their association with serious illness. Indicators of serious illness were positive blood cultures, related death within 1 month of ED visit, need for surgery or other invasive procedure, hospitalization for 4 or more days, IV antibiotics for 3 or more days, and a second ED visit within 72 hours for a related condition.

Results.—Follow-up information was available for 470 of 489 eligible patients, including 354 who were admitted and 116 who were discharged.

TABLE 5.—Logistic-Regression Analysis of Clinical Features Associated With Serious Illness

Clinical Feature	OR	95% CI	P
Temperature			
103°F or higher	7.27	1.62–32.55	<0.01*
102°–102.9°F	1.74	0.82–3.71	0.15
101°–101.9°F	1.56	0.86–2.83	0.14
100°–100.9°F	1.00		
Respirations			
30 or more	3.32	1.34–8.23	<0.01*
20–29	1.54	0.88–1.54	0.13
Fewer than 20	1.00		
WBC count ($\times 10^9$)			
20 or more	19.58	2.57–148.72	0.01*
11.0–19	1.90	1.13–2.19	0.015*
Fewer than 11	1.00		
Infiltrate	2.55	1.29–5.03	0.01*
Pulse			
120 or more	3.09	1.08–5.83	0.04*
100–119	1.45	0.82–2.54	0.20
Fewer than 100	1.00		

* Statistically significant.
(Courtesy of Marco CA, Schoenfeld CN, Hansen KN, et al: Fever in geriatric emergency patients: Clinical features associated with serious illness. *Ann Emerg Med* 26:18–24, July 1995.)

At least 1 indicator of serious illness was present in 356 patients, 334 of whom were admitted. In multivariate analysis, clinical features independently associated with serious illness were maximum temperature of at least 103°F, leukocytosis of 11.0 × 10⁹/L or greater, respiration rate of 30 or greater, heart rate of 120 or greater, and the finding of an infiltrate on chest radiography (Table 5). Pneumonia and urinary tract infection accounted for nearly half of the final diagnoses (25% and 22%, respectively), and sepsis/bacteremia for 18%. Most of these elderly patients (84.2%) recovered and returned to their baseline levels of function.

Conclusions.—Fever, an important sign of disease in all age groups, often indicates the presence of serious illness among geriatric ED patients. Hospital admission should be considered for all geriatric patients with fever, especially when the clinical features identified here are present. The absence of abnormal clinical findings, however, does not necessarily rule out serious illness.

▶ Although many older persons with serious infectious illness are afebrile when initially seen, those who are seen in the ED with fever often pose a management dilemma for physicians. This case-series of persons aged 65 years or older who had fever in the ED emphasizes the importance of this presentation. More than three fourths of these individuals had serious illness as defined by several criteria, caused most often by pneumonia, urinary tract infection, or sepsis. Moreover, the authors were able to identify clinical predictors of serious illness, especially a temperature of 103°F or greater, a pulse of 120 or greater, a respiratory rate of 30 or greater, a white blood cell count of 11.0 × 10⁹/L or greater, or an infiltrate on chest radiography. However, almost half of those with serious illness had no identifiable predictor. Thus, it appears that the vast majority, if not all, of older individuals who are seen in the ED with fever should be hospitalized. As new methods of health care delivery (e.g., direct admission to nursing homes for subacute care, home hospitalization) are developed and tested, these may become alternatives to hospitalization.

D.B. Reuben, M.D.

Hospital Admission Risk Profile (HARP): Identifying Older Patients at Risk for Functional Decline Following Acute Medical Illness and Hospitalization

Sager MA, Rudbeg MA, Jalaluddin M, et al (Univ of Wisconsin, Madison; William S Middleton Mem Veterans Hosp, Madison, Wis; Univ of Chicago; et al)

J Am Geriatr Soc 44:251–257, 1996　　　　　　　　　　　　　　1–19

Background.—Among the elderly, hospitalization for acute illness is often correlated with the development of disability. Currently, there is no agreement about who is at risk of becoming functionally disabled. An instrument for stratifying patients during admission based on their risk of having new disabilities develop in activities of daily living (ADL) was designed and validated.

Methods.—Four university and 2 private acute care hospitals participated in the prospective study. A cohort of 448 patients was studied to develop the instrument, called the Hospital Admission Risk profile. Another cohort (379 patients) was studied to validate it. All patients were 70 years or older and were hospitalized for acute medical illness between 1989 and 1992. Patients were examined on admission, at discharge, and 3 months after discharge.

Findings.—Three patient characteristics independently predicted functional decline in the first cohort: increasing age, lower admission Mini-Mental Status Examination scores, and lower pre-admission instrumental ADL function. On the basis of a scoring system developed for each predictor variable, patients were assigned to low-, intermediate-, and high-risk categories. In the first cohort, the rate of ADL decline at discharge was 17% for the low-risk group, 28% for the intermediate-risk group, and 56% for the high-risk group. The corresponding figures for the validation cohort were 19%, 31%, and 55%. Patients at low risk were significantly more likely to recover ADL function and avoid placement in a nursing home in the 3 months after discharge.

Conclusions.—The Hospital Admission Risk profile is a simple instrument that can be used to identify elderly patients at risk of functional decline after hospitalization for an acute illness. This instrument will be useful for identifying patients who may benefit from comprehensive discharge planning, specialized geriatric care, and experimental interventions to prevent or decrease the development of disability in hospitalized elderly patients.

▶ This article describes a number of easily measured predictors of functional decline in the elderly after hospitalization. It builds on the well-confirmed observation that older patients who are hospitalized for acute illness often have disability develop at the time of discharge or shortly thereafter.

The objectives of this study were to identify patient characteristics that are measurable at the time of hospital admission and are associated with the loss of ADL function; to use these patient characteristics to develop a practical instrument that would identify high- and low-risk patients at the time of admission; to test the ability of the instrument to identify patients with differing degrees of functional impairment in a prospective study of hospitalized older adults; to determine the extent to which these high- and low-risk patients recover to pre-admission levels of ADL function 3 months after discharge; and finally to evaluate the influence of discharge diagnoses and hospital length of stay on functional decline in both the high- and low-risk patients.

Three patient characteristics were identified as predictors of loss of ADL function: increasing age, cognitive impairment, and pre-admission disability in instrumental ADL functions.

Of interest is that patients in the high-risk category also were less likely to recover their ADL functions 3 months postdischarge. This is important because this information might be used to identify individuals in whom interventions targeted at preventing this postdischarge decline are clearly available. The investigators emphasize that the development of disability is an interplay between these patient characteristics and the illness itself and, perhaps even more important, the process of care. In this study, no diagnostic category was significantly associated with functional decline. If this observation is confirmed, then targeting criteria that rely on specific diagnosis or geriatric conditions may be less efficient in prospectively identifying patients for geriatric intervention.

There are a number of limitations to this study. First, the observations are only generalizable to general medical patients living in the community before hospitalization, and included only those with medical illnesses. Second, the study relied on patients' self-report of ADL function, which in itself might well have reduced the predictive discrimination of the risk factors.

Perhaps the most valid use of the Hospital Admission Risk profile would be in discharge planning—identifying patients for special inpatient care and planning interventions directed at both inpatient and postdischarge rehabilitative efforts.

J.C. Beck, M.D.

Predictive Validity of a Postal Questionnaire for Screening Community-Dwelling Elderly Individuals at Risk of Functional Decline
Hébert R, Bravo G, Korner-Bitensky N, et al (Hôpital d'Youville, Sherbrooke, PQ, Canada; Jewish Rehabilitation Hosp, Laval, PQ, Canada)
Age Ageing 25:159–167, 1996   1–20

Background.—Effective screening of community-dwelling elderly individuals could help identify those at risk for functional decline, thereby allowing early interventions that could reduce dependency and morbidity while increasing active life expectancy. The postal questionnaire is 1 such screening method, whereby all elderly individuals living in a defined area receive a simple questionnaire designed to identify at-risk individuals. The capability of a postal questionnaire to predict functional decline in community-dwelling elderly individuals was determined.

Participants and Methods.—A representative sample of 842 community-dwelling elderly individuals older than 75 years of age received a 21-item postal questionnaire. One month later, all individuals were contacted by a nurse for an in-home interview that included an evaluation of functional independence. Twelve months later, participants were again reevaluated by the same nurse.

Results.—The postal questionnaire was returned by 736 of the eligible participants (mean age, 79.9 years), 655 of whom participated in the first in-home interview. At the 1-year mark, 607 participants were available for reevaluation. During the course of the 12-month period, 43 individuals had died, 13 were institutionalized, and 109 had experienced a significant reduction in functional autonomy, giving an annual occurrence of functional decline of 27.2%. Participants who experienced functional decline were significantly older, more depressed, cognitively impaired, and dependent at the first interview compared with those who had no decline. These individuals also had been hospitalized more often and were more likely to have received home services during the course of the 12-month follow-up. Age and 14 of the questions were associated with a significant relative risk. Surprisingly, participants living alone were noted to be at a lower risk of functional decline. The relative risk associated with not responding to the questionnaire was 2.1.

Six of the 14 items were identified as independent predictors of functional decline on stepwise logistic regression analyses. These included not living alone, taking more than 3 medications per day, having problems with hearing, having problems with seeing, using ambulatory aids, and having problems with memory. Age and the remaining 8 questions did not significantly improve the prediction of functional decline. Additional analyses were performed using a 6-item postal questionnaire, and 56% of the population was identified as being at risk for functional decline with 75% sensitivity and 52% specificity.

Conclusions.—A postal questionnaire offers an effective and reliable means of screening elderly community-dwelling individuals to determine their risk of functional decline.

▶ This study describes a 6-item postal questionnaire that identifies elderly individuals who are truly in need of interventions to prevent functional decline. The authors point out that the first step in a preventive program is to identify a subgroup of the total elderly population who have the highest risk of functional decline in a subsequent year. The 6 items are as follows: (1) Do you live alone?; (2) Do you take more than 3 different medications every day?; (3) Do you regularly use a cane, a walker, or a wheelchair to move about?; (4) Do you see well; (5) Do you hear well?; and (6) Do you have problems with your memory? It is of interest that, in this study, living alone is not a risk factor for functional decline but a marker for better health, which confirms previous observations in the Aberdeen Survey.[1, 2]

J.C. Beck, M.D.

References

1. Taylor RC, Ford GG: The elderly at risk: A critical examination of commonly identified risk groups. *J R Coll Gen Pract* 33:699–705, 1983.
2. Ford G, Taylor R: Risk groups and selective case finding in an elderly population. *Soc Sci Med* 17:647–655, 1983.

Relationship of Age and Calcitonin Gene-related Peptide to Postprandial Hypotension

Edwards BJ, Perry HM III, Kaiser FE, et al (St Louis Univ, Mo; St Louis VA Med Ctr, Mo; Pfizer Inc, Groton, Conn)
Mech Ageing Dev 87:61–73, 1996   1–21

Objective.—Many falls in elderly individuals occur after meals, perhaps because of a drop in blood pressure related to carbohydrates in the meal. The mechanism of this postprandial hypotension is unknown. The vasodilatory peptide calcitonin gene-related peptide (CGRP) is released in response to carbohydrate loading. Its possible role in the occurrence of postprandial hypotension was investigated.

Methods.—Levels of CGRP were measured in 29 community-dwelling adults during an oral glucose tolerance test. The participants, who ranged in age from 20 to 83 years, were classified as young, middle-aged, or old. Heart rate and blood pressure responses were measured as well.

Results.—Systolic blood pressure declined by more than 15 mm Hg after glucose loading in 5 individuals, 4 of whom were older than 60 years. One of these individuals had temporary lightheadedness. On linear regression analysis, the oldest individuals showed a significant association between changes in CGRP, systolic blood pressure, and mean blood pressure. The change in CGRP was significantly greater for older individuals with a blood pressure drop of 15 mm Hg or more. No association between the changes in CGRP and blood pressure was noted in the young or middle-aged individuals.

Conclusions.—Increased levels of CGRP are linked to reduced blood pressure, and older individuals are more susceptible to these changes. Thus, CGRP may be involved in the pathogenesis of postprandial hypotension; other vasodilatory peptides may play a role as well. Further research is needed to clarify the role of CGRP in postprandial hypotension, particularly among the frail elderly.

▶ Postprandial hypotension has been known for almost 70 years; more recently, multiple studies have been done to further document this problem in older individuals. These studies have focused on community-dwelling elderly, particularly in older institutionalized individuals. The pathophysiologic mechanisms responsible for this well-documented fall in blood pressure after a meal in some individuals still require further investigation. The proposed hypotheses include an impaired sympathetic reflex reactivity to splanchnic vasodilation, interface between insulin and the sympathetic nervous system, or both.

It is of interest that this phenomenon has only been convincingly shown by oral glucose administration. This observation in itself raises the issue of whether 1 of the many vasoactive gut peptides may be involved in this abnormality. This article gives early evidence of a possible role of a CGRP as an explanation of the mechanism of this hypotension. This peptide is widely distributed in perivascular nerves and appears to have a role in the regulation of arterial blood flow. Numerous studies have shown an increase in the blood flow in the superior mesenteric, celiac, and renal arteries. In this study using a limited number of experimental individuals, CGRP level increased significantly in response to a glucose load both in the middle-aged group, as well as in the elderly, although the latter group seemed to show less effect in response to an oral glucose load.

It is interesting that in this study, individuals with a significant drop in blood pressure had the greatest change in CGRP levels and that the association was more pronounced in the older group. The study also is important because it clearly showed a total lack of correlation between insulin levels and hypotension, which suggests that other humoral agents play a role.

It is unfortunate that the investigators did not measure atrial natriuretic peptide, because this peptide is known to be released by glucose and there is moderately good evidence that the hypotensive response to atrial natriuretic peptide is greater in older individuals. This small study thus suggests that CGRP is 1 of the possible mediators of postprandial hypotension in older individuals, but clearly a larger number of individuals need to be studied. Such studies would be greatly enriched with the additional measurement of atrial natriuretic peptide.

J.C. Beck, M.D.

A Multidisciplinary Intervention to Prevent the Readmission of Elderly Patients With Congestive Heart Failure

Rich MW, Beckham V, Wittenberg C, et al (Washington Univ, St Louis, Mo)
N Engl J Med 333:1190–1195, 1995   1–22

Objective.—For individuals older than 65 years, congestive heart failure is the most common reason for hospitalization, and the rate of admission to treat this condition has been increasing. The impact of behavioral factors—such as poor treatment compliance and social isolation—on early readmission suggests that many admissions for congestive heart failure could be prevented. The ability of a multidisciplinary treatment approach to reduce the rate of readmission for congestive heart failure was studied among high-risk elderly patients.

Methods.—The prospective, randomized trial included 282 patients aged 70 years or older who had congestive heart failure and 1 or more risk factors for early admission: history of heart failure, 4 or more hospitalizations in the previous 5 years, or congestive heart failure caused by acute myocardial infarction or uncontrolled hypertension. The patients were randomized to receive either conventional care or a nurse-directed, multidisciplinary intervention. The intervention included comprehensive patient and family education, a prescribed diet, social services consultation and planning for early discharge, medication review, and intensive follow-up. The goals of follow-up were to reinforce the previous teaching, to make sure the patient was complying with medications and diet, and to identify recurrent symptoms that might be treatable on an outpatient basis. The patients were followed up for 90 days for hospital readmission. Quality of life and costs of care were also assessed.

TABLE 2.—Readmission and Death Within 90 Days of Initial Discharge From the Hospital

VARIABLE	CONTROL GROUP (n = 140)	TREATMENT GROUP (n = 142)	DIFFERENCE† (%)	P VALUE
Patients readmitted (no. of times)				
≥1	59 (42.1)	41 (28.9)	−31.5	0.03
≥2	23 (16.4)	9 (6.3)	−61.4	0.01
No. of readmissions	94	53	−44.4	0.02‡
For CHF	54	24	−56.2	0.04‡
Not for CHF	40	29	−28.5	NS
Hospital days				
All	865	556	−35.7	Not applicable
Per patient	6.2 ± 11.4	3.9 ± 10.0	−36.6	0.04‡
Deaths from any cause	17 (12.1)	13 (9.2)	−24.6	NS
In hospital	2 (1.4)	6 (4.2)	—	NS
After discharge	15 (10.7)	7 (4.9)	—	NS
Survival without readmission	75 (53.6)	91 (64.1)	+19.6	0.09
Death without readmission	6 (4.3)	10 (7.0)	—	NS

* Plus-minus values are means ± SD. Values followed by a number in parentheses are numbers of patients and percentages of the group.
† Percent differences were calculated by dividing the absolute percent difference between groups by the control-group percentage.
‡ By the Wilcoxon rank-sum test.
Abbreviations: CHF, congestive heart failure; *NS*, not significant.
(Reprinted by permission of *The New England Journal of Medicine*. Rich MW, Beckham V, Wittenberg C, et al: A multidisciplinary intervention to prevent the readmission of elderly patients with congestive heart failure. *N Engl J Med* 333:1190–1195, 1995. Copyright 1995, Massachusetts Medical Society.)

Results.—Sixty-four percent of patients in the intervention group and 54% of those in the control group survived to 90 days without readmission, a nonsignificant difference. Twenty-nine percent of patients in the intervention group vs. 42% of those in the control group required readmission (risk ratio, 0.56). The study intervention reduced the number of readmissions for heart failure significantly, by 56%. There was also a nonsignificant (29%) reduction in the number of readmissions for other causes. The percentage of patients having more than 1 readmission was 6% in the intervention group vs. 16% in the control group, (risk ratio, 0.39) (Table 2). A subgroup analysis showed more improvement in quality-of-life scores for patients in the intervention group. The intervention was also associated with an overall cost of care of $460 less, mainly because of fewer hospital admissions.

Conclusions.—The multidisciplinary intervention for congestive heart failure described in this study can significantly reduce the need for early readmission for elderly patients. The intervention is also associated with a significant improvement in quality of life and a significant reduction in the costs of care. If the intervention were implemented on a widespread basis, it could significantly reduce overall health care costs.

▶ Congestive heart failure is the most common admitting diagnosis for hospitalization among older individuals, and approximately one third to one half are readmitted within 3–6 months after initial hospitalization. Readmissions for congestive heart failure were reduced by 56% and readmissions for other causes by 28% through a nurse-directed, multidisciplinary intervention that consisted of intensive education about congestive heart failure and its treatment, individualized dietary instruction given by a dietitian, consultation with social service personnel to facilitate discharge planning, review of medications by a geriatrics cardiologist, and an intensive home-visit and telephone follow-up program. Moreover, quality-of-life scores improved and the overall cost of care was less in the treatment group. Unfortunately, many of the services provided in this innovative program would not be covered by fee-for-service Medicare. Hence, most likely the dissemination of these findings will be confined to at-risk capitated Medicare contractors.

D.B. Reuben, M.D.

A Trial of Annual In-Home Comprehensive Geriatric Assessments for Elderly People Living in the Community
Stuck AE, Aronow HU, Steiner A, et al (Univ of California, Los Angeles; Veterans Affairs Geriatric Research, Education, and Clinical Ctr, Sepulveda, Calif; Senior Health and Peer Counseling, Santa Monica, Calif; et al)
N Engl J Med 333:1184–1189, 1995   1–23

Background.—The increasing number of elderly individuals who are disabled will create increased demands on health care and social services. Preventive home visits for geriatric assessment have the potential to modify risk factors for disability but formal studies of in-home preventive services yielded variable results. The impact of annual, in-home comprehensive geriatric assessments and follow-up on the rate of disability among community-dwelling elderly individuals was evaluated.

Methods.—The 3-year, randomized, controlled trial included 414 individuals in 1 California county who were 75 years of age or older and living at home. Each was assigned to an intervention or control group. Individuals in the intervention group were visited at home by gerontologic nurse practitioners in each year of the study. The nurses collaborated with geriatricians to evaluate the subjects' problems and risk factors for disability, to make specific recommendations, and to provide health education which emphasized reducing the risk factors for disability. The subjects were encouraged to actively participate in their care and to discuss their problems with their physicians. Subjects in the control group received their usual medical care. The intervention was assessed for its effects in preventing disability, defined as the need for assistance with basic or instrumental activities of daily living, and in preventing nursing home admissions.

Results.—After 3 years, 12% of survivors in the intervention group vs. 32% of survivors in the control group required assistance with basic activities of daily living, for an adjusted odds ratio of 0.4. There was no significant difference in the number of subjects who needed help with instrumental activities of daily living. Permanent nursing home admission was required by 4% of the individuals in the intervention group vs. 10% of those in the control group; there was no difference in acute care hospital or short-term nursing home admissions. After the first year of the study, the subjects in the intervention group made significantly more physician visits than those in the control group: mean number of visits in year 3 was 1.27 and 0.92, respectively. The intervention cost approximately $6,000 per each year of disability-free life gained.

Conclusions.—Annual, comprehensive in-home geriatric assessments seem to prevent disability and reduce nursing home admission for community-living elderly individuals. It is uncertain which specific elements of the program tested have the most influence.

▶ Despite little evidence-based data from the United States to support outpatient comprehensive geriatric assessment, studies from other countries have suggested that in-home preventive services administered by an interdisciplinary team may be beneficial. In this randomized clinical trial, a program using nurse practitioners to conduct annual home assessments for unselected older (age 75 years or older) persons reduced the likelihood of requiring assistance in performing basic activities of daily living and being permanently admitted to a nursing home at 3 years. Although the number of physician visits during the second and third years of the study was more for subjects in the intervention group, the cost of the intervention for each year of disability-free life gained was modest ($6,000). The study challenges the widely held tenet that comprehensive geriatric assessment must be reserved for those older individuals who meet "targeting" criteria that identify those who are at most need for this service. It also emphasizes the need for follow-up by the team and subsequent revision of the initial care plan.

D.B. Reuben, M.D.

▶ This important randomized, controlled trial shows that annual in-home, comprehensive geriatric assessments performed by nurse practitioners not associated with the patient's primary care provider had positive outcomes on deterioration of basic activities of daily living but not instrumental activities of daily living. The intervention resulted in less frequent long-term stays in nursing homes but did not result in a decrease in the use of acute hospitals or short-term nursing home admissions. The study did not show a significant increase in the use of in-home supportive services.

These are important data and provide support for the value of this form of in-home comprehensive geriatric assessment performed by nurse practitioners. It is quite curious that there was less deterioration of the basic activities of daily living than instrumental activities of daily living, as this is not intuitive. It is not clear how the study impacted on the primary care providers involved in the patient's care, as only some of these individuals were notified and then only when a major problem was identified. Nevertheless, I think these are the kind of programs that I suspect will proliferate rapidly and especially in managed care settings. I suspect the outcomes would be considerably better if the innervation was tightly connected to the primary care providers. This, however, remains to be proved. I hope this study will be replicated.

A similar paper in the same issue of *The New England Journal of Medicine*[1] describes a randomized controlled trial of a nurse-directed, multidisciplinary intervention showing improved quality of life and decreased hospital admission rates for patients with severe congestive heart failure. The intervention featured a major educational effort and home visits as well as careful phone contact to insure compliance and provide oversight for care. Both of these papers improve our knowledge of the importance of multidisciplinary care for home visits to improve outcome in select patients.

J.R. Burton, M.D.

Reference

1. Rich MW, Beckham V, Whittenberg C, et al: A multidisciplinary intervention to prevent the readmission of elderly patients with congestive heart failure. *N Engl J Med* 333:1190–1195, 1995.

Physician Implementation of and Patient Adherence to Recommendations From Comprehensive Geriatric Assessment
Reuben DB, Maly RC, Hirsch SH, et al (Univ of California, Los Angeles; SysteMetrics, Santa Barbara, Calif; Mount Sinai Med Ctr, New York; et al)
Am J Med 100:444–451, 1996   1–24

Background.—Comprehensive geriatric assessment (CGA) is a promising but controversial intervention. Patients are screened and targeted for the intervention, strategies are recommended, and the patient and physician implement the recommendations. The benefits of CGA have not been demonstrated consistently, however, often because of low rates of implementation. A group of older individuals selected for outpatient CGA consultation was followed for physician implementation and patient adherence to recommended interventions.

Patients and Methods.—Participants were recruited through a program that screens community-dwelling older individuals for functional impairment, falls, depressive symptoms, and urinary incontinence. During the study, 150 of 820 screened individuals failed the screen and agreed to receive CGA; 139 completed follow-up interviews. Patients and the 115 physicians who provided their primary care received 1 of 3 interventions designed to increase implementation and adherence. Each of these interventions had a physician education component and a patient education and empowerment component. Patients were interviewed to determine adherence rates.

Results.—Individuals receiving CGA had a mean age of 76 years and received a mean of 3.8 recommendations. Most individuals were white (95%), female (71%), and lived alone (55%). The most common specific conditions for which recommendations were made were urinary incontinence and depression. The 3 intervention types did not appear to differ significantly in implementation and adherence. Recommendations described as "most important" by the CGA had the highest rates of implementation (83%) and adherence (81.8%). Recommendations for HMO patients had higher rates of physician implementation than recommendations for patients in other categories. Men had a higher rate of adherence than women. Adherence was lower when a patient had a greater number of recommendations, but higher among patients who had a greater number of identified problems.

Conclusions.—Low-cost adherence interventions, consisting of telephone calls and letters, was helpful in achieving high rates of implementation and adherence to recommendations of CGAs. Health benefits of the interventions will depend on accurate screening, value of the recommendations, and quality of care.

▶ A limiting factor to the effectiveness of CGA has been the inability of CGA teams to implement their recommendations. This lack of adherence by primary care physicians and their patients has been particularly problematic in consultative models of CGA and in ambulatory settings.

In this case-series of 139 individuals who received a 1-time outpatient CGA consultation and an adherence intervention aimed at both the primary care physician and the patient, adherence rates for major recommendations were high. The patient component focused on information sharing and patient empowerment to change physician behavior. However, this intervention was much less successful at implementing self-care recommendations, especially those requiring lifestyle modification or counseling. This study suggests that a relatively low-cost adherence intervention may improve the effectiveness of CGA but may not be enough to prompt major lifestyle changes.

D.B. Reuben, M.D.

Evaluation of Outpatient Geriatric Assessment: A Randomized Multisite Trial
Silverman M, Musa D, Martin DC, et al (Univ of Pittsburgh, Pa; Univ Ctr for Social and Urban Research, Pittsburgh, Pa; Shadyside Hosp, Pittsburgh, Pa)
J Am Geriatr Soc 43:733–740, 1995   1–25

Background.—The concept of multidisciplinary geriatric assessment and management has been studied extensively during the past 20 years. However, previous research has been limited by various methodological problems. The process and outcome of outpatient consultative geriatric assessment was compared with results of traditional community care. The study focused on the identification of common geriatric syndromes, the resulting health status of participants 1 year after randomization, health services utilization in the intervening years, patient satisfaction with care, and caregiver well-being.

Methods.—Four hundred forty-two elderly individuals with a health problem or recent change in health status were recruited to the randomized, controlled, 1-year trial. Patients were seen at 1 of 4 hospital-based ambulatory geriatric clinics or community physicians' offices.

Findings.—Compared with traditional community care, geriatric assessment enabled the identification of a significantly greater number of patients with cognitive impairment, depression, and incontinence. Greater improvement in anxiety levels at 1 year was documented in the group undergoing geriatric assessment. Caregivers of the elderly patients undergoing geriatric assessment also evidenced less stress at 1 year. The geriatric assessment and traditional care groups had comparable outcomes in mortality, nursing home admissions, cognitive health, functional health, or health services utilization. The geriatric assessment group showed some evidence of greater patient satisfaction.

Conclusions.—Consultative outpatient geriatric assessment resulted in significant improvements in the diagnosis of health problems common to the elderly, such as cognitive impairment, depression, and incontinence. There were also positive psychological and emotional benefits for patients and their caregivers.

▶ There have been well over 100 studies published on comprehensive geriatric assessment, and the reader might well ask: Why yet another report in this volume? I believe that this very carefully executed study is the fifth outpatient study reported in the literature, and it identifies some new areas of possible benefit. However, like the other studies of assessment in the ambulatory setting, it yields equivocal results with respect to health status, functional status, health services utilization, etc. The benefit was primarily on several psychosocial outcomes, including anxiety, patient satisfaction, and family caregivers. The convincing evidence of a benefit to family caregivers confirms one previous observation in this domain by Silliman et al., who also reported that geriatric assessment was beneficial in relieving caregiver stress.[1] Perhaps the major critique of this study, which I believe to be an effectiveness study in the real world of practice, is that there was no follow-up in terms of whether the recommendations made as a result of the assessment were actually implemented by the patients and their health providers.

J.C. Beck, M.D.

Reference

1. Silliman RA, McGarvey ST, Raymond PM, et al: The senior care study: Does inpatient interdisciplinary geriatric assessment help the family caregivers of acutely ill older patients? *J Am Geriatr Soc* 38:461–466, 1990.

Screening for Common Problems in Ambulatory Elderly: Clinical Confirmation of a Screening Instrument

Moore AA, Siu AL (Univ of California, Los Angeles; Mount Sinai School of Medicine, New York)
Am J Med 100:438–443, 1996

1–26

Introduction.—Functional deficits are better able to predict patient outcomes after hospitalization than admitting diagnoses. Existing instruments for measuring health status and function in elderly patients have not been useful for physicians in clinical practice. An instrument was developed and tested to determine if nonphysician office staff could effectively evaluate the functional ability of ambulatory elderly patients seen in physicians' offices.

Methods.—A literature review was conducted to identify problems that typically contribute to functional disability. Easy-to-administer screening measures were developed for 8 problems often missed during traditional physical examination: malnutrition/weight loss, visual impairment, hearing loss, cognitive impairment, urinary incontinence, depression, physical disability, and reduced leg mobility. A research assistant administered the screening to patients before they were seen by a geriatrician. These physicians were blinded to results of the screening performed by the research assistant. Results of the screening were compared with the geriatrician's evaluation. This was considered the gold standard. Geriatricians were then allowed to see the screening results and were given the opportunity to revise the original assessment. The sensitivity, specificity, and predictive value of the blinded and unblinded geriatric assessments were compared.

Results.—The mean age of the 109 patients in the study population was 79 years. The screening package (Table 1) took 8–12 minutes to administer. The interrater agreement per item ranged from 77% to 100%. Sensitivities were 0.65–0.93 (blinded) and 0.70–0.95 (unblinded). Specificities were 0.50–0.95 (blinded) and 0.64–0.95 (unblinded). The prevalence rate for the functional deficits measured ranged from 21% to 72%. The positive predictive values for items in the screening tool ranged from 0.60 and 0.91. The negative predictive values for same ranged between 0.77 and 0.96. Depending on the educational and skill level of the employee doing these screenings, it was estimated that the direct cost per patient screened in a clinical practice would be $1 to $7.

Conclusion.—The screening instrument developed to assess functional status in elderly patients in a clinical practice was inexpensive, short, and easy to use. Its validity and reliability were good. In a clinical setting, this tool could help physicians focus on the problems that commonly compromise the health and functioning of elderly patients.

▶ As pressure mounts for physicians to increase their productivity, concerns have been raised about the ability to provide comprehensive care within a shorter amount of time. Several recent efforts have been made to reduce the burden of work for the physicians by delegating some of their

TABLE 1.—Screening Package Characteristics

Problem	Screening Measure	Positive Screen	Supporting Data
Vision	2 Parts: Ask: "Do you have difficulty driving, or watching television, or reading, or doing any of your daily activities because of your eyesight? If yes, then: Test each eye with Snellen chart while patient wears corrective lenses (if applicable)	Yes to question and inability to read greater than 20/40 on Snellen chart.	Question: derived from some of the most reliable items on the Boston Activities of Daily Vision Scale; test-retest reliability is 0.8; Snellen chart: "gold" standard.
Hearing	Use audioscope set at 40 dB. Test hearing using 1,000 and 2,000 Hz.	Inability to hear 1,000 or 2,000 Hz in both ears or either of these frequencies in one ear.	In physicians' offices: sensitivity = 0.94; specificity = 0.72.
Leg mobility	Time the patient after asking: "Rise from the chair. Walk 20 feet briskly, turn, walk back to the chair and sit down."	Unable to complete task in 15 seconds.	Modified version of the "Up & Go"; inter-rater and test-retest reliability = 0.99; good correlations with other measures of gait and balance (−0.6 to −0.8).
Urinary incontinence	2 Parts: Ask: "In the last year, have you ever lost your urine and gotten wet?" If yes, then ask: "Have you lost urine on at least 6 separate days?"	Yes to both questions.	83% agreement between patient response and urologic assessment.
Nutrition/weight loss	2 Parts: Ask: "Have you lost 10 lbs. over the past 6 months without trying to do so?" Weigh the patient.	Yes to the question or weight <100 lb.	Question: relative risk of death = 2.0* (NHEFS); weight: PPV of malnutrition = 0.99.

Memory	Three-item recall.	Unable to remember all three items after 1 minute.	Likelihood ratios: recalls all 3 = 0.06; recalls 2 = 0.5; recalls <2 = 3.1.
Depression	Ask: "Do you often feel sad or depressed?"	Yes to the question.	Sensitivity = 0.78; specificity = 0.87.
Physical disability	Six questions: "Are you able to … : "Do strenuous activities like fast walking or bicycling?" "Do heavy work around the house like washing windows, walls, or floors?" "Go shopping for groceries or clothes?" "Get to places out of walking distance?" "Bathe, either a sponge bath, tub bath, or shower?" "Dress, like putting on a shirt, buttoning and zipping, or putting on shoes?"	Yes to any of the questions.	Coefficient of scalability 0.86; coefficient of reproducibility 0.96; test-retest reliability 0.88; good correlation with other measures of physical function 0.63–0.89.

* Personal communication from Tamara B. Harris, M.D.

Abbreviations: NHEFS, National Health Epidemiologic Follow-up Study; *PPV,* positive predictive value.

(Reprinted by permission of the publisher from Moore AA, Siu AL: Screening for common problems in ambulatory elderly: Clinical confirmation of a screening instrument. *American Journal of Medicine* 100:438–443, Copyright 1996 by Excerpta Medica, Inc.)

traditional tasks to office staff. Two years ago, Miller et al. reported a screening procedure that used individual instruments that had, by and large, been validated in other studies.[1] That battery required 21 minutes of an office assistant's time. Moore and Siu here report an even briefer screen that requires 10 minutes to administer and covers many of the common syndromes affecting older persons. These instruments, and others that will undoubtedly be developed, may prove extremely useful in ensuring that geriatric problems are not overlooked. However, their value depends on proper implementation and appropriate action based on the results of the screen. Practitioners or health care systems must be willing to invest the costs to release office staff to perform the screens, or hire additional staff to administer them. Moreover, clinicians must know how to respond when screening indicates a potential problem, including the appropriate subsequent diagnostic and therapeutic steps.

D.B. Reuben, M.D.

Reference

1. Miller DK, Brunworth D, Brunworth DS, et al: Efficiency of geriatric case-finding in a private practioner's office. *J Am Geriatr Soc* 43:533–537, 1995.

A Controlled Trial to Improve Care for Seriously Ill Hospitalized Patients: The Study to Understand Prognoses and Preferences for Outcomes and Risks of Treatments (SUPPORT)
Knaus WA, for The SUPPORT Principal Investigators (Univ of Virginia, Charlottesville)
JAMA 274:1591–1598, 1995   1–27

Introduction.—There is a new focus on obtaining realistic predictions of the results of life-sustaining treatments and on improving patient-physician communication regarding end-of-life decisions. Increased communication and better understanding of prognoses and patient preferences could reduce the time needed to make treatment decisions, time spent in undesirable states before death, and resource utilization. This hypothesis was tested in the Study to Understand Prognoses and Preferences for Outcomes and Risks of Treatments (SUPPORT).

Methods.—A phase I, prospective observational study of 4,301 seriously ill hospitalized patients confirmed the presence of barriers to optimal patient management and deficits in patient-physician communication. Based on these findings, thus, a phase II study was performed to determine whether the SUPPORT interventions were able to improve the decision-making process and to reduce the frequency of the mechanically supported, prolonged process of dying. Four thousand eight hundred four patients and their physicians were randomized by specialty group into intervention and control groups. In the intervention group, physicians received estimates of the likelihood of 6-month survival, the outcomes of

CPR, and functional disability at 2 months. Patient preferences were assessed by a trained research nurse who had multiple contacts with the patient and family as well as with the physician and hospital staff. The nurse also sought to enhance understanding of outcomes, attention to pain control, advance care planning, and patient-physician communication.

Results.—In the phase I study, although 31% of patients preferred that CPR be withheld, fewer than half of their physicians were aware of this preference. About half of do-not-resuscitate (DNR) orders were not written until 2 days before the patient died. Thirty-eight percent of deaths occurred after at least 10 days in the ICU, and half of conscious patients were in moderate-to-severe pain at least half the time before they died, according to family reports.

In the phase II study, the SUPPORT interventions made no difference in patient-physician communication. For example, approximately 60% of both groups failed to discuss their CPR preferences. Neither was there any improvement in the incidence or timing of DNR orders; physician knowledge of patients' resuscitation preferences; number of days in the ICU or percentage of patients receiving mechanical ventilation or becoming comatose before death; or reported pain level. Hospital resource use was also unaffected by the interventions.

Conclusion.—There are ongoing problems with the care provided to seriously ill patients in the hosptial. No improvements in care or patient outcomes were noted with implementation of the SUPPORT interventions. The results suggest that increased patient-physician communication may be insufficient to alter usual practice surrounding end-of-life decisions. Progress in this area may require increased commitment on the part of individuals and society, as well as more aggressive interventions.

▶ Seriously ill hospitalized patients are responsible for a large component of health care costs, often for care that does not result in substantial improvement in survival or quality of life. Moreover, many persons do not want aggressive treatments that may simply prolong life when cure or a return to usual functional capacity is not possible. However, communication between patient and physician to express personal preferences regarding treatments such as CPR, intubation and mechanical ventilation, and transfer to ICUs are infrequently discussed.

In preparation for this multisite trial, a multidisciplinary intervention was designed specifically to improve communication and understanding regarding prognosis. This intervention was then tested in a clinical trial at 5 teaching hospitals with the intent of improving 5 outcomes: (1) whether DNR orders were written and the timing of these; (2) patient and physician agreement on CPR preferences; (3) days spent in an ICU receiving mechanical ventilation or in a comatose state before death; (4) frequency and severity of pain; and (5) hospital resource use.

Although there was a slight increase in the number of patient-physician DNR agreements, no other outcomes demonstrated benefit from the intervention. Even with the intervention, fewer than half of the patients reported discussing their preferences with their physicians; furthermore, almost half of those who had no discussions said they would have liked to discuss CPR. It is clear that discussions about preferences regarding aggressiveness of care are among the most difficult for physicians to initiate. Given the importance of such planning for patients, perhaps this topic should be addressed earlier and more systematically throughout the training of all physicians.

D.B. Reuben, M.D.

Exercise Rehabilitation Programs for the Treatment of Claudication Pain: A Meta-Analysis
Gardner AW, Poehlman ET (Univ of Maryland, Baltimore; Baltimore Veterans Affairs Med Ctr, Md)
JAMA 274:975–980, 1995   1–28

Introduction.—Intermittent claudication occurs at an annual incidence of 20 per 1,000 individuals 65 years of age or older. Disabling symptoms are expected to occur in 1.3 million elderly individuals every 2 years for the next 50 years. Treatment for claudication consists of drug therapy, which is expensive and minimally effective, and surgery, which has risks of cardiovascular complications. Exercise rehabilitation is a noninvasive, inexpensive, and effective method of treating symptoms of intermittent claudication. A meta-analysis was conducted to identify the components of exercise rehabilitation programs that were the most effective in providing improvements in claudication pain symptoms.

Methods.—A search of the English-language literature was conducted to locate published studies on exercise rehabilitation programs for patients with intermittent claudication. To be considered for inclusion, studies had to use treadmill testing before and after an exercise program as part of the assessment. Studies were excluded if times or distances walked before onset of pain and maximal pain were not reported. The duration and mode of exercise, program length, pain end point used during the exercise session, and level of supervision were recorded for each study. Patient characteristics, walking times and distances to onset of pain, and treadmill protocol intensity were also recorded.

Results.—Twenty-one studies met the criteria for study inclusion; 18 were noncontrolled and nonrandomized, and 3 were randomized trials. The mean duration of exercise and program length was 39.1 minutes per session (3.1 sessions per week) and 21.8 weeks, respectively, for the 18 noncontrolled trials. For the randomized trials, the mean duration of exercise was 30 minutes per session (3 sessions per week) for 30.3 weeks. In the nonrandomized trials, a significant increase from baseline in the distance walked to the onset of pain was noted, as was a significant increase in the distance to maximal pain. For the randomized trials, patients in exercise groups also experienced significant increases in distance to onset of pain and to onset of maximal pain as compared with control patients.

Individual components of the exercise programs were evaluated for their independent effects on claudication pain. Exercise duration of 30 minutes or longer, exercise frequency of 3 sessions or more per week, programs of 26 weeks or longer, walking as the exercise used, and near-maximal pain as an end point for each training session were each found to result in significantly greater improvements in distance to onset of pain and distance to maximal pain. A large percentage of the variance observed in increases in distance to onset of pain and to maximal pain could be explained by use of pain as an end point during exercise, program length, or type of exercise used. Age was found to correlate with improvement, with older patients experiencing greater improvement as compared with younger patients.

Conclusions.—Participation in exercise rehabilitation programs resulted in increases of 120% to 180% in distance to onset of pain and to maximal claudication pain in patients with peripheral vascular disease. Use of near-maximal pain as an end point during exercise sessions, program duration of 6 months or more, and use of walking as the exercise were found to be the components of the rehabilitation program that were most responsible for patients' improvements.

▶ Peripheral arterial disease is one of the leading causes of morbidity in elderly individuals, whereas cardiovascular and cerebral vascular disease are leading causes of mortality. Drug treatment for peripheral arterial disease has had equivocal results. Surgery is expensive and is not applicable in a substantial number of older persons. There is a great deal of uncertainty as to whether exercise rehabilitation is effective and, on this basis, this paper describes a meta-analysis of 21 studies. There seems to be no question that exercise rehabilitation improved both distances to onset of pain and to maximal claudication.

The most important component of exercise appears to be the use of near-maximal claudication pain as the end point. The second most effective component is the length of the exercise program, and the meta-analytic data suggest that the program should be of no less than 6 months' duration. Finally, the mode of exercise is also of importance; rehabilitation programs involving walking only appeared to be more effective than those that involve other forms of exercise as well. From a practicing physician's point of view, good medical care for patients seen with intermittent claudication should include an optimal exercise program based on these 3 principles.

J.C. Beck, M.D.

Nifedipine: Dose-Related Increase in Mortality in Patients With Coronary Heart Disease

Furberg CD, Psaty BM, Meyer JV (Bowman Gray School of Medicine, Winston-Salem, NC; Univ of Washington, Seattle)

Circulation 92:1326–1331, 1995   1–29

Introduction.—Previous meta-analyses have shown no evidence of improved survival of coronary patients treated with any of the 3 main groups of calcium antagonists. Indeed, the calcium antagonists are associated with a slight increase in the mortality risk in these patients. The impact of the dose level was investigated in a new meta-analysis of randomized trials of nifedipine, and the likely mechanisms of action underlying the increased mortality were reviewed.

Methods.—The results of 16 randomized secondary-prevention clinical trials of nifedipine that had mortality data were analyzed. These trials included 8,350 patients who were treated with doses of nifedipine ranging from 30 to 120 mg/day. The relationship between nifedipine and mortality was analyzed across all trials and by dose.

Results.—Nifedipine treatment was associated with a relative risk of mortality of 1.16, indicating a statistically significant adverse effect. However, the relative risk of mortality varied substantially with the dose level. The mortality rates of the nifedipine-treated patients were similar to those of control groups in trials using doses between 30 and 50 mg/day. The relative risk of mortality increased to 1.18 in trials using doses of 60 mg/day and to 2.83 in trials using doses of 80 mg/day. The potentially harmful effects associated with nifedipine treatment included a proischemic effect, a negative inotropic effect, an effect on rhythm, a prohemorrhagic effect, and hypotension.

Discussion.—The risk of mortality associated with nifedipine treatment is strongly dose-dependent, indicating that patients who have stable or unstable angina and survivors of acute myocardial infarction should not be treated with moderate or high doses of nifedipine. It is likely that the nifedipine-induced increase in sympathetic activity is the mechanism of action underlying the reported harmful effects of treatment. These findings may also pertain to other short-acting dihydropyridines, underscoring the need for adequate study of the long-term safety of treatment with calcium antagonists.

▶ There have been a multiplicity of meta-analyses addressing the relationship between calcium antagonists in myocardial infarction and unstable angina and mortality. I believe this is the first paper that, in its meta-analysis, related the mortality data to the dose level of nifedipine. The data are summarized in the abstract, but it is clear that there is a strong and direct relationship between mortality and the dose of nifedipine. Any doses, greater than 60 mg/day lead to an almost threefold risk of death. There are some suggestions from the data that there may be a threshold effect at these high doses, but I do not believe that the data available in this paper are convincing. Although it is important that the effects of nifedipine on morbidity and mortality in hypertension be addressed as a separate issue, I think one must conclude that the use of these agents in higher doses should probably be restricted until adequate safety information is available. The paper also does not address the issue of the long-acting forms of this series of drugs; these data are badly needed.

J.C. Beck, M.D.

A Comparison of Low-Molecular-Weight Heparin Administered Primarily at Home With Unfractionated Heparin Administered in the Hospital for Proximal Deep-Vein Thrombosis

Levine M, Gent M, Hirsh J, et al (McMaster Univ, Hamilton, Ont, Canada; Hamilton Civic Hosps Research Centre, Ont, Canada; Hamilton Regional Cancer Centre, Ont, Canada; et al)
N Engl J Med 334:677–681, 1996   1–30

Background.—For most patients with acute proximal deep vein thrombosis (DVT), the initial hospital treatment consists of IV standard (unfractionated) heparin. Several characteristics of low–molecular weight heparins, including their longer plasma half-life, better bioavailability after subcutaneous administration, and more predictable anticoagulant response, could permit patients with proven DVT to be treated at home rather than in the hospital. Hospital treatment with IV standard heparin and home treatment with subcutaneous low–molecular weight heparin were compared.

Methods.—A total of 500 patients with acute proximal DVT were randomly assigned to receive either in-hospital treatment with IV standard heparin in a continuous infusion (253 patients) or low–molecular weight heparin given primarily at home (247 patients). The home treatment regimen consisted of enoxaprin, 1 mg/kg, given subcutaneously twice daily. Patients assigned to low-molecular weight heparin were permitted to return home immediately, and patients who were already hospitalized when they started taking low–molecular weight heparin were discharged early. Warfarin treatment started on the second day for all patients.

Results.—The rate of recurrent thromboembolism was 5.3% in the low–molecular weight heparin group vs. 6.7% in the standard heparin group, for an absolute difference of 1.4% (95% confidence interval, −3.0–5.7). Major bleeding occurred in 5 patients in the low–molecular weight heparin group and in 3 patients in the standard heparin group. The mean hospital stay after randomization was 1.1 days in the low–molecular weight heparin group compared with 6.5 days in the standard heparin group, and nearly half of the former group did not require hospitalization.

Conclusions.—Many patients with proximal DVT can be safely treated at home with subcutaneous low–molecular weight heparin. This treatment is convenient for the patient and reduces costs substantially for the health care system.

▶ See comment following Abstract 1–31.

Treatment of Venous Thrombosis With Intravenous Unfractionated Heparin Administered in the Hospital as Compared With Subcutaneous Low-Molecular-Weight Heparin Administered at Home

Koopman MMW, for the Tasman Study Group (Academic Med Ctr, Amsterdam; Slotervaart Hosp, Amsterdam, Istituto di Semeiotica Medica, Padua, Italy; et al)

N Engl J Med 334:682–687, 1996   1–31

Background.—The standard in-hospital treatment for patients with deep-vein thrombosis consists of an IV course of unfractionated heparin, with dose adjustments to prolong the activated partial-thromboplastin time to the length desired. However, fixed-dose subcutaneous low–molecular weight heparin, which can be given on an outpatient basis, appears to be as safe and effective. The 2 treatments were compared in symptomatic outpatients with proximal-vein thrombosis but no signs of pulmonary embolism.

Methods and Findings.—By random assignment, 198 patients were given adjusted-dose IV standard heparin in the hospital, and 202 received fixed-dose subcutaneous low–molecular weight heparin at home. Thromboembolism recurred in 8.6% of the patients receiving standard heparin and 6.9% of those receiving low–molecular weight heparin. Major bleeding occurred in 2% and 0.5% of patients, respectively. Both groups showed improvement in quality of life. Patients given low–molecular weight heparin had better physical activity and social functioning. Thirty-six percent of those receiving low–molecular weight heparin were never hospitalized. Forty percent were discharged early. The number of days spent in the hospital was reduced by 67%.

Conclusions.—Outpatient treatment with fixed-dose subcutaneous low–molecular weight heparin in the treatment of proximal-vein thrombosis is effective and safe. Such treatment does not adversely affect physical or mental well-being, and it decreases costs.

▶ These 2 papers (Abstracts 1–30 and 1–31), appearing simultaneously, were selected because they convincingly demonstrate that low–molecular weight heparin can be safely and effectively used to treat patients with deep-vein thrombosis at home. They represent a multicenter Canadian study and a multicenter European-Australasian study, respectively.

Current practice with respect to the treatment of deep-vein thrombosis has been the use of IV standard (unfractionated) heparin for a minimum of 5 days in a dose-adjusted schedule to increase the activated partial-thromboplastin time into a desired range. Oral anticoagulant therapy has usually been started concomitantly and continued for 3 months. The outcomes from this approach have clearly demonstrated their effectiveness, but the major limitation has been that patients required hospital admission, thus exposing them to all the risks associated with hospitalization.

Previous work has clearly demonstrated that depolymerization of heparin yields low–molecular weight heparins that have a number of advantages over the standard heparin. These include a better bioavailability, a longer half-life, and a much more predictable anticoagulant activity period. In-hospital studies have demonstrated that fixed doses of subcutaneous low–molecular weight heparin are as effective as the adjusted doses of IV standard heparin.[1-5] These 2 randomized trials convincingly demonstrate in large populations of patients that the use of low–molecular weight heparin at home is feasible with an effectiveness that is equal to that of the traditional treatment regimen and, in the study of Koopman et al., is not associated with any reduction in quality of life. In fact, there was a clear demonstration of less impairment of physical activity and social functioning. This new regimen either averted hospitalization or reduced the average hospital stay. The increased need for ambulatory and home health services did not offset this decreased use of institutional resources.

These results, I believe, have major implications because each year approximately 250,000 Americans have needed to be hospitalized for 5–10 days of IV heparin therapy. However, there are 3 potential hazards that must be dealt with: (1) Because the clinical diagnosis of deep-vein thrombosis is unreliable, the disease must be confirmed objectively to avoid unnecessary treatment; (2) there must be an adequate assessment of risk factors for venous thromboembolism; and (3) community facilities must be prepared to provide proper anticoagulant therapy before the treatment of this disorder is moved from the hospital to the community.

J.C. Beck, M.D.

References

1. Prandoni P, Lensing AWA, Buller HR, et al: Comparison of subcutaneous low-molecular-weight heparin with intravenous standard heparin in proximal deep-vein thrombosis. *Lancet* 339:441-445, 1992.
2. Hull RD, Raskob GE, Pineo GF, et al: Subcutaneous low-molecular-weight heparin compared with continuous intravenous heparin in the treatment of proximal-vein thrombosis. *N Engl J Med* 326:975-982, 1992.
3. Lopaciuk S, Meissner AJ, Filipecki S, et al: Subcutaneous low molecular weight heparin versus subcutaneous unfractionated heparin in the treatment of deep vein thrombosis: A Polish multicenter trial. *Thromb Haemost* 68:14–18, 1992.
4. Lindmarker P, Homstrom M, Granqvist S, et al: Comparison of once-daily subcutaneous Fragmin with continuous intravenous unfractionated heparin in the treatment of deep vein thrombosis. *Thromb Haemost* 72:186–190, 1994.
5. Lensing AWA, Prins MH, Davidson BL, et al: Treatment of deep venous thrombosis with low-molecular-weight heparins: A meta-analysis. *Arch Intern Med* 155:601–607, 1995.

Axial Bone Mass in Older Women

Orwoll ES, for the Study of Osteoporotic Fractures Research Group (Portland Veterans Affairs Med Ctr, Ore; Kaiser Permanente Ctr for Health Research, Portland, Ore; Univ of California, San Francisco; et al)

Ann Intern Med 124:187–196, 1996   1–32

Background.—There is substantial evidence that bone mineral density (BMD) decreases in women with increasing age, particularly after menopause. This decrease in BMD is associated with an increased risk of fracture. Factors associated with axial BMD in the spine and proximal femur were evaluated.

Methods.—During a 2-year period, 9,704 nonblack women aged 65 years or older were studied. Bone mineral density of the lumbar spine, femoral neck, intertrochanteric region, trochanter, and the Ward triangle was measured with dual-energy x-ray absorptiometry. The women completed a questionnaire addressing family and reproductive history, medications, calcium intake, physical activity, weight, knee height, and height loss since the age of 25 years. They were also assessed for muscle strength and gait speed. The significance of associations between BMD and the assessed variables suggest ways to better identify risk for fracture.

Results.—A reduced BMD at all sites was associated with increasing age and was most strongly predicted by weight. There were positive associations between BMD and overall height and knee height. Both spinal and femoral BMD increased with earlier menarche and later menopause and with current use of oral estrogen. The benefits of estrogen use decreased progressively after discontinuation. A family history of hip fracture was associated with reduced spine and femoral BMD. Calcium and vitamin-D intake were positively associated with BMD, as were strength, walking speed, and the level of physical activity. There were negative correlations between BMD and tobacco use, caffeine intake, and glucocorticoid or anticonvulsant treatment and a positive association between BMD and alcohol consumption and thiazide diuretic use. The multivariable regression models explained 21% to 25% of the variation in femoral and spinal BMD.

Conclusions.—Several factors are predictive of bone mass, including family and reproductive history, nutritional factors, medication use, and exercise. Examination of these factors can improve the estimation of fracture risk.

▶ Many attempts have been made to find the determinants of BMD, but most of these have involved relatively small selected populations; thus the relative importance of many of the proposed factors have been difficult to assess and often controversial. This paper was selected because of certain unique features, including the study's large size, the careful delineations of the variables studied, and the large amount of additional information that is available about the study cohort. There are several variables including weight, height, estrogen exposure, non–insulin-dependent diabetes mellitus, and thiazide use that were consistently associated with greater bone mass. A positive effect of calcium intake was clearly present at both femoral and radial sites and at the spine in the bivariate models. In contrast, a family history of fracture had a negative effect at all skeletal sites, and aging was associated with lower BMD in all areas except the spine, where artifact may have obscured this trend.

One of the surprising observations was that nonthiazide diuretics were related to higher bone mass, an association that persisted even when participants who had ever taken thiazides were omitted from the analysis. The association of BMD with diuretics with differing mechanisms of action prompts further study of their mechanism of action. The data also suggest that excessive thinness should be discouraged and physical activity should be encouraged.

There are a number of limitations of this study: (1) the study population was made up of independently living volunteers of which a special population may have been selected; (2) the study was cross-sectional in design; and (3) some of the information was obtained by recall.

J.C. Beck, M.D.

Gastric Emptying in Parkinson's Disease: Patients With and Without Response Fluctuations
Djaldetti R, Baron J, Ziv I, et al (Beilinson Med Ctr, Petah Tiqva, Israel; Elias Sourasky Med Ctr, Tel Aviv, Israel; Tel Aviv Univ, Israel)
Neurology 46:1051–1054, 1996   1–33

Background.—Interest in gastrointestinal dysfunction in patients with Parkinson's disease (PD) is increasing, especially regarding its involvement in oral levodopa absorption in patients with response fluctuations. Gastric motility in patients with PD was investigated with a radionuclide gastric-emptying method, and findings were correlated with disease severity and response fluctuations.

Methods.—Thirty patients with PD underwent radionuclide` gastric-emptying investigation with the use of a standard technetium-99m colloid-labeled solid meal. Fifteen patients were fluctuators with "delayed-on" and "no-on" phenomena, and 15 were nonfluctuators. Fasting patients received the standard meal. Gastric emptying was monitored with a gamma camera positioned over the stomach, recording data for 1 hour.

Findings.—Compared with normal control subjects, patients with PD had prolonged gastric emptying measured after 60 minutes. Gastric retention at 1 hour was increased in patients with fluctuations, compared with those without fluctuations. Patients with response fluctuations also had significantly delayed half-time emptying.

Conclusions.—Delayed gastric emptying is common in patients with PD, being more marked in those with response fluctuations. The stomach is an important target organ, affected by the basic pathology of PD, chronic drug use, or both.

▶ There is increasing interest in gastrointestinal dysfunction in PD because it may be involved in oral levodopa absorption in patients with response fluctuations. Previous studies have showed a high frequency of gastric atony and reduced gastric motility in PD, but these studies usually have been reported in abstract form only.

This study investigated gastric motility in patients with PD with a radio-nuclide gastric-emptying technique and correlated the findings with disease severity and response fluctuations. The results showed that impairment of gastric motility occurs in about 70% of patients with PD and is especially severe in those with response fluctuations. Of interest was that patients with "delayed-on" and "no-on" subtypes of response fluctuations had significantly longer retention times of food in the stomach than did those without response fluctuations. This finding strongly supports the argument that these response fluctuations are caused by peripheral pharmacokinetic mechanisms, particularly delayed gastric emptying, which retards or prevents levodopa absorption.

The site of the effect that explains this delayed gastric emptying is still unclear. Some evidence suggests a local lesion in the myenteric plexuses, whereas other evidence suggests an effect comparable to downregulation associated with prolonged levodopa use.

It is of interest that no correlation was found between disease severity or the duration of the PD and the presence of gastric impairment in this study. It also is important to emphasize that 6 patients with long-standing disease had normal gastric emptying.

J.C. Beck, M.D.

Mortality Following Conjugal Bereavement and the Effects of a Shared Environment
Schaefer C, Quesenberry CP, Jr, Wi S (Kaiser Found Research Inst, Oakland, Calif)
Am J Epidemiol 141:1142–1152, 1995   1–34

Background.—Conjugal bereavement has been associated with an increased risk of mortality among surviving spouses. However, the duration of that increased risk and the effects of age, sex, socioeconomic status, and preexisting health problems or health-related behaviors have not been thoroughly investigated. These issues were explored.

Methods.—A cohort of 12,522 spouse pairs completed a questionnaire and underwent a physical examination between 1964 and 1973. All were members of a prepaid health care plan in northern California. The cohort was followed through 1987.

Findings.—The spouses of 1,453 men and 3,294 women died between 1964 and 1987. Thirty percent of bereaved men and 15% of bereaved women died during that time. In a proportional hazards analysis, death rates after bereavement were significantly increased for both sexes after adjusting for age, education, and other mortality predictors. The greatest relative risk (RR) of death occurred 7–12 months after the death of a spouse. Women had an RR of 1.9 during this period. The effect of bereavement among men interacted with previous health status. Men with few health problems had an RR of 2.12, and men with many health problems had an RR of 1.56 7–12 months after the death of their wife. The RR declined after the first year of bereavement among both sexes but continued to exceed 1.0 for more than 2 years after the spouse's death. There appeared to be no effect of a shared unfavorable environment on mortality after bereavement.

Conclusions.—The increase in mortality after the death of a spouse appears to be real, rather than an artifact of selection or unmeasured covariates. This phenomenon merits further research, as it is one of the few well documented examples of how social environment profoundly affects human health.

▶ This large prospective study gives new insight into the relationships explaining the increased mortality after conjugal bereavement. Although the study supports and extends previous findings of the increased risk of mortality after conjugal bereavement, its strength lies in the size of the study, the fact that it was prospective, and that the study had data on health habits and the health status of both spouses before bereavement. Because the study was a secondary analysis, it was free from any selection bias and it made use of newer statistical models including proportional hazard models, which virtually eliminates previous critiques of differential lengths in follow-up.

The study clearly demonstrates that the effects of a shared environment do not explain the increased risk of mortality, thus necessitating abandonment of a major previous belief. In addition, controlling for a variety of risk factors present before bereavement clearly demonstrates that these risk factors do not explain the increased risk of mortality. Finally, these results together with past studies convincingly demonstrate that the increased mortality is a real one and not an artifact. I believe it thus deserves further study as an excellent example of a major change in social environment affecting human health. Such a study might give major insights into the mechanisms by which this is brought about.

J.C. Beck, M.D.

Geriatric Syndromes: Hearing, Vision, Pressure Sores, Benign Prostatic Hyperplasia, and Malnutrition

Central Auditory Dysfunction, Cognitive Dysfunction, and Dementia in Older People
Gates GA, Cobb JL, Linn RT, et al (Univ of Washington, Seattle; Boston Univ; Erie County Med Ctr, Buffalo, NY)
Arch Otolaryngol Head Neck Surg 122:161–167, 1996   1–35

Objective.—Participants in the Framingham Heart Study underwent auditory testing and were scored on the Mini-Mental State Examination (MMSE) to determine the relation between auditory dysfunction and cognitive dysfunction in older individuals. The value of central auditory test abnormalities to predict cognitive decline or the onset of clinical dementia was also assessed.

Methods.—Central auditory testing was performed for 1,026 study members at the eighteenth biennial examination. Participants ranged in age from 63 to 95 years. Abnormal results were noted in 18.2% of 816 individuals who received the Synthetic Sentence Identification with Ipsilateral Competing Message (SSI-ICM), in 10.7% of 941 who took the Staggered Spondaic Word test, and in 1.4% of 1,009 who took the Performance-Intensity function of Phonetically Balanced Words. Two subscores of the MMSE were created for this analysis: the visual subscore, defined as the sum of responses to questions with predominantly visual input; and the auditory subscore, defined as the sum of responses to all other items that depended solely on auditory cues. Those with abnormal findings on the MMSE underwent detailed neuropsychological testing. Auditory test results were recorded for better and worse ears and compared with MMSE scores and with the onset of clinical dementia during the subsequent 6 years.

Results.—Clinical dementia developed in 41 of 1,509 individuals who completed basic audiometric tests and the MMSE; 20 of the 41 underwent central auditory testing at examination 18. Nineteen of 20 were classified as having probable Alzheimer's disease, and 1 had dementia caused by brain injury. Of the 19 individuals with probable Alzheimer's disease, 4 also had a stroke during follow-up, and 3 had Parkinson's disease diagnosed. The worse ear SSI-ICM score was significantly related to concurrent MMSE raw score, subsequent onset of dementia, and subsequent decline in the MMSE score. As expected, the relation between the SSI-ICM score and the MMSE was principally with the auditory parts of the MMSE.

Conclusions.—Central auditory dysfunction may be an early marker for senile dementia. Individuals with very poor SSI-ICM scores in 1 ear had a relative risk of 6 for subsequent clinical dementia or cognitive decline; the relative risk was 12.5 for those with scores less than 50% in both ears. Measures of peripheral and central auditory functions are recommended as part of standard evaluations for the older population.

▶ In elderly individuals, hearing loss can be related to either peripheral (sensorineural) or central factors. Although presbycusis is the most common cause of hearing loss in older individuals, impaired central auditory processing is also important in this age group. The relationship between hearing loss and dementia has been difficult to establish because the dementing process may interfere with adequate auditory evaluation; conversely, impaired auditory function may interfere with adequate cognitive testing.

This study using the Framingham Heart Study cohort provides additional insight into this relationship. The investigators administered tests of both peripheral and central auditory function and monitored subsequent changes in MMSE score as well as incident diagnoses of dementia. Their principal finding was that central hearing dysfunction preceded the development of declines in MMSE scores and the diagnosis of dementia. The study is limited by the small number of subjects (*n* = 20) of the sample who had dementia develop during the follow-up period. Nevertheless, these results help expand our inventory of the symptoms associated with early dementia.

D.B. Reuben, M.D.

Cataract Surgery in One Eye or Both: A Billion Dollar Per Year Issue
Javitt JC, Steinberg EP, Sharkey P, et al (Georgetown Univ, Washington, DC; Johns Hopkins Univ, Baltimore, Md; Johns Hopkins Med Inst, Baltimore, Md; et al)
Ophthalmology 102:1583–1593, 1995   1–36

Background.—Most outcome studies of cataract surgery, the most frequent surgical procedure among Medicare beneficiaries, have focused on the changes occurring after the first eye undergoes the operation. There have been no studies assessing the benefits—both visual and quality of life—of having cataract surgery in both eyes. The relative effects of second-eye cataract surgery on functional impairment, satisfaction, and vision problems were assessed.

Methods.—Seventy-five ophthalmologists in 3 United States cities were asked to enroll 14 consecutive patients who were scheduled to undergo first-eye cataract surgery. The patients were interviewed at enrollment and again at 4 and 12 months after first-eye cataract surgery. A special preoperative interview was also conducted in patients whose second-eye surgery was to take place before the 4-month interview. In addition to a 14-question assessment of visual function (the VF-14), each interview included questions about symptoms related to cataract, visual problems, and satisfaction with vision.

Results.—Of 772 patients enrolled, 669 gave interview data from enrollment to 12 months. Thirty-six percent had cataract surgery in the second eye during that year. Improvement in the VF-14 score was 61% greater for patients who underwent second-eye cataract surgery, compared with those who had cataract surgery in only 1 eye. This difference was related not only to the direct effect of the second-eye surgery but also to a decline in visual function in the 1-eye surgery group from 4 to 12 months postoperatively. The patients who had surgery for both eyes also reported 27% greater decline in visual problems and 24% greater improvement in satisfaction with vision. Older patients and those whose vision was worse at baseline tended to obtain the most benefit from second-eye surgery.

Conclusions.—Cataract surgery on the second eye has important benefits in addition to those of first-eye cataract surgery. The second operation is associated with significant reductions in functional impairment and trouble with vision and increased satisfaction with vision. The indication for cataract surgery in the second eye should be impairment in the patient's functional ability that is related to the cataract and that is of concern to the patient.

▶ Cataract surgery, the most frequently performed surgical procedure performed on older persons, has improved visual function and quality of life, according to observational studies. Because the disease is frequently bilateral, the additional benefit of a second procedure to remove cataracts in the second eye remains an economically important but unanswered question. From patients enrolled in the National Study of Cataract Outcomes, the investigators interviewed 164 of 243 subjects (who had surgery in both eyes) after their first surgery but before their second surgery. These subjects and an additional 426 who had surgery in only one eye were interviewed 12 months after entry into the study. Those who had bilateral surgery had worse initial vision and visual function but demonstrated substantially greater improvement in visual function and satisfaction with vision. Advancing age, better baseline visual functioning, and the presence of other eye diseases were associated with less improvement of visual function; second eye surgery remained independently predictive of improved visual function at 12 months. The authors interpret these changes to improvement as a result of the second eye surgery as well as decline in function in the eye that did not undergo surgery. These findings underscore the importance of binocular vision in older persons. Unfortunately, it also means that any move to deny second cataract extractions to Medicare beneficiaries would also likely compromise visual function and lead to consequent medical and functional complications in this population.

D.B. Reuben, M.D.

Cigarette Smoking and Risk for Progression of Nuclear Opacities
West S, Muñoz B, Schein OD, et al (Johns Hopkins Univ, Baltimore, Md; Univ of Melbourne, Australia)
Arch Ophthalmol 113:1377–1380, 1995   1–37

Background.—Cigarette smoking has been associated with an increased risk of cataracts. The relationships between smoking and the 5-year incidence of new nuclear opacities as well as the progression of nuclear opacities were explored prospectively in a cohort of Chesapeake Bay watermen.

Methods.—Four hundred forty-two men aged 30 years or older were included in the analysis. All had paired, gradable lens photographs of at least 1 eye in 1985 and 1990. Two readers graded the photographs using the Wilmer Institute scheme. Severity ranged in decimal units between 0 and 4. Smoking histories were obtained by personal interview in 1985 and 1990.

Findings.—Opacity incidence and progression increased with age. Current and former smoking was not significantly correlated with the incidence of a nuclear opacity. Men who were current smokers in 1985 had a 2.4-fold greater risk of progression of nuclear opacities of less than grade 3 to grade 3 or worse compared with nonsmokers and exsmokers, after adjustment for age, initial opacity status, and alcohol use. Each pack-year between 1985 and 1990 was significantly correlated with an 18% increase in the risk of progression. The effect of quitting smoking between 1985 and 1990 on the risk of progression could not be analyzed, as only 39 men quit in that period.

Conclusions.—These findings support the association of smoking with the risk of nuclear opacities. The role of smoking is especially clear in progression in current smokers. Further research is needed on the precise mechanism by which smoking damages the lens.

▶ This paper serves as a follow-up to one study on the association between smoking and risk of cataracts in the Chesapeake Bay watermen that appeared early in the YEAR BOOK series.[1] As summarized in the abstract, there is a significant association between smoking and progression of cataracts. This strongly suggests that smoking is a promoting factor for nuclear opacification. Unfortunately, there were only 39 persons in the sample who quit in the intervening period so that no significant data were available on the impact of quitting smoking. The data also demonstrate that the association is with current smokers and is dose related. This clearly suggests that quitting smoking might reduce the risk of nuclear opacity, and these findings are consistent with the findings of the original study, which was a cross-sectional epidemiologic study.

J.C. Beck, M.D.

Reference

1. West S, Muñoz B, Emmett EA, et al: Cigarette smoking and risk of nuclear cataracts. *Arch Ophthalmol* 107:1166–1169, 1989.

Alcohol Use and Age-Related Maculopathy in the Beaver Dam Eye Study
Ritter LL, Klein R, Klein BEK, et al (Univ of Wisconsin, Madison)
Am J Ophthalmol 120:190–196, 1995   1–38

Background.—Age-related maculopathy is a major cause of visual loss in persons older than 65 years. However, there currently are no public health strategies or medical interventions to prevent the development or progression of this entity. Alcohol intake, a modifiable behavior, may increase oxidant stress or affect mechanisms that protect against oxidative damage. The association between history of alcohol intake and age-related maculopathy was investigated.

Methods.—A total of 4,926 Beaver Dam, Wisconsin, residents aged 43–84 years participated in the study. The subjects completed a standardized questionnaire on their alcohol intake in the preceding year. They were then examined, and age-related maculopathy status was determined on stereoscopic color fundus photographs.

Findings.—Drinking beer in the preceding year was associated with greater odds of increased retinal pigment degeneration and exudative macular degeneration after adjustment for other variables. There was no correlation between current intake of wine or liquor and early or late age-related maculopathy.

Conclusions.—Beer consumption appears to be associated with greater odds of having exudative macular degeneration. It is unknown whether this relationship is the result of a toxic effect specific to beer or of other, unknown confounding variables.

▶ Age-related maculopathy remains a major cause of visual loss for which interventions are, at best, marginal. This has resulted in a search for modifiable risk factors, and there are only a few epidemiologic studies examining a possible relationship between alcohol ingestion and age-related maculopathy.[1, 2] It is of interest that only beer drinking appears to be associated with age-related maculopathy. On the basis of the results of this large epidemiologic study, beer drinkers are more likely to be men and either past or current smokers, and they are more likely to drink large quantities. Controlling for smoking history and sex did not alter the basic findings, which suggests that there are unmeasured factors in beer or noxious substances that may contribute to the development of maculopathy.

The major limitation of this study is that it is cross-sectional and, thus, the exact relationship within the association remains undecided. Hopefully, as this is an ongoing study, further longitudinal studies of this population will be made.

J.C. Beck, M.D.

References

1. Maltzman BA, Mulvihill MN, Greenbaum A: Senile macular degeneration and risk factors: A case-control study. *Ann Ophthalmol* 11:1197–1201, 1979.
2. The Eye Disease Case-Control Study Group: Risk factors for neovascular age-related macular degeneration. *Arch Ophthalmol* 110:1701–1708, 1992.

Randomized Clinical Trial of Ascorbic Acid in the Treatment of Pressure Ulcers
ter Riet G, Kessels AGH, Knipschild PG (Univ of Limburg, The Netherlands)
J Clin Epidemiol 48:1453–1460, 1995   1–39

Introduction.—Previous studies have suggested that taking ascorbic acid (AA), the reduced form of vitamin C, at a dose of 10–20 mg/day enhances healing of incisional or punch biopsy wound. One commonly cited clinical trial suggested that an AA dose of 500 mg twice daily nearly doubled the healing rate of pressure ulcers. These 2 AA doses were compared as an adjunct to standard therapy for pressure ulcers.

Methods.—The multicenter, blinded, randomized trial included 88 patients from 11 nursing homes and 1 hospital. They were randomized to receive AA at a dose of either 10 mg or 500 mg twice daily. The results were assessed by intention-to-treat analysis in terms of wound survival, healing rates of wound surfaces, and clinimetric changes during a 12-week treatment period.

Results.—Wound closure rate was not different between the 2 dose groups, with a Cox hazard ratio of 0.78 for the higher-dose group. Mean surface reduction rates were 0.21 cm^2/week in the 500 mg/day group and 0.27 cm^2 /week in the 10 mg/day group. The higher dose had no favorable effect on relative healing rates or healing velocities, nor on either of 2 clinimetric indexes.

Conclusions.—High-dose AA supplementation does not seem to enhance the healing of pressure ulcers. Although scurvy can delay wound healing, this problem is prevented by an AA dose of 10–20 mg/day.

▶ Despite the effectiveness of frequent positioning and other nursing measures in preventing pressure ulcers, these continue to be common complications of hospitalizations and nursing home stays. After pressure ulcers develop, a variety of treatments, ranging from beds designed to reduce pressure to topical dressings, have been widely used. Vitamin C has generally been added as an adjunct based on earlier research conducted on hospitalized patients, many of whom were vitamin-C deficient. This randomized clinical trial conducted primarily at 11 nursing homes ensured that control group subjects were not vitamin-C deficient by providing a very low dose of vitamin-C to prevent scurvy (20 mg/day) and then tested the additional benefit of 500 mg twice daily. The investigators found no benefit from the higher dose overall, nor in subgroup analyses examining those subjects with ulcers of smaller vs. larger surface area, those with differing amounts of spontaneous movements, and those with different baseline plasma vitamin-C concentrations. Although the sample size of the study was small, the estimate of effect did not suggest that a larger sample size would have made any difference. Thus, it appears that vitamin-C can be safely omitted from the armamentarium of treatments for pressure sores.

D.B. Reuben, M.D.

The Efficacy of Terazosin, Finasteride, or Both in Benign Prostatic Hyperplasia

Lepor H, for the Veterans Affairs Cooperative Studies Benign Prostatic Hyperplasia Study Group (VA Med Ctr, New York; New York Univ; VA Med Ctr, Perry Point, Md; et al)
N Engl J Med 335:533–539, 1996   1–40

Introduction.—Drugs are now available that relieve the symptoms of benign prostatic hyperplasia, thus offering an alternative to surgical treatment of the disorder. The 2 drug options are finasteride, a 5α-reductase inhibitor, and long-lasting α$_1$-adrenergic–antagonist agents such as terazosin. The safety and efficacy of finasteride, terazosin, and the combination of both drugs in patients with symptomatic benign prostatic hyperplasia were compared.

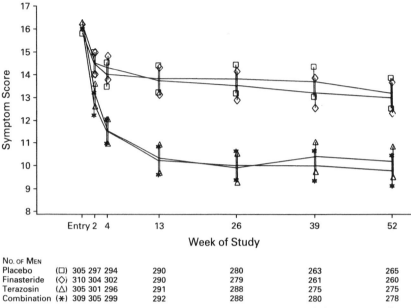

No. of Men

Placebo	(□)	305 297 294	290	280	263	265
Finasteride	(◇)	310 304 302	290	279	261	260
Terazosin	(△)	305 301 296	291	288	275	275
Combination	(✳)	309 305 299	292	288	280	278

FIGURE 1.—American Urological Association symptom scores in men with benign prostatic hyperplasia, according to treatment group. Scores are expressed as adjusted means and 95% confidence intervals. The results of primary pairwise comparisons (with Bonferroni's adjustment) are as follows: finasteride and terazosin, $P < 0.001$; finasteride and combination therapy, $P < 0.001$; and terazosin and combination therapy, $P = 1.00$. The results of secondary pairwise treatment comparisons are as follows: finasteride and placebo, $P = 0.63$; terazosin and placebo, $P < 0.001$; and combination therapy and placebo, $P < 0.001$. (Reprinted by permission of *The New England Journal of Medicine*. Lepor H, for the Veterans Affairs Cooperative Studies Benign Prostatic Hyperplasia Study Group: The efficacy of terazosin, finasteride, or both in benign prostatic hyperplasia. *N Engl J Med* 335:533–539, 1996. Copyright 1996, Massachusetts Medical Society.)

Patients and Methods.—Eligible patients were aged 45–80 years, had a mean score of at least 8 on the American Urological Association Symptom Index, a mean peak urinary-flow rate of no more than 15 mL/sec and no less than 4 mL/sec, with a minimal voided volume of 125 mL, and a mean residual volume after voiding of less than 300 mL. A total of 1,229 men from outpatient clinics at Veterans Affairs medical centers entered the study; 305 were randomly assigned to receive placebo, 310 to receive finasteride (5 mg daily), 305 to receive terazosin (10 mg daily), and 309 to receive a combination of the active drugs. Patients were evaluated at baseline and at 10 visits during a year of follow-up. Primary outcome variables were American Urological Association symptom scores and peak urinary-flow rates.

Results.—The 4 treatment groups were comparable in mean age (65 years), racial distribution (79% to 81% white), and baseline clinical variables. The 222 men who did not complete a year of treatment were equally distributed among groups, but significantly fewer withdrew from placebo because of adverse effects. Compliance with medication was high in all groups. Symptom scores decreased a mean of 2.6 points from baseline in the placebo group, 3.2 points in the finasteride group, 6.1 points in the terazosin group, and 6.2 points in the combination therapy group (Fig 1). After 1 year, the placebo group showed an increase in peak urinary-flow rates of 1.4 mL/sec; the finasteride group, 1.6 mL/sec; the terazosin group, 2.7 mL/sec; and the combination therapy group, 3.2 mL/sec. Finasteride was no more effective than placebo in improving either outcome measure. Only finasteride and combination therapy were associated with significant decreases in prostatic volume.

Conclusions.—Both symptom scores and urinary-flow rates were significantly improved in men with benign prostatic hyperplasia who were treated with terazosin. The combination of terazosin and finasteride was no more effective than terazosin alone, and finasteride alone offered no more benefits than placebo.

▶ During the past several years there has been an increasing trend toward medical management of benign prostatic hyperplasia using 1 of 2 approaches: 5 α-reductase inhibition or α₁-adrenergic antagonism. These 2 approaches emphasize different aspects of the pathophysiology of the disorder. The former blocks formation of intracellular androgens, whereas the latter relaxes smooth muscle in the prostate. In previous studies, both have been shown to be effective; however, until this trial, the combination of the 2 drugs had never been examined, nor had they been compared directly 1 against each other.

This 4-arm factorial design compared finasteride (a 5 α-reductase inhibitor), terazosin (an α₁- adrenergic antagonist), the combination of the 2, and placebo.

The findings were surprising in that terazosin with or without finasteride improved symptoms and peak urinary-flow rates, but finasteride alone did not; moreover the combination conferred no advantage beyond terazosin alone. One possible explanation is that the men included in this study had smaller prostates than those in previous studies in which the efficacy of finasteride had been demonstrated. Thus, it may be most prudent to treat men with symptoms and smaller prostates with terazosin alone and perhaps try finasteride for those with larger prostates; whether combination therapy in men with larger glands confers additional benefit remains to be determined.

D.B. Reuben, M.D.

Low Cholesterol Concentrations in Free-Living Elderly Subjects: Relations With Dietary Intake and Nutritional Status
Goichot B, Schlienger J-L, Grunenberger F, et al (CHU Hautepierre, Strasbourg, France; Hôpital Central, Strasbourg, France)
Am J Clin Nutr 62:547–553, 1995 1–41

Introduction.—There is epidemiologic evidence that a low serum cholesterol level is associated with an increased risk of death from noncardiovascular conditions. Low cholesterol is described in various pathologic states as well as in elderly patients who are institutionalized, but it has not been directly implicated as a pathogenetic factor.

Objective.—The prevalence and origin of hypocholesterolemia were examined in 380 free-living individuals 65 years of age or older who were participating in a dietary survey. Three-day food records were solicited.

Findings.—Hypocholesterolemia, defined as a total serum cholesterol value below 1.4 g/L, was identified in only 12 individuals. The 9 affected men had lower high-density lipoprotein cholesterol (HDL-C) levels than other men, as well as lower levels of apolipoprotein A-1, apolipoprotein B, prealbumin, and thyroid hormones. Total energy intake did not differ significantly. Statistical comparisons were not feasible in the 3 woman with low total cholesterol levels. In both men and women, prealbumin was most predictive of the total cholesterol level. Body mass index was the chief predictor of HDL-C.

Conclusion.—Hypocholesterolemia is not a frequent finding in free-living elderly individuals, but, when it is present, it does reflect impaired health. The role of nutrient factors as a determinant of hypocholesterolemia appears to be minimal.

▶ Serum cholesterol appears to demonstrate a U-shaped relationship to mortality. High serum cholesterol may be genetically or nutritionally mediated. Much less is understood about the pathogenesis of hypocholesterolemia. Although some evidence supports the role of cytokines[1] and continued inflammation as a cause, it is also possible that there is a nutritional component.

In this community-based sample of older individuals in the east of France, a number of measures of nutritional status were taken, including a 3-day food record, which was reviewed by a dietitian. The study found that hypocholesterolemia was rare (prevalence less than 4%) and did not appear to be related to overall energy, protein, or cholesterol intake. However, hypocholesterolemia was associated with low levels of prealbumin, free thyroxine, and free triiodothyronine. The major shortcoming of the study was the sample size; the study identified only 12 subjects with hypocholesterolemia, including only 3 women. Nevertheless, it provides further evidence that hypocholesterolemia may be better regarded as an indicator of a disease process rather than a dietary deficiency.

D.B. Reuben, M.D.

Reference

1. Ettinger WH, Tamara H, Verdery RB, et al: Evidence for inflammation as a cause of hypocholesterolemia in older people. *J Am Geriatr Soc* 43:264-266, 1995.

A Cross-sectional Validation Study of the FICSIT Common Data Base Static Balance Measures

Rossiter-Fornoff JE, Wolf SL, Wolfson LI, et al (Washington Univ, St Louis, Mo; Emory Univ, Atlanta, Ga; Univ of Connecticut, Farmington; et al)
J Gerontol 50A:M291–M297   1–42

Background.—Much research on balance has focused on postural sway and limits of stability as proxies for balance. In the current research, a composite measure of static balance status based on ability to maintain balance over a decreasing base of support was developed. No special equipment is needed for these maneuvers, which require little time. The construction of a composite balance measure and its test-retest reliability and construct validity were reported.

Methods.—Data from Frailty and Injuries: Cooperative Studies of Intervention Techniques (FICSIT) were used. Scales combining ability to maintain balance in parallel, semitandem, tandem, and one-legged stances were constructed using Fisher's method. Reliability was inferred from the stability of the measure during 3–4 months and construct validity by cross-sectional correlations.

Findings.—Test-retest reliability during 3–4 months was good, with a correlation coefficient of 0.66. The low correlation of the FICSIT-3 scale with age, its moderate to high associations with physical function measures, and 3 balance assessment systems provided evidence of the validity of this scale. Balance in a wide variety of health statuses was discriminated by the FICSIT-4 scale. The 3-test scale had a marked ceiling effect in community samples.

Conclusions.—The FICSIT-3 scale measures static balance, or a person's ability to maintain posture over a limited base of support. The balance scale showed good consistency of results when retested during several months as well as good construct validity. The FICSIT-3 appears to be reliable in a general population.

▶ This study represents an interesting by-product of the FICSIT study. It describes the development of a composite measure of static balance, which requires no specialized equipment and little time to perform, thus making it a useful maneuver in generalist physician's offices. The composite measure of static balance addresses the ability of an older person to maintain balance over a diminishing base of response and the authors describe 2 versions: the FICSIT-3 and FICSIT-4 scales. The FICSIT-4 version evolved because the scores suggested a ceiling effect in community dwelling elderly, and with the addition of a fourth item—one-legged standing time—performance was improved with highly functioning persons. Additional work is necessary to fully explore the usefulness of this procedure. The data presented are adequate, I believe, to recommend its use as a procedure to better understand the cause of falling in older persons who report this problem or are at risk for it.

J.C. Beck, M.D.

Falls in the Elderly: A Prospective Study of Risk Factors and Risk Profiles

Graafmans WC, Ooms ME, Hofstee HMA, et al (Vrije Universiteit, Amsterdam; Academisch Ziekenhuis Vrije Universiteit, Amsterdam)

Am J Epidemiol 143:1129–1136, 1996   1–43

Background.—Falls among the elderly can result in injury, social isolation, and psychological difficulty. Important risk factors for falls include impairment in mobility and cognition and the use of medication. Risk factors and risk profiles were prospectively studied.

Methods.—Falls among 354 individuals aged 70 years and older were registered during a 28-week period in 1992. All individuals were living in homes or apartments for the elderly in the Amsterdam area.

Findings.—One hundred twenty-six individuals (36%) had a total of 251 falls. Fifty-seven of them had 2 or more falls. Mobility impairment was associated with falls, with an odds ratio (OR) of 2.1, and was especially associated with recurrent falls (OR, 5.0). Dizziness on standing also was associated with falls and recurrent falls, with ORs of 2.1 for each. Several risk factors were associated with recurrent falls only, including history of stroke (OR, 3.4), poor mental state (OR, 2.4), and postural hypotension (OR, 2.0). When all of the aforementioned risk factors were present, an elderly individual had an 84% probability of recurrent falls in a 28-week period, compared with 3% when none of these risk factors were present. The probability of recurrent falls ranged from 11% to 29% when predicted by number of falls occurring the previous year. Neither falls nor recurrent falls were strongly associated with physical activity, the use of high-risk medication, or the use of vitamin D_3, which was allocated randomly to the participants.

Conclusions.—The risk profiles established in this study predicted a large range of probabilities of falls, especially recurrent falls. Impairment of mobility was the major risk factor. Improving mobility may help prevent recurrent falls.

▶ Falls remain a major problem in the elderly; they cause injuries, primarily fractures; a fear of falling; and social isolation. Previous studies have shown that mobility impairment, cognitive impairment, and use of medication are important risk factors for falls.

This study, a prospective one carried out in Amsterdam, carefully identified falls and examined the role of potential risk factors in both single falls and recurrent falls. The authors subsequently combined these factors to form risk profiles. The study analyzed 2 different outcome measures in an institutionalized population that appears to be comparable to that of a residential care facility in this country. The 2 outcome measures were at least 1 fall vs. none and recurrent falls vs. 1 fall or less. The study shows that a history of stroke, postural hypotension, disabilities of the lower extremities, and impaired cognitive function increases the risk of recurrent falls; it also shows that the mobility items were more strongly related to recurrent falls than to single falls.

It is interesting that the use of medication in this study did not reveal a strong relationship with falls or recurrent falls, in striking contrast to many other studies.[1-4] It is difficult to determine the reason for this difference, although this group of authors used medications at baseline, whereas most other studies have identified medication use at the time of the fall.

The most important message of this and other studies[5, 6] is that recurrent falls may be especially amenable to preventive strategies. Mobility impairment is the strongest risk factor and perhaps the easiest to change in a prevention program that includes exercise, and recent studies have showed its effectiveness in terms of averting falls, but none have showed its effectiveness in the prevention of fractures.

J.C. Beck, M.D.

References

1. Grisso JA, Kelsey JL, Strom BL, et al: Risk factors for falls as a cause of hip fracture in women: The Northeast Hip Fracture Study Group. *N Engl J Med* 324:1326–1331, 1991.
2. Tinetti ME, Speechley M, Ginter SF: Risk factors for falls among elderly persons living in the community. *N Engl Med* 319:1701–1707, 1988.
3. Prudham D, Evans JG: Factors associated with falls in the elderly: A community study. *Age Ageing* 10:141–146, 1981.
4. Granek E, Baker SP, Abbey H, et al: Medications and diagnoses in relation to falls in a long-term care facility. *J Am Geriatr Soc* 35:503–511, 1987.
5. Tinetti ME, Baker DI, McAvay G, et al: A multifactorial intervention to reduce the risk of falling among elderly people living in the community. *N Engl J Med* 331:821–827, 1994.
6. MacRae PG, Feltner ME, Reinsch S: A 1-year exercise program for older women: Effects on falls, injuries, and physical performance. *J Aging Phys Activity* 2:127–142, 1994.

Endocrinology and Metabolism

Individual Sulfonylureas and Serious Hypoglycemia in Older People

Shorr RI, Ray WA, Daugherty JR, et al (Vanderbilt Univ, Nashville, Tenn)
J Am Geriatr Soc 44:751–755, 1996   1–44

Introduction.—Older patients with diabetes are at increased risk for hypoglycemia associated with the therapeutic use of sulfonylureas. Little is known, however, about the relative safety of individual sulfonylureas in this patient population. A retrospective study of diabetic Medicaid enrollees examined the rate of serious hypoglycemia among users of oral hypoglycemic drugs and compared the risk of hypoglycemia associated with individual sulfonylureas.

Methods.—Potential cohort members were all enrollees in the Tennessee Medicaid program, aged 65 years and older, who used oral hypoglycemic drugs between 1985 and 1989. The sulfonylureas studied and their estimated daily doses were chlorpropamide (250 mg), tolazamide (250 mg), tolbutamide (500 mg), acetohexamide (500 mg), glyburide (5 mg), and glipizide (10 mg). Medical records were reviewed to identify all episodes of serious hypoglycemia that occurred outside the hospital and led to an emergency department visit, hospitalization, or death. Chlorpropamide, the agent most often not recommended for use in older adults, was selected as the reference drug to estimate risk for hypoglycemia.

Results.—A total of 422 of 549 potential events were available for review; 255 met the study definition for serious hypoglycemia. Patients with serious hypoglycemia had a mean age of 78 years; 84% were women and 47% were white. Common symptoms at presentation were lethargy (32%) and loss of consciousness (48%). The most common treatment (85%) was IV dextrose, and 70% of patients showed immediate improvement. Catastrophic complications such as stroke (3 patients) or death (2 patients) were rare. The risk for serious hypoglycemia was increased among new users of sulfonylureas (during the first 30 days of exposure after 1 year without exposure to the drugs) and those taking more than the median dose. The crude rate (per 1,000 person-years) of serious hypoglycemia was highest for glyburide (16.6) and lowest for tolbutamide (3.5). The risk was similar for chlorpropamide and glyburide users, and lower for users of tolbutamide, tolazamide, and glipizide (Table 1).

Discussion.—There was considerable variation in the risk for serious hypoglycemia among older patients treated with sulfonylureas. The risk was highest among users of chlorpropamide and glyburide and lowest among those treated with tolbutamide. These findings occurred in all demographic and exposure strata.

TABLE 1.—Exposure, Events, and Rate of Severe Hypoglycemia Associated With Sulfonylurea Use Among Older Tennessee Medicaid Enrollees, 1985–1989

Agent	Person-Years (%)	Serious Hypoglycemia	Possible Hypoglycemia	Missing Records	Other Events	Rate* (95% CI)
Chlorpropamide	6089 (29)	93	14	41	41	15.3 (12.2,18.4)
Glyburide	5669 (27)	94	16	46	39	16.6 (13.2,19.9)
Glipizide	2907 (14)	25	0	15	24	8.6 (5.2,12.0)
Tolazamide	2720 (13)	25	3	10	11	9.2 (5.6,12.8)
Tolbutamide	2538 (12)	9	2	8	6	3.5 (1.2,5.9)
Acetohexamide	792 (4)	9	1	7	10	11.4 (3.9,18.8)
Total	20715 (100)	255	36	127	131	12.3 (10.8,13.8)

* Serious hypoglycemia per 1,000 person-years.
Abbreviation: CI, confidence interval.
(Courtesy of Shorr RI, Ray WA, Daugherty JR, et al: Individual sulfonylureas and serious hypoglycemia in older people. *J Am Geriatr Soc* 44(7):751–755, 1996.)

▶ Diabetes is among the more common diseases affecting older persons; it is present in about 1 of every 9 individuals aged 65 years or older. Almost all have non–insulin-dependent diabetes, and many are treated with oral hypoglycemic agents, either with or without insulin. Because of its long duration of action and risk of hypoglycemia, chlorpropamide has been avoided in favor of shorter-acting agents.

In this study of elderly Medicaid recipients, the authors compared different oral agents regarding their potential to cause "serious" hypoglycemia, defined as a blood glucose level below 50 mg/dL, leading to hospitalization, emergency department admission, or death. Their findings confirmed the increased risk of serious hypoglycemia among users of chlorpropamide but also among users of glyburide, a second-generation sulfonylurea that has a shorter half-life than chlorpropamide. Although newer oral agents, such as metformin, may offer better glycemic control without the risk of hypoglycemia, many older persons cannot take this drug because of impaired renal function. Accordingly, sulfonylureas will likely remain a major therapeutic choice for the next several years. Judicious choice of which sulfonylurea to use may help avoid serious hypoglycemia.

D.B. Reuben, M.D.

Natural History of Peripheral Neuropathy in Patients With Non-Insulin-Dependent Diabetes Mellitus
Partanen J, Niskanen L, Lehtinen J, et al (Univ of Kuopio, Finland)
N Engl J Med 333:89–94, 1995   1–45

Introduction.—Up to 7.5% of patients with non–insulin-dependent diabetes mellitus (NIDDM) reportedly have clinical neuropathy at the time of diagnosis, and the likelihood of sustaining concurrent neuropathy appears to increase with time; however, little is known about the incidence or natural history of this condition. To determine the long-term risk of diabetic polyneuropathy and the factors affecting that risk, a cohort of patients with NIDDM and control subjects underwent 10 years of follow-up with regular evaluation of peripheral nerve function.

Methods.—Examination of patients and controls was done at baseline (shortly after diagnosis of diabetes mellitus), after 5 years, and after 10 years. Clinical criteria, including the presence of pain and paresthesias and electrodiagnostic studies such as nerve conduction velocity and response-amplitude values, were used in the evaluation of polyneuropathy. Eighty-six patients with NIDDM and 121 controls survived to the end of the follow-up.

Results.—The prevalence of definite or probable polyneuropathy at baseline was 8.3% among patients with NIDDM and 2.1% among control subjects. Paresthesias and lack of an Achilles-tendon reflex were more common in patients with NIDDM; these patients also had slower nerve conduction velocity in sensory and motor nerves. After 10 years, the prevalence of polyneuropathy among patients with NIDDM increased to

41.9%, whereas that among controls was 5.8%. Patients with NIDDM who experienced poor glycemic control were more likely to have polyneuropathy than those with better glycemic control. Regardless of glycemia status, low serum concentrations of insulin before and after oral administration of glucose were associated with polyneuropathy.

Conclusions.—As the trial progressed, the frequency of polyneuropathy in patients with NIDDM, as opposed to controls, increased, suggesting a cumulative effect of neuropathic factors. Poor glycemic control appears to be an important risk factor for the development or worsening of polyneuropathy, but controlled intervention studies are required for confirmation. Glycemic control was also related to axonal damage. Axonal degeneration (as indicated by decreasing sensory amplitude values) appeared to be more important than demyelination (as indicated by the slowing of nerve conduction velocities) as a cause of diabetic polyneuropathy in these patients. Clinical and electrodiagnostic criteria can be used to diagnose polyneuropathy in patients who have NIDDM. Patients with NIDDM who have diminished insulin secretion may gain neuroprotective benefit from early insulin therapy.

▶ This carefully executed study is the first to give detailed insight into the natural history of neuropathy in NIDDM. The data presented suggest a cumulative effect of the neuropathic factors with time. It is of real interest that the neurophysiologic studies identify axonal degeneration as the major cause of the diabetic polyneuropathy. This is supported by the decreased amplitudes of sensory and motor responses as a prominent feature, rather than by the mere slowing of nerve conducting velocities. The relationship to both glycemic control and serum levels of insulin is of major clinical importance. The hypoinsulinemia might suggest that patients with NIDDM who have neuropathy be given insulin early for its well-known neural protective effects.

J.C. Beck, M.D.

Veterans Affairs Cooperative Study on Glycemic Control and Complications in Type II Diabetes (VA CSDM): Results of the Feasibility Trial
Abraira C, Emanuele NV, Colwell JA, et al (Dept of Veterans Affairs Cooperative Studies Program, Hines, Ill)
Diabetes Care 18:1113–1123, 1995   1–46

Background.—The feasibility of effectively sustaining intensive drug treatment in patients with non–insulin-dependent diabetes mellitus (NIDDM) has not been established. Nor have the relative risks and benefits of intensive insulin treatment in this patient population been clearly defined. Standard and intensive therapy in a group of men with NIDDM requiring insulin because of sustained hyperglycemia were compared.

Methods.—One hundred fifty-three men (mean age, 60 years) treated at 5 centers were enrolled in a prospective, feasibility study. The patients had

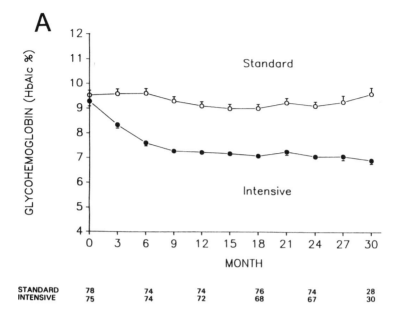

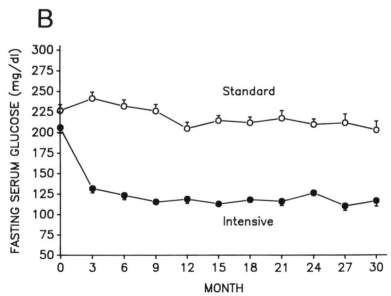

FIGURE 1.—**A**, mean (±SE) glycosylated hemoglobin (HbA$_{1c}$) in patients with non–insulin-dependent diabetes mellitus who were receiving standard or intensive therapy. The difference between treatments was statistically significant at all points beyond the baseline ($P < 0.001$). The number of patients evaluated appears below the graph. **B**, mean fasting serum glucose in patients treated with standard or intensive therapy. The difference between the 2 groups beyond baseline was statistically significant until the end of the study ($P < 0.0001$). (Courtesy of Abraira C, Emanuele NV, Colwell JA, et al: Veterans Affairs Cooperative Study on glycemic control and complications in type II diabetea (VA CSDM): Results of the feasibility trial. *Diabetes Care* 18:1113–1123, 1995.)

received a diagnosis of diabetes a mean of 7.8 years earlier. By random assignment, the patients received standard insulin treatment or intensive treatment designed to achieve near-normal glycemia and a clinically significant separation of glycohemoglobin from the standard arm. Intensive therapy consisted of an evening insulin injection, the same injection adding daytime glipizide, 2 injections of insulin alone, multiple daily injections, and daily self-monitoring. The mean follow-up was 27 months.

Findings.—After 6 months, the mean hemoglobin A_{1c} (Hba_{1c}) in the patients receiving intensive treatment was at or below 7.3% and remained 2% lower than that of the patients receiving standard therapy for the rest of the study. Most of the reduction in the mean HbA_{1c} in the patients undergoing intensive therapy was achieved by a single injection of evening intermediate insulin alone or with the daytime glipizide. By the end of the study, 64% of these patients were administering 2 or more insulin injections daily in an attempt to attain normal HbA_{1c}. However, the additional benefit from more than 1 injection of insulin per day was small. The incidence of severe hypoglycemia was only 2 events per 100 patients per year. The occurrence of severe hypoglycemia and changes in weight, blood pressure, and plasma lipids did not significantly differ between groups. Sixty-one new cardiovascular events occurred in 40 patients. Ten patients died, 6 from cardiovascular causes (Fig 1).

Conclusions.—Intensive stepped insulin treatment effectively maintains near-normal glycemic control for more than 2 years in patients with NIDDM who have failed to achieve glycemic control with drug therapy. This treatment produces no excessive severe hypoglycemia, weight gain, hypertension, or dyslipidemia. In this group of patients with NIDDM, the rate of cardiovascular events is high. The risk–benefit ratio of intensive therapy for hyperglycemia in patients with NIDDM requiring insulin needs to be determined in a long-term, prospective study.

▶ Diabetes is among the most common diseases affecting older persons and its optimal management in this age group is controversial. Data from the Diabetes Control and Complications Trial indicate the benefit of blood glucose control in younger patients with type I diabetes. The benefit of such control in older persons with type II diabetes has not been established, although several observational studies have suggested improved cardiovascular,[1] cerebral vascular,[2] and visual[3] outcomes among those with better metabolic control. On the other hand, the risks and consequences of hypoglycemia are substantial in this age group.

In this feasibility study conducted at 5 Department of Veterans Affairs medical centers, older men (average age, 60 years) were treated with a stepped approach that ranged from 1 evening injection of insulin to multiple daily injections in an attempt to reduce the HbA_{1c} by at least 1.5%. Most subjects required 2 or more shots each day, but the average decrease was 2.1%. The biggest improvement in metabolic control occurred in the first 2 steps of therapy (which required no more than 1 injection per day). More intensive regimens added little benefit. Severe hypoglycemia was uncommon but mild or moderate hypoglycemic episodes occurred in virtually all subjects treated with the intensive regimen. This study provides justification for a multisite trial to determine whether better metabolic control of type II diabetes can prevent complications of this disease.

D.B. Reuben, M.D.

References

1. Kuusisto J, Mykkanen L, Pyorala K, et al: NIDDM and its metabolic control predict coronary heart disease in elderly subjects. *Diabetes* 43:960–967, 1994.
2. Kuusisto J, Mykkanen L, Pyorala K, et al: Non–insulin-dependent diabetes and its metabolic control are important predictors of stroke in elderly subjects. *Stroke* 25:1157–1164, 1994.
3. Morisaki N, Watanabe S, Kobayashi J, et al: Diabetic control and progression of retinopathy in elderly patients: Five-year follow-up study. *J Am Geriatr Soc* 42:142-145, 1994.

Prospective Study of Small LDLs as a Risk Factor for Non–Insulin Dependent Diabetes Mellitus in Elderly Men and Women
Austin MA, Mykkänen L, Kuusisto J, et al (Univ of Washington, Seattle; Univ of Kuopio, Finland; Univ of Texas Health Sciences Ctr, San Antonio)
Circulation 92:1770–1778, 1995   1–47

Background.—Patients with non–insulin-dependent diabetes mellitus (NIDDM) have an excess risk of atherosclerosis. However, the presence of conventional risk factors does not fully explain this increased risk. Previous research has suggested that the increased atherogenicity of the prediabetic phase may contribute to the risk of coronary heart disease before overt diabetes develops. Prospective studies are needed to determine whether low-density lipoprotein (LDL) subclass phenotype B precedes NIDDM onset. The role of small, dense LDL as a risk factor for incident NIDDM was investigated in a nested case-control study of Finnish men and women.

Methods.—Two hundred four elderly men and women in Kuopio were included in the study. Two to 14% polyacrylamide gels were produced to characterize LDL subclasses by size. The subjects were followed up for 3.5 years.

Findings.—In a logistic regression analysis, subjects in LDL subclass phenotype B—a predominance of small LDL—had a more than two-fold increase in risk for the development of NIDDM during follow-up. This relationship was independent of age, sex, glucose intolerance, and body mass index but not of fasting triglyceride or insulin levels. A 5Å increase in LDL diameter was correlated with a 16% decline in NIDDM risk. Also, a composite variable of LDL diameter and triglyceride and high-density lipoprotein cholesterol levels was correlated with the development of NIDDM.

Conclusions.—In older men and women, the presence of small, dense LDL more than doubles the risk for NIDDM development. Small LDL appears to contribute to the risk of coronary heart disease in prediabetic individuals.

▶ This paper further clarifies the previously described association between small, dense LDL and NIDDM in both women and men. This prospective study demonstrates that small, dense LDL levels increase the risk for NIDDM more than twofold in the prediabetic state. In seems independent of family history of diabetes, hypertension, medication use, and waist-to-hip ratio but not independent of fasting triglyceride or insulin levels. In a principal-component analysis, 3 lipoproteins (increased plasma triglycerides, decreased high-density lipoprotein (HDL) cholesterol, and small, dense LDLs) were also associated with the development of NIDDM. The analysis would also suggest that these small LDL particles contribute to the risk of atherosclerosis among prediabetic individuals. It is of interest that in a small study[1] patients with NIDDM treated with gemfibrozil showed significant decreases in triglycerides and increases in HDL cholesterol and changes in LDL toward larger, less buoyant particles. This observation would suggest a large intervention trial to further explore whether a comparable strategy might reduce the onset of NIDDM in individuals who show the LDL risk factor.

J.C. Beck, M.D.

Reference

1. Lahdenpera S, Tilly-Kiesi M, Vuorinen-Markkola H, et al: Effects of gemfibrozil on low-density lipoprotein particle size, density distribution, and composition in patients with type II diabetes. *Diabetes Care* 16:584-592, 1993.

Testosterone Administration to Elderly Men Increases Skeletal Muscle Strength and Protein Synthesis
Urban RJ, Bodenburg YH, Gilkison C, et al (Univ of Texas, Galveston; Shriners Burns Inst, Galveston)
Am J Physiol 269:E820–826, 1995   1–48

Objective.—As men age, they lose muscle and strength, regardless of their physical activity level. The aging-related reductions in muscle function are correlated with serum testosterone concentrations. This response could involve the growth hormone insulin-like growth factor I (IGF-I) system, which has well-known anabolic effects in humans. The effects of testosterone on muscular strength and muscle protein synthesis were investigated in elderly men.

Methods.—The study included 6 healthy men (mean age, 67 years), each with a serum testosterone concentration of 480 ng/dL or less. They received serum testosterone injections every week for 4 weeks. The goal of the injections was to maintain the serum total testosterone concentration between 500 and 1,000 ng/dL, comparable to the range in young men.

Testosterone's effects on skeletal muscle protein synthesis, strength, and the IGF-I system were examined.

Results.—The subjects' estradiol and prostate-specific antigen concentrations increased and their high-density lipoprotein (HDL) concentrations decreased significantly during testosterone administration. There were significant increases in strength of the right and left hamstring and quadriceps muscles, as measured by isokinetic dynamometer, but no increase in muscle endurance. A significant increase in the fractional synthetic rate of muscle protein, as assessed by stable isotope infusion, was also noted. Total RNA was obtained from muscle for ribonuclease protection assays. These tests indicated significant increases in mRNA concentrations of IGF-I and significant decreases in mRNA concentrations of IGF binding protein-4.

Conclusions.—Short-term administration of testosterone to elderly men increases skeletal muscle protein synthesis and muscle strength. The intramuscular IGF-I system seems to play a role in these effects. Because increasing muscle strength could prevent falls and improve quality of life for elderly men, physiologic administration of testosterone—analogous to estrogen replacement in postmenopausal women—could have significant benefits in this age group.

▶ The search for agents to restore the muscle strength that decreases with aging has led to the administration of trophic hormones and secretagogs, including human growth hormones and dihydroepiandrosterone-sulfate. With aging, serum testosterone levels decrease and are correlated with decreased muscle function. In this small pretest-posttest study of healthy men (mean age, 67 years), the investigators administered weekly IM injections of testosterone titrated to maintain serum levels between 500 and 1,000 ng/dL for 4 weeks, comparable to those of younger men. They found that muscle strength increased significantly in the hamstring and quadricep groups although there was no change in endurance or thigh muscle volume. There was also evidence of increased muscle protein synthesis, although the peripheral GH-IGF-I system did not change, molecular evidence of changes in the intramuscular IGF-I system were noted. Despite these encouraging findings, several concerns were raised, including statistically significant increases in prostatic specific antigen levels and decreases in HDL cholesterol. Although the clinical implications of this study are quite preliminary, there may yet be a role for testosterone replacement therapy in elderly men.

D.B. Reuben, M.D.

Growth Hormone Replacement in Healthy Older Men Improves Body Composition but Not Functional Ability

Papadakis MA, Grady D, Black D, et al (Univ of California, San Francisco; Dept of Veterans Affairs Med Ctr, San Francisco; San Francisco Gen Hosp)
Ann Intern Med 124:708–716, 1996   1–49

Background.—In young adults with hypopituitarism, growth hormone replacement improves muscle volume, isometric strength, and exercise capacity. The muscle weakness and functional decline that occur with aging may be caused partly by reduced growth hormone secretion. The effects of growth hormone replacement on functional ability in older men were investigated.

Methods.—Fifty-two healthy men (age range, 70–85 years) were enrolled in the randomized, controlled, double-blind trial. All had well-preserved functional ability but low baseline insulin-like growth factor 1 levels. The men received growth hormone, 0.03 mg/kg of body weight, or placebo 3 times per week for 6 months.

Findings.—The patients receiving growth hormone had a mean lean mass increase of 4.3% at 6 months, compared with a 0.1% decrease in patients receiving placebo. Fat mass decreased by a mean 13.1% in patients given growth hormone and by 0.3% in those given placebo. Knee and hand grip strength, as well as systemic endurance, did not differ significantly between groups. Mean Trails B scores improved by 8.5 sec in the growth hormone group and decreased by 5 sec in the placebo group. Forty-eight incidents of side effects occurred in 26 growth hormone recipients, compared with 14 incidents in 26 placebo recipients. Twenty-six percent of the men receiving growth hormone needed dose reductions.

Conclusions.—Lean tissue mass increased and fat mass decreased among healthy older men given physiologic doses of growth hormone for 6 months. However, there was no improvement in functional ability. Adverse effects were common. Thus, growth hormone should not be given to preserve or improve functional ability in healthy elderly men with well-preserved functional abilities.

▶ Among the physiologic changes that occur with aging, decreases in growth hormone and insulin-like growth have been of particular interest because of the potential for replacement therapy. In this randomized clinical trial, community-dwelling older men, whose baseline insulin-like growth hormone concentrations were within the lowest tenth percentile, received replacement growth hormone for 6 months. The authors found that growth hormone replacement was associated with improvements of body composition (e.g., replacement of fat mass by lean body mass and slight increase in bone density), but they were unable to demonstrate improvements in muscle strength (e.g., knee extension, hand grip). There were no changes in endurance as measured by maximal oxygen consumption or functional status as measured by Physical Performance Test scores.

Although these findings are somewhat disappointing, this study does not provide final answers about the use of growth hormone replacement in elderly individuals for several reasons. First, the population studied was highly functional; a more frail population may have experienced greater gains. Second, such therapy may need to be coupled with an exercise program (and nutritional repletion for those who are malnourished) to fully achieve the potential gains from changing body composition. And third, the duration of the trial was likely too short to demonstrate any preventive effect on functional decline. Nevertheless, as the authors note, side effects were frequent and may be a limiting factor. Several additional studies of growth hormone and growth hormone secretagogue replacement are currently in progress and should shed additional light on the topic.

D.B. Reuben, M.D.

▶ This paper is important in that it addresses certain of the outcome events, body composition and function, for which human recombinant growth hormone is under study in older subjects. Clearly, growth hormone administration alters body composition: increasing lean body mass and decreasing fat mass. Several studies now show either a minor impact or no impact on bone mass after as long as 1 year of treatment.[1] Growth hormone appears more effective in increasing bone mass in growth hormone deficient individuals but only after approximately 24 months of treatment. In terms of muscle mass, growth hormone is a weak second to exercise in increasing muscle bulk. Side effects constitute the major deterrant to long-term administration of growth hormone.

However, these equivocal results have not slowed the search for growth hormone–related factors that may have improved anabolic action without side effects. Currently under study are both peptide and non-peptide growth hormone secretagogues that stimulate the release of pituitary growth hormone and elevate insulin-like growth factor 1.[2] Unlike recombinant growth hormone, these agents can be administered orally. I am skeptical that the overall growth hormone effect will be much different when stimulated by a pituitary release factor as contrasted with direct administration of growth hormone.

J.R. Shapiro, M.D.

References

1. Holloway L, Butterfield RI, Hintz RL, et al: Effects of hGH on metabolic indices, body composition and bone turnover in healthy elderly women. *J Clin Endocrinol Metab* 79:470–479, 1994.
2. Tuilpakov AN, Bulatov AA, Peterkova VA, et al: Growth hormone (GH)–releasing effects of synthetic peptide GH-releasing peptide-2 and GH-releasing hormone (1-29NH2) in children with GH insufficiency and idiopathic short stature. *Metabolism* 44:1199–1204, 1995.

Homocysteine Metabolism and Risk of Myocardial Infarction: Relation With Vitamins B₆, B₁₂, and Folate

Verhoef P, Stampfer MJ, Buring JE, et al (Agricultural Univ, Wageningen, The Netherlands; Brigham and Women's Hosp, Boston; Harvard Med School, Boston; et al)

Am J Epidemiol 143:845–859, 1996   1–50

Background.—Increased levels of plasma homocysteine have been found to be an independent risk factor for vascular disease. The relation of the risk of myocardial infarction with fasting plasma homocysteine and vitamins, important cofactors in homocysteine metabolism, was investigated in a case-control study.

Methods.—One hundred thirty patients hospitalized for myocardial infarction for the first time and 118 population control subjects were enrolled in 1982 and 1983. A food-frequency questionnaire was administered to estimate dietary intakes of vitamins B_6, B_{12}, and folate.

Findings.—The geometric mean plasma homocysteine level was 11% higher in patients than in controls, after adjustment for sex and age. There was no clear excess of patients with very increased levels. The age- and sex-adjusted odds ratio was 1.35 for each 3 μmol/L increase in plasma homocysteine. The odds ratio was unaffected after adjustment for several other risk factors. However, the confidence interval was greater and the *P* value for trend was less significant.

Dietary and plasma concentrations of vitamin B_6 and folate were reduced in patients in comparison with controls. These vitamins were inversely related to the risk of myocardial infarction, independent of other potential risk factors. Vitamin B_{12} was unassociated with myocardial infarction, although methylmalonic acid levels were significantly higher in the patients. When the average levels of several homocysteine metabolites among patients and controls were compared, homocysteine remethylation impairment was found to be the main cause of high homocysteine levels in patients. Plasma folate and (to a lesser degree) plasma vitamin B_{12}, but not plasma vitamin B_6, were inversely associated with plasma homocysteine, even at high-normal levels.

Conclusions.—Plasma homocysteine was again shown to be an independent risk factor for myocardial infarction. Folate was the most important determinant of plasma homocysteine in the current population, even in those with apparently adequate nutritional intake of this vitamin.

▶ This article was selected because it adds further epidemiologic evidence to the increasingly attractive hypothesis that plasma homocysteine is an independent risk factor for coronary artery disease. The graded effect suggests that lowering the plasma homocysteine might have important public health effects for a large adult population. It also supports the view that providing adequate dietary folate intake or folate supplements might be an important step toward normalizing homocysteine levels. This effect has been shown to occur within a few weeks,[1] even in individuals with genetically caused hyperhomocysteinemia.

The issue of whether such an intervention would reduce the risk of coronary artery disease can only be determined by randomized trials relating intake and status to the incidence of coronary heart disease. It raises the practical question whether the recommended daily allowance of folate should be restored to its previously recommended value of 400 μg/day from the present recommended 200 μg/day.

J.C. Beck, M.D.

Reference

1. Brattstrom LE, Israelsson B, Jeppsson JO, et al: Folic acid: An innocuous means to reduce plasma homocysteine. *Scand J Clin Lab Invest* 48:215–221, 1988.

Osteoporosis

Risk Factors for Osteoporotic Fractures in Elderly Men

Nguyen TV, Eisman JA, Kelly PJ, et al (Garvan Inst of Med Research, Sydney, Australia; Vincent's Hosp, Sydney, Australia)

Am J Epidemiol 144:255–263, 1996   1–51

Introduction.—The problem of osteoporosis in aging women has received considerable attention, but few studies have included men. The pattern for age-related bone loss and the incidence and potential risk factors for osteoporotic fractures in men were examined.

Methods.—Dubbo, a small city located 400 km northwest of Sydney, was chosen for an epidemiologic study of osteoporosis because the age and sex distribution of its population closely resembles that of the larger Australian population. Potential risk factors for osteoporotic fractures were assessed in 820 men aged 60 years or older in 1989. A questionnaire administered at study entry gathered data on age, lifestyle factors, physical activity, and history of falls and fractures. Baseline bone mineral density (BMD) was measured in the lumbar spine and femoral neck of 752 (91%) men. Follow-up continued until 1994.

Results.—The men were divided into 5 age groups: 60–64 years, 65–69 years, 70–74 years, 75–79 years, and 80 years or older. Advancing age was associated with declines in weight, height, physical activity index, and quadriceps strength, and an increase in body sway. Although lumbar spine BMD was stable or increased throughout the later decades, mean BMD decreased with age at the femoral neck and at Ward's triangle and trochanteric areas. Femoral neck BMD was inversely correlated with age and smoking but positively related to weight, dietary calcium intake, and quadriceps strength. Similar trends were seen in a second BMD determination, obtained in 442 men at an average of 2.5 years after baseline studies. The rate of multiple falls increased from 3.9% in men aged 60–64 years to 9% in those aged 75 years and older. The incidence of atraumatic fractures and of multiple fractures increased significantly with age. Independent risk factors for fracture in multivariate analysis were lower baseline femoral neck BMD, quadriceps strength, and body sway.

Conclusions.—The incidence of fractures increases with age in men as well as in women, but a more powerful predictor of fracture risk is BMD, particularly at the femoral neck. Most fractures result from falls, and risk factors for falling include quadriceps weakness, impaired postural stability, shorter height, and a history of previous fractures and/or falls. A higher level of physical activity is protective against the risk of fractures in men.

▶ Risk factors for osteoporosis among women have been studied extensively, and recent longitudinal data have clarified the role of sociodemographic, lifestyle, and health factors[1]; however, considerably less is known about factors associated with the development of low bone density and osteoporotic fractures among men. This cohort study in Dubbo, Australia, followed 820 men aged 60 years or older for 5 years. Risk factors for decline in femoral neck bone mass as measured by densitometry included age and weight change, but factors predicting changes in the lumbar spine could not be identified. Risk factors for fracture included baseline femoral neck bone density, quadriceps strength, and body sway.

This study confirms some but not all the risk factors that have been identified in women. Moreover, many of these factors are modifiable through exercise and pharmacotherapy to increase bone density. Although the findings of this study represents a substantial advance in our knowledge about osteoporosis in men, unfortunately its population included virtually all white men. Risk factors for osteoporosis in nonwhite men (and women) still remain to be identified.

D.B. Reuben, M.D.

Reference

1. Cummings SR, for the Study of Osteoporotic Fractures Research Group: Risk factors for hip fracture in white women. *N Engl J Med* 332:767–773, 1995.

Late Physical and Functional Effects of Osteoporotic Fracture in Women: The Rancho Bernardo Study
Greendale GA, Barrett-Connor E, Ingles S, et al (Univ of California, Los Angeles; Univ of California San Diego, La Jolla, Calif)
J Am Geriatr Soc 43:955–961, 1995   1–52

Background.—The cumulative number of hip fractures in the United States is projected to double by 2040. Research has shown that hip fracture leads to substantial impairment in the ability to perform activities of daily living, which may affect a person's ability to live independently. The relationship between osteoporotic fractures and problems with selected physical and functional activities in elderly women was investigated.

Methods.—A total of 1,010 women aged 55 and older (mean age, 72.6 years) who lived in the community were included in the study. This sample represented 80% of women participating in a study of osteoporosis between 1988 and 1991.

Findings.—One hundred sixty minimal trauma fractures occurred for the first time between 1972 and 1991. The fracture site was the wrist in 62 patients, rib in 29, hip in 25, and spine in 23. The mean interval since fracture was 6.7 years. Experiencing any osteoporotic fracture was significantly correlated with a 1.7-fold to three-fold increase in problems bending, lifting, reaching, walking, climbing stairs, and descending stairs. There was also a significant association between any fracture and a 1.9-fold to 6.7-fold increase in problems dressing, cooking, shopping, and performing heavy housework. Compared with the relative odds of physical limitation related to any osteoporotic fracture, hip fractures had an odds ratio of 3.6 for problems walking and of 4.1 for descending stairs. Spine fractures were more strongly associated with problems bending, with an odds ratio of 3.1; lifting, 3.4; and descending stairs, 4.2.

Conclusions.—Osteoporotic fracture appears to have a marked long-term effect on physical and functional ability. Although the differences in the relative odds of impairment and the variation in activities affected by different fracture types provide evidence that these relationships are causal, longitudinal follow-up studies are needed to confirm this.

▶ This paper addresses the impact of a variety of skeletal fractures related to osteoporosis on function in older women using the Rancho Bernardo Study cohort. It is well known that more than half of patients with hip fracture do not regain prefracture levels in their basic activities of daily living and three quarters of them do not regain prefracture levels in their independent activities of daily living. However, little information is available on vertebral, wrist, and other fractures. Of special importance is the observation that functional impairments were similar for osteoporotic fractures of the hip and spine, and that the degree of impairment associated with fractures of the wrist was much greater than had been anticipated by previous studies. In the latter instance, older women with wrist fractures had trouble climbing and descending stairs, as well as limitations in shopping and cooking.

There are a number of limitations to this study which include the following: (1) The study is cross-sectional and it is impossible to sort out the causal relationship, although with both vertebral and wrist fractures, this is much less of a problem; (2) the population that was studied are "the survivors" in that they were still living independently; (3) the entire study population did not have radiographs of the vertebral spine, and, thus, there may have been a selection bias in this subset; and (4) because these women were white, well educated, and upper middle class, the generalizability may be in doubt, although, as the authors point out, the predictive validity of self-report scales has been demonstrated.

J.C. Beck, M.D.

Effect of Oral Alendronate on Bone Mineral Density and the Incidence of Fractures in Postmenopausal Osteoporosis

Liberman UA, for the Alendronate Phase III Osteoporosis Treatment Study Group (Tel Aviv Univ, Petah-Tikva, Israel)
N Engl J Med 333:1437–1443, 1995   1–53

Background.—Alendronate has been shown to inhibit osteoclast-mediated bone resorption in animals and patients with osteoporosis at daily doses that do not affect bone mineralization. In multicenter, randomized, double-blind, placebo-controlled dose-ranging studies, the efficacy of continuous treatment with oral alendronate at 3 doses in postmenopausal women with osteoporosis was evaluated.

Methods.—Postmenopausal women with osteoporosis who were between the ages of 45 and 80 years and living in 8 countries were randomly assigned to receive either placebo or daily oral alendronate at doses of 5, 10, or 20 mg for 3 years. At baseline and after 3 years, bone mineral density of the lumbar spine, femoral neck, trochanter, forearm, and total body was measured by dual-energy x-ray absorptiometry. Vertebral fractures and the progression of vertebral deformities were assessed with annual lateral spine films. Height was measured every 3 months.

Results.—The treatment groups had similar baseline characteristics and risk factors for fracture. The bone mineral density of the spine, femoral neck, trochanter, and total body increased significantly during all 3 years with all 3 doses of alendronate, but decreased significantly in the placebo group (Fig 1). There were significantly greater increases in bone mineral density with the 10-mg dose than with the 5-mg dose of alendronate; the 10-mg dose was as effective as the 20-mg dose. New vertebral fractures occurred in 6.2% of the placebo group and 3.2% of the combined alendronate groups. The risk of new vertebral fractures was decreased with all doses of alendronate. There was an increase in the Spine Deformity Index of 33% in the alendronate groups and of 41% in the placebo group. At 3 years, the mean loss of height was 35% less in the alendronate group than in the placebo group, which was a difference of 0.7 mm annually. There was also a trend toward fewer nonvertebral fractures in the alendronate groups. There were no significant differences in adverse effects associated with placebo or alendronate treatment.

Conclusion.—Daily oral alendronate treatment for 3 years induced significant increases in bone mineral density and decreases in risk of vertebral fracture, vertebral deformities, and loss of height, suggesting increased bone strength in both the appendicular and the axial skeleton.

▶ Osteoporosis is a major cause of morbidity and disability among older persons, particularly women. The pharmacologic options for prevention and treatment of postmenopausal osteoporosis have been extremely limited. One class of medications that has demonstrated some promise, the bisphosphonates, inhibits bone resorption by osteoclasts. Previous studies of etidronate have demonstrated some initial benefits.[1]

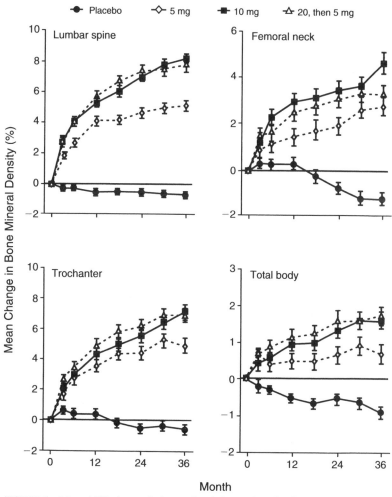

FIGURE 1.—Mean (±SE) changes in bone mineral density from baseline values in women with postmenopausal osteoporosis receiving alendronate or placebo for 3 years. Data are shown for bone mineral density (measured by dual-energy x-ray absorptiometry) of the spine, femoral neck, trochanter, and total body. Data for the alendronate group are shown according to the dose: 5 or 10 mg/day for 3 years or 20 mg/day for 2 years followed by 5 mg/day in year 3. (Reprinted by permission of The New England Journal of Medicine. Liberman UA, for the Alendronate Phase III Osteoporosis Treatment Study Group: Effect of oral alendronate on bone mineral density and the incidence of fractures in postmenopausal osteoporosis. *N Engl J Med* 333:1437–1443, 1995. Copyright 1995, Massachusetts Medical Society.)

Alendronate, a new bisphosphonate that can be given daily, was tested in 2 multicenter dose-ranging studies that were used to demonstrate its efficacy. At the 10-mg dose, the drug increased bone mineral density of the spine (8.8%), the femoral neck (5.9%), the trochanter (7.8%) and the total body (2.5%) at 36 months. Moreover, the groups receiving the drug had significantly fewer vertebral fractures (3.2% vs. 6.2% in the control group).

The drug was well tolerated with similar discontinuation rates in the alendronate and control groups. If these benefits are sustained and translate into reduced fractures of the hip, the introduction of alendronate (and, likely, other bisphosphonates that are currently in testing phases) will be a major advance in the treatment of osteoporosis.

D.B. Reuben, M.D.

Reference

1. Harris ST, Watts NB, Jackson RD, et al: Four-year study of intermittent cyclic etidronate treatment of postmenopausal osteoporosis: Three years of blinded therapy followed by one year of open therapy. *Am J Med* 95:557–567, 1993.

Vitamin D Supplementation and Fracture Incidence in Elderly Persons: A Randomized, Placebo-Controlled Clinical Trial

Lips P, Graafmans WC, Ooms ME, et al (Vrije Universiteit, Amsterdam, The Netherlands)
Ann Intern Med 124:400–406, 1996
                                                                                    1–54

Background.—Previous research has suggested that vitamin-D supplementation may decrease the incidence of hip fractures. However, interventions to increase bone mineral density do not necessarily result in increased bone strength. Studies of the effect of vitamin D supplementation should use hip fracture as the outcome criterion. The effect of vitamin-D supplementation on the incidence of hip fractures and other peripheral bone fractures was investigated.

Methods.—The prospective, double-blind trial included 1,916 women and 662 men age 70 years or older. By random assignment, the study participants were given vitamin D_3, 400 IU in 1 tablet daily, or placebo for as long as 3.5 years. Follow-up lasted for as long as 4 years.

Findings.—Dairy products accounted for 868 mg/day of mean dietary calcium intake. In the third year of the study, the vitamin-D group had a mean serum 25-hydroxyvitamin D 25(OH)D concentration of 60 nmol/L, compared with 23 nmol/L in the placebo group. During follow-up, 48 placebo recipients and 58 vitamin-D recipients had hip fractures. Seventy-seven subjects given vitamin D and 74 given placebo had other peripheral fractures.

Conclusions.—Vitamin-D supplementation did not reduce the incidence of hip fractures and other peripheral fractures in this cohort. Possibly, the effect of vitamin-D supplementation on the incidence of fractures may be evident only in populations that are older and frailer than the one studied here.

▶ Vitamin-D deficiency is common in older individuals, particularly among those who live in climates with limited sun exposure and those with diets poor in this vitamin. Moreover, replacement of vitamin D in nursing home residents has been demonstrated to decrease hip fractures[1] and increase bone density among community-dwelling older individuals.[2] The findings of this large, randomized clinical trial must dampen the enthusiasm for routine supplementation of vitamin D because there was no benefit on hip or peripheral fractures in the treated vs. placebo groups. As the authors note, the dietary calcium intake and average age of participants this study was higher and younger, respectively, than in another trial[1] which showed benefit of such replacement. Thus, it seems that selective rather than universal vitamin-D supplementation is most effective. The precise population who will benefit, however, has yet to be defined; given the minimal side effects and relatively low cost of vitamin-D supplementation, it is probably better to err on the side of over- rather than undertreating those for whom the benefit is uncertain.

D.B. Reuben, M.D.

References

1. Chapuy MC, Arlot ME, Duboeuf F, et al: Vitamin D₃ and calcium to prevent hip fractures in elderly women. *N Engl J Med* 327:1637–1642, 1992.
2. Ooms ME, Roos JC, Besemer PD, et al: Prevention of bone loss by vitamin D supplementation in elderly women: A randomized double-blind trial. *J Clin Endocrinol Metab* 80:1052–1058, 1995.

Combined Therapy With Estrogen and Etidronate Has an Additive Effect on Bone Mineral Density in the Hip and Vertebrae: Four-Year Randomized Study
Wimalawansa SJ (Royal Postgraduate Med School, London)
Am J Med 99:36–42, 1995   1–55

Introduction.—Giving estrogen or etidronate can increase bone mineral density in postmenopausal women. The potential added benefits of giving hormone replacement therapy (HRT) along with cyclically administered etidronate were studied. The possibility of eliminating the mineralization defects associated with etidronate was evaluated as well.

Methods.—The study sample comprised 58 postmenopausal women referred for advice on prevention of osteoporosis. All had undergone natural menopause no more than 5 years earlier and had bone mineral density values within the normal range for women between 30 and 40 years of age. Their mean dietary calcium intake was 770 mg/day.

The patients were randomized into 4 groups. Those in group 1 received percutaneously administered 17β-estradiol (17β-E₂), at 2.5 g/day, equivalent to 1.5 mg of 17β-E₂ daily; oral micronized progesterone, 200 mg/day for 12 days each month; and elemental calcium, 1.0 g/day. Group 2 patients received intermittent cyclically administered etidronate sodium (ICE), 400 mg/day for 14 days, followed by 10 weeks of elemental calcium, 1.0 g/day. Patients in group 3 received a combination of HRT, ICE, and calcium, and those in group 4 received 1 g of calcium only daily. The patients did not take calcium on the days they received etridonate. Bone mineral density and biochemical indicators of bone turnover were measured at baseline and after 2 and 4 years of treatment.

Results.—In group 1, vertebral bone mineral density increased by 4% at 2 years and by 7% at 4 years, and femoral bone mineral density increased by 2% and 4%, respectively. The patients in group 2 had a similar increase in vertebral bone mineral density, but only a modest increase in femoral bone mineral density. In group 3, the combined treatment group, vertebral bone mineral density increase by 6% at 2 years and 11% at 4 years. Increases in femur bone mineral density were 5% and 7%, respectively. Increases at both sites were significantly greater than in groups 1 and 2. Bone loss occurred at both sites in patients who received calcium only (4% in the vertebrae and 5% in the femur at 4 years) and even more so in patients who refused any treatment. The patients receiving combination therapy had normal bone histomorphometric findings, whereas 3 of 9 patients treated with ICE and calcium were found to have definite osteomalacia on biopsy.

Conclusions.—In postmenopausal women, ICE and HRT have additive effects on the bone mineral density in the vertebrae and hips. Although HRT plus calcium supplementation also has a positive effect on bone mineral density, the magnitude of the effect is less than that of combination therapy. This study is the first to document the effects of etidronate in women who have recently gone through menopause. Unless combined with HRT, ICE plus calcium is neither safe nor effective in this patient group.

▶ This was the first study to demonstrate the effects of ICE in early postmenopausal women; all previous studies having been conducted in older women with established osteoporosis. Furthermore, it demonstrates an additive effect of combined treatment, which is pronounced and confirmed by iliac crest bone biopsy. An important observation is that the well-described adverse effects of ICE on bone mineralization are eliminated when the agent is combined with HRT. A study such as this one—done in a relatively small number of patients but nevertheless extending over 4 years—deserves to be repeated in a large, randomized trial. One of the major outcome measures in such a study would be the reduction in rates of fracture and maintenance of function.

J.C. Beck, M.D.

Health Care Economics

State Health Care Expenditures Under Competition and Regulation, 1980 Through 1991
Melnick GA, Zwanziger J (RAND, Santa Monica, Calif)
Am J Public Health 85:1391–1396, 1995   1–56

Introduction.—With the shift of health care reform to the states, the decision now is between a regulatory or a competitive approach to policy. The competitive model is demonstrated by 1982 California legislation that

TABLE 2.—Comparison of Cumulative Growth in Real Total Per Capita Health Expenditures and in Selected Components of Health Expenditures: 1980 through 1991

	Total	Expenditure Category, % Growth		
		Hospital Services	Physician Services	Drugs
United States	63.0	54.0	82.0	65.0
California	39.0	27.0	58.0	41.0
Maryland	59.0	34.1	107.3	117.0
Massachusetts	70.2	44.9	151.8	114.7
New Jersey	86.4	84.6	92.0	88.3
New York	85.4	56.5	104.6	85.4

(Courtesy of Melnick, GA, Zwanziger J: State health care expenditures under competition and regulation, 1980 through 1991. *Am J Public Health* 85:1391–1396, 1995. Copyright American Public Health Association.)

allowed the formation of contractual preferred provider health plans, many of which require price concessions and utilization review. The regulatory approach provides for regulation by a government agency of prices and provider payments. Cost and price results from rate regulation states of Maryland, New Jersey, New York, and Massachusetts were compared with results of the competitive approach of California.

Methods.—State expenditures were compared using per capita health expenditures in hospital services, physician services, retail drugs, and the sum of these components. A multivariate analysis of California hospital net revenues was performed to determine whether reductions in hospital expenditures had been sustained.

Results.—California had the lowest growth in all measures compared (Table 2). The difference between the least competitive and most competitive hospitals in California declined steadily between 1980 and 1990 (Fig 2). By 1990, hospitals in the most competitive markets collected an average of 1.62% less revenues than hospitals facing the least competitive influence.

Comments.—Empirical evidence shows that competition did not lead to cost shifting in the California model. However, the data used to generate these results covered only 70% of total health care expenditures and did not examine possible cost shifting in other areas such as long-term care. To establish that competition was responsible for lower expenditure growth, trends in hospital revenue growth were compared between both the most competitive and the least competitive markets. California results showed that price competition caused the most competitive hospitals to limit increases and to maintain those limitations over time and throughout the system rather than simply in the hospital sector alone. The current merger trend could undermine the gains resulting from the increasing competitive environment. Although California had the lowest growth rate in expenditures, it also has an increasing percentage of the population without insurance. Future studies will need to examine the effect that this uncompensated population has on expenditure results and on the quality and access ramifications of this new competitive environment.

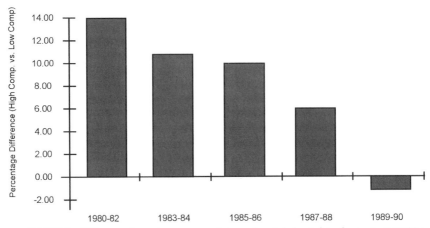

FIGURE 2.—Differences in total net revenue between hospitals located in the most competitive markets and those located in the least competitive markets: California, 1980 through 1990. Results are based on a variance components regression model that controlled for differences in hospital characteristics (ownership, teaching status, output levels, case mix), demographic characteristics of the hospital's market, financial impact of the Medicare PPS program, competitiveness of the physician markets operating in the hospital's market, and individual year effects. (Courtesy of Melnick GA, Zwanziger J: State health care expenditures under competition and regulation, 1980 through 1991. *Am J Public Health* 85:1391–1396, 1995. Copyright American Public Health Association.)

▶ I selected this paper to call attention to the fact that there is some evidence that would permit states interested in establishing their own health plans to arrive at decisions about whether they use the competitive or the regulatory approach. Decisions about this often are accompanied by more heat than light. The study compares the state of California with its far advanced competitive model with national data, as well as with data from 4 states that adopted the regulatory approach. It addresses expenditures for hospital services, physician services, and drugs, as well as total expenditure. The evidence presented suggests that California health expenditures showed the slowest rise and that this could not be accounted for by shifts from the hospital sector to other sectors. These data, if confirmed by additional studies, would support the competitive model. It is important to emphasize that the apparent beneficial effect on health care expenditures could be abolished if mergers and consolidations continue at their present pace.

There are a number of limitations to this study of which the most important include the fact that only 70% of the health care expenditures are accounted for in this study. In addition, no data are presented on whether the apparent beneficial effect could be accounted for by an increase in the number of uninsured persons during the comparable time period. Finally, there are no data as to whether the cost savings reported had any impact on accessibility to care or on quality of care.

J.C. Beck, M.D.

Ethics

Physician-assisted Suicide and Euthanasia in Washington State: Patient Requests and Physician Responses

Back AL, Wallace JI, Starks HE, et al (Veterans Affairs Puget Sound Health Care System, Seattle; Univ of Washington, Seattle)
JAMA 275:919–925, 1996   1–57

Purpose.—In the ongoing debate regarding physician-assisted suicide and euthanasia, many basic questions remain unanswered. Little is known about how often physicians receive these requests and how they respond. Washington State physicians were surveyed to address these issues.

Methods.—An anonymous questionnaire was mailed to 1,453 physicians, including a random 25% sample of primary care physicians and all physicians in certain subspecialties, including oncology, cardiology, neurology, and geriatrics. The physicians were asked whether they had ever received any requests for physician-assisted suicide. Those who responded affirmatively were asked to provide case descriptions, including their responses to the requests.

Results.—The response rate was 57%. Twelve percent of the respondents had received at least 1 explicit request for physician-assisted suicide, and 4% had received requests for euthanasia. A total of 207 case descriptions were obtained. Cancer, neurologic disease, and AIDS were the most commonly involved diagnoses. When asked about their perceptions of the patients' concerns, the physicians cited worries about loss of control, being a burden, being dependent on others, and loss of dignity. Patients with physical symptoms were more likely to receive help from the physicians, who rarely sought advice from their colleagues about these cases. Thirty-eight of 156 patients requesting physician-assisted suicide received a prescription, which led to death in 21 patients. Fourteen of 58 patients who requested euthanasia received injected medications and died.

Conclusions.—Many physicians have had patients ask about physician-assisted suicide and euthanasia. Physicians sometimes honor these requests, even though physician-assisted suicide and euthanasia are currently illegal. Further study is needed to provide information relevant to the ongoing debate about physician-assisted death.

▶ The debate regarding euthanasia and physician-assisted suicide is gaining increasing intensity and is, at the moment, primarily focused on the issue of morality. Very little empirical data exists. I selected this article because it is one of the first to give insight into the frequency of these requests, the major concerns of the individuals requesting either one of these procedures, and how physicians respond to requests of this type.

This empirical study documents the frequency of patient requests, the physicians' perception of patient concerns, and the scope of physician evaluation. It reveals that patient requests for physician-assisted death are not rare; that patient concerns underlying these requests are often nonphysical, in contrast to present beliefs; that physicians do not consult each other often about these cases; and that physicians occasionally provide physician-assisted death. Clearly, more studies of this type are needed—to further inform by ethical reflection so that the debate may be a more informed one.

J.C. Beck, M.D.

2   Long-term Care

Introduction

The tradition in this chapter has been to define long-term care in broad terms. Therefore, articles appear in this chapter that apply to any aspect of the health care of the elderly that is provided for extended periods. This approach clearly results in overlap with other chapters. Nevertheless, I have elected to keep such articles in this chapter with the thought that it may be helpful to the reader by creating consistency in the editorial comments.

The job of selecting articles, quite frankly, has become more difficult every year. New and important knowledge is accumulating rapidly. This year, the chapter is broken down into subsections about urinary incontinence, comprehensive geriatric assessment, infections, ethical issues (including advance directives, physician-assisted suicide, and the use of restraints), miscellaneous nursing home issues, prostate disease, and miscellaneous issues. Significant advances in these many areas can be reviewed by a quick perusal of the chapter.

This year especially there is increasing public discussion of ethics. Physician-assisted suicide is in the news every week, and two studies related to this important and critical issue are presented. Physicians must come to terms with physician-assisted suicide and provide leadership for the public—whichever side of the issue they fall. Also, advances in comprehensive geriatric assessment performed in the home are abstracted to provide several examples of new ways of delivering health care. A variety of studies that reflect advances in managing infections, restraints, and incontinence in nursing homes also have been selected for medical directors and directors of nursing in long-term care facilities.

I hope the chapter will provide a quick overview of some of the significant advances in long-term care that occurred in the past year.

John R. Burton, M.D.

Urinary Incontinence

Detection of Urinary Incontinence During Ambulatory Monitoring of Bladder Function by a Temperature-Sensitive Device

Eckford SD, Finney R, Jackson SR, et al (Southmead Hosp, Bristol, England)
Br J Urol 77:194–197, 1996   2–1

Background.—In the assessment of incontinent patients, it is essential to reliably demonstrate incontinence. Although long-term ambulatory monitoring (LTAM) is being used increasingly, it is more difficult to record incontinence in mobile patients. An engineering technology, diode temperature sensors, was evaluated as a method of evaluating incontinent patients with LTAM by detecting small temperature differences between leaked urine and the perineum.

Methods.—A 6-diode device spanning 5 cm was placed under the top layer of tissue in a light perineal pad. A single diode, placed on the reverse side of the pad, was the reference diode for detecting changes. The diodes were attached to an amplifier/digitizer and recorder. Fifty-one incontinent women and 23 continent controls wore the pads with the device for an ambulatory/exercising cycle of LTAM. The findings of the device were compared with changes in pad weight to determine the accuracy of the device.

Results.—A temperature differential between urine and the perineum was recorded in all positions except sitting cross-legged. Using the pad-test result as the reference, the temperature-sensitive device had a sensitivity of 95.2% and a specificity of 90.6%. However, the volume of leaked urine did not correlate with the area under the temperature-time curve.

Conclusions.—The temperature-sensitive device detecting temperature differences between leaked urine and the perineum is a reliable method of detecting episodes of urinary incontinence during LTAM studies, although the volume of leaked urine cannot be quantified with this method. Because the device records when voiding occurs, it is possible to differentiate between voluntary and involuntary detrusor contractions at the time of voiding.

▶ This study represents a novel method of detecting urinary incontinence in women. The device is a thermal sensor that takes advantage of the difference between perineal and urine temperatures. The device appears to be unobtrusive. It has a sensitivity of 95% and a specificity of 91% compared with the perineal pad-weighing technique.

This device, when available commercially, may be a useful aid to help clinicians quantify the number of episodes of urinary incontinence in women. It would be a valuable way to monitor the effects of therapeutic endeavors.

J.R. Burton, M.D.

Nocturnal Enuresis in Community-Dwelling Older Adults

Burgio KL, Locher JL, Ives DG, et al (Univ of Alabama, Birmingham; Univ of Pittsburgh, Pa)
J Am Geriatr Soc 44:139–143, 1996

2–2

Introduction.—Although enuresis is common in children, it typically resolves spontaneously and is uncommon in adults. However, there are few data on the prevalence of nocturnal enuresis among older adults. Similarly, the causes of enuresis have been widely studied in children but not in older adults. It has been hypothesized that the normal pattern of excreting twice as much urine during the day as at night is reversed in both enuretic children and older adults. The prevalence and characteristics, as well as potential predicting factors, of nocturnal enuresis were investigated in independent, community-dwelling older adults.

Methods.—A total of 3,870 noninstitutionalized older adults between the ages of 65 and 79 were interviewed, using the Health Risk Appraisal (HRA), which included questions on involuntary loss of urine, treatment of incontinence, demographic factors, medical history, use of alcohol, social support, and sleep patterns.

Results.—Of the 3,870 participants, 1,090 reported incontinence and 80 reported nocturnal enuresis. The prevalence of nocturnal enuresis was 2.1% overall, 2.9% in women, and 1% in men. Compared with participants with daytime incontinence only, those with enuresis had significantly more severe incontinence (Fig 1), which was more likely to have required treatment, and which had a less successful treatment outcome. Nocturnal

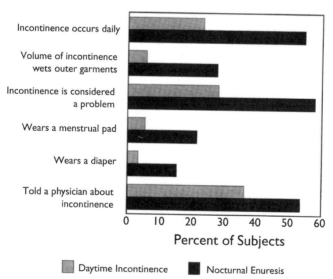

FIGURE 1.—Indicators of incontinence severity in subjects with nocturnal enuresis vs. daytime incontinence alone. (Courtesy of Burgio KL, Locher JL, Ives DG, et al: Nocturnal enuresis in community-dwelling older adults. *J Am Geriatr Soc* 44(2):139–143, 1996.)

enuresis was more likely to occur in subjects with mixed stress and urge daytime incontinence than in subjects with only stress incontinence or urge incontinence. Enuresis was significantly associated with congestive heart failure and the frequent use of sleep medication.

Conclusions.—Nocturnal enuresis is uncommon in older adults, occurring with a prevalence of approximately 2%. However, this type of incontinence is more severe, has a greater impact on the patient, and is less responsive to treatment than other types of incontinence. The close association between nocturnal enuresis and the symptoms of congestive heart failure suggests that enuresis is caused by daytime fluid accumulation and the mobilization of excess fluid during sleep. Therefore, more research on the patterns and regulation of urine production may yield improved treatment methods.

▶ There are very few data on nocturnal enuresis in adults. This very large and carefully done study of this problem is, therefore, quite valuable. Among community-dwelling elders, urinary incontinence was found in 28% of subjects. This prevalence has been reported in other surveys also.

Nocturnal enuresis is uncommon. But, it does seem to be a marker for more severe urinary incontinence. Those subjects with nocturnal urinary incontinence responded less well to a variety of therapies. Consistent with the proposed theory of nocturnal enuresis is that individuals with this problem were more likely to have symptoms of congestive heart failure. Indeed, the nocturnal mobilization of fluid may explain the enuresis.

J.R. Burton, M.D.

Measuring the Psychosocial Impact of Urinary Incontinence: The York Incontinence Perceptions Scale (YIPS)
Lee PS, Reid DW, Saltmarche A, et al (York Univ, Toronto; Sunnybrook Health Sciences Centre, Toronto; Victorian Order of Nurses, Peterborough, Ont, Canada)
J Am Geriatr Soc 43:1275–1278, 1995   2–3

Background.—Despite documentation in the medical literature of the negative aspects of incontinence, few standardized instruments are available for assessment of the psychosocial aspects of this problem. Research has identified that factual knowledge about incontinence, beliefs about its control, coping, personal efficacy, acceptance, and perceived family impact are issues central to pscyhosocial effect. The York Incontinence Perception Scale (YIPS) was developed as a tool for measuring the psychosocial aspects and management of urinary incontinence. The internal consistency and validity of this scale were examined.

Methods.—Participants included 101 women aged 29–98 years (mean, 67.4 years) with a diagnosis of urinary incontinence and living in rural Southern Ontario. Participants were referred to the study by themselves, their families, their family physicians, or an outside agency. The women

APPENDIX 1.—York Incontinence Perceptions Scale

1. How much control do you now feel you have over your incontinence?

1	2	3	4	5	6	7
none						a great deal

2. How well do you now accept your incontinence?

1	2	3	4	5	6	7
not at all well						very well

3. How well do you now cope with your incontinence?

1	2	3	4	5	6	7
not at all well						very well

4. How much do you now feel you know about urinary incontinence?

1	2	3	4	5	6	7
none						a great deal

5. Please rate the amount of sleep that you now are able to have with your incontinence.

1	2	3	4	5	6	7
none						a great deal

6. Please rate how effective your efforts now are in reducing your incontinence.

1	2	3	4	5	6	7
not at all effective						very effective

7. Please rate your general quality of life now.

1	2	3	4	5	6	7
low						high

8. Please rate the effect your incontinence has on your family now.

1	2	3	4	5	6	7
very negative						very positive

(Courtesy of Lee PS, Reid DW, Saltmarche A, et al: Measuring the psychosocial impact of urinary incontinence: The York Incontinence Perceptions Scale (YIPS). *J Am Geriatr Soc* 43(11):1275–1278, 1995.)

were randomly assigned to receive either no intervention or one-to-one counseling in behavioral techniques for self-management of incontinence. The daily number of incontinence episodes and fluid intake were recorded. The Incontinence Impact Questionnaire (IIQ: measures the self-perceived influence of incontinence on ability to participate in activities) was given before and after the trial. The YIPS (Appendix 1) was administered as part of the overall assessment at the end of the study (week 25). Participants also completed the Aids to Living Scale and single-item ratings of amount of leakage, continence status, and overall health status.

Results.—Treatment and control groups did not differ at baseline in terms of average number of episodes of incontinence, continence impact (IIQ), or education. Treated participants reported a more positive adjustment on the YIPS than did controls at the conclusion of the treatment period. This adjustment was concordant with the reduced incidence of incontinence in the treated women. Internal consistency of the YIPS was high. Lower frequency of incontinence and self-ratings of improvement in amount of leakage, improved continence status, and overall health status were correlated with positive adjustment on the YIPS. No differences in YIPS scores were found among participants with different diagnostic subgroups of incontinence.

Conclusions.—The YIPS is brief, easy to administer, and internally consistent and appears to be sensitive to differences in continence status between those receiving significantly effective treatment vs. no intervention. Further studies should include a pretest administration of the YIPS.

▶ This study documents and validates a urinary incontinence perception scale. The psychological impact of incontinence may be profound. This scale appears to have promise in allowing investigators and clinicians to monitor the psychosocial impact of a patient's urinary incontinence and its response to treatment.

J.R. Burton, M.D.

Pyuria Among Chronically Incontinent But Otherwise Asymptomatic Nursing Home Residents
Ouslander JG, Schapira M, Schnelle JF, et al (Univ of California, Los Angeles; Jewish Home for the Aging, Los Angeles)
J Am Geriatr Soc 44:420–423, 1996 2–4

Background.—Symptomatic and asymptomatic urinary tract infections are common among nursing home residents. The diagnosis may be difficult, as even those with symptomatic infections typically have nonspecific symptoms. Pyuria has been used to determine whether to prescribe antimicrobial treatment. However, the accuracy of pyuria as a marker for bacteriuria has not been studied. A study of asymptomatic, chronically incontinent nursing home residents provided data from urinalyses and cultures to evaluate the relationship between pyuria and bacteriuria.

Methods.—Urine specimens were obtained by a clean catch technique from 231 incontinent nursing home residents. The specimens were tested for leukocyte esterase with a dipstick method, then cultured. Microscopic analyses determined the levels of pyuria, defined as more than 10 white blood cells per high field of spun urine.

TABLE 1.—Relationship of Pyuria to Bacteriuria ($n = 124$)

Level of Pyuria	Bacteriuria: No. of Specimens	
	Present	Absent
All specimens		
>20	38	28
11–20	16	14
0–10	37	81
Females		
>20	26	20
11–20	15	11
0–10	29	51
Males		
>20	12	8
11–20	1	3
0–10	8	30

(Courtesy of Ouslander JG, Schapira M, Schnelle JF, et al: Pyuria among chronically incontinent but otherwise asymptomatic nursing home residents. *J Am Geriatr Soc* 44(4):420–423, 1996.)

TABLE 2.—Accuracy of Leukocyte Esterase Dipstick Test Compared With Microscopic Urinalysis Performed by a Clinical Laboratory ($n = 214$)

Leukocyte Esterase	Pyuria: No. of Specimens	
	Present	Absent
All specimens		
Positive	80	57
Negative	16	61
Females		
Positive	61	45
Negative	11	35
Males		
Positive	19	12
Negative	5	26

(Courtesy of Ouslander JG, Schapira M, Schnelle JF, et al: Pyuria among chronically incontinent but otherwise asymptomatic nursing home residents. *J Am Geriatr Soc* 44(4):420–423, 1996.)

Results.—There was an overall prevalence of 45% for pyuria and 43% for bacteriuria. Pyuria was observed in 59% of the specimens with bacteriuria and 34% of the specimens without bacteriuria (Table 1). Bacteriuria was observed in 56% of the specimens with pyuria and 31% of the specimens without pyuria. As a marker for bacteriuria, pyuria had a sensitivity of 59%, a specificity of 66%, a positive predictive value of 56%, and a negative predictive value of 69% overall. The values were somewhat higher in men than in women. In the diagnosis of pyuria, the leukocyte esterase dipstick test had a sensitivity of 83%, a specificity of 52%, and positive predictive value of 58%, and a negative predictive value of 79% (Table 2). These values were somewhat higher in women than in men.

Conclusions.—There is a high prevalence of pyuria among nursing home residents, and it is often present in patients without bacteriuria. Therefore, using pyuria as a marker for bacteriuria in asymptomatic patients may lead to unnecessary antimicrobial treatment. More study is needed to determine the diagnostic value of pyuria in symptomatic patients and the significance of sterile pyuria.

▶ This study provides new knowledge about pyuria among incontinent nursing home residents. Pyuria is common, and it occurs both in the presence and absence of bacteriuria. Its presence cannot be used as proof of a symptomatic urinary tract infection or one that should be treated. The leukocyte esterase screening test for pyuria is reasonably sensitive but very poorly specific.

These and other data reinforce the premise that there is no value in a screening urinalysis in an elderly patient, especially those in nursing homes. Such a test should be ordered only when a specific clinical question is being addressed and when a clinical decision will be made based on its results. Even when considering the diagnosis of a urinary tract infection, a urinalysis that is negative for pyuria does not rule out bacteriuria or a symptomatic infection. The bottom line is simple. A urinalysis is of little help in the evaluation of nursing home residents with urinary incontinence.

J.R. Burton, M.D.

Collagen Injection for Intrinsic Sphincteric Deficiency in Men
Aboseif SR, O'Connell HE, Usui A, et al (Univ of Texas, Houston; Univ of California, San Francisco)
J Urol 155:10–13, 1996   2–5

Introduction.—In 1993, the Food and Drug Administration approved the use of collagen for the treatment of intrinsic sphincteric deficiency. Glutaraldehyde cross-linked collagen is a highly purified suspension of bovine dermal collagen associated with minimal inflammatory response and no tendency to migrate. An early experience with collagen injections in the treatment of male urinary incontinence caused by intrinsic sphincteric deficiency was described.

Patients.—Eighty-eight men, aged 54–82 years (mean age, 68 years), with mild-to-severe intrinsic sphincter deficiency were treated. Urinary incontinence secondary to intrinsic sphincteric deficiency was caused by prostatectomy in 85 men, trauma in 1, myelodysplasia in 1, and chondroma of the sacral roots in 1. All men had been incontinent for 1 year and had failed to respond to medical treatment.

Procedure.—All patients underwent skin testing with 0.1 mL of glutaraldehyde cross-linked collagen and were observed for 4 weeks. Except for 15 patients who required general anesthesia, all injections were given with the patient under local anesthesia (1% lidocaine). Under direct vision, collagen was injected slowly and submucosally, proximal to the external sphincter on both sides, until urethral mucosa coaptation was achieved (Fig 2). The end point for treatment was either cure or administration of 5 injections at intervals for 1 month.

Outcome.—The mean follow-up was 10 months. The mean number of treatments was 3.5, and the mean total volume of collagen injected was 25 mL. The patients were subdivided into 2 groups based on the response to collagen injection. Group 1 included 61 patients (85%) with normal bladder compliance who gained some benefit from collagen therapy, including 42 who became completely dry (47%) and 19 (19%) who had substantial improvement but who required 1–3 pads per day. Group 2 included 27 patients with severe incontinence who required more than 4 pads per day before treatment. Of these, 14 consistently used fewer pads (but still more than 3 per day) after treatment and 13 showed no improvement. The 2 groups were similar in age, duration of incontinence, volume of collagen used, and number of injections given. Worse response to

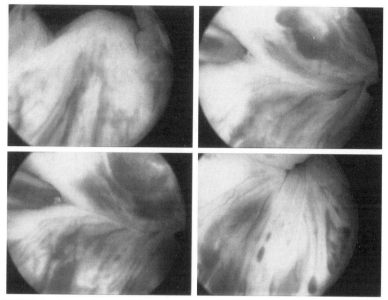

FIGURE 2.—Sequential images show increasing coaptation as collagen is injected. (Courtesy of Aboseif SR, O'Connell HE, Usui A, et al: Collagen injection for intrinsic sphincteric deficiency in men. *J Urol* 155:10–13, 1996.)

collagen therapy was associated with more severe pretreatment incontinence status, concomitant detrusor abnormalities, and the cause of the sphincteric deficiency. There was no significant morbidity; only 11% of patients required clean intermittent catheterization for 24–48 hours.

Conclusions.—Transurethral injection of collagen is effective and safe in carefully selected patients who have intrinsic sphincteric deficiency. Many patients who respond to treatment have previously undergone only uncomplicated radical retropubic prostatectomy without another procedure and have normal bladder function.

▶ I am increasingly impressed with the effectiveness of using collagen injections for treatment of urinary incontinence resulting from intrinsic sphincter deficiency in men. This study reports the outcome in 88 highly selected men who had been incontinent for at least 1 year. Most were incontinent after prostatectomy. The authors demonstrate nearly a 70% marked or better improvement with an average follow-up of 10 months. It will be necessary to see longer follow-up data but, nonetheless, these are impressive results and are accomplished with relatively minimal side effects. These results are better than those previously reported, and they likely reflect the increasing experience of this group of urologists.

Figure 2 shows the endoscopic view of the effect of the collagen injections. Clinicians should recall that it is always best to initiate behavioral therapies and/or other medical therapies before consideration of referral to a urologist for an invasive procedure. If, or when, a referral is made for consideration of collagen injection, it should be to someone who is greatly experienced in this procedure. There are still too few data to make any recommendations regarding women who may benefit from this procedure.

J.R. Burton, M.D.

Oxybutynin With Bladder Retraining for Detrusor Instability in Elderly People: A Randomized Controlled Trial
Szonyi G, Collas DM, Ding YY, et al (Univ College London)
Age Ageing 24:287–291, 1995   2–6

Purpose.—Oxybutynin is a commonly used supplement to bladder retraining for patients with urinary incontinence resulting from detrusor instability. Oxybutynin, a tertiary amine with detrusor effects, also acts as a local anesthetic and smooth muscle relaxant. Although oxybutynin appears ineffective for institutionalized elderly individuals, it has not been studied for use in the frail but independent-living elderly population. This population was the subject of a randomized controlled trial using oxybutynin plus bladder training for detrusor instability.

Methods.—The randomized, double-blind, parallel-group study included 60 frail elderly patients (mean age, 82 years) who were living independently in the community. All received bladder retraining and were randomized to receive either oxybutynin, 2.5 mg twice daily, or placebo. All patients kept a bladder chart throughout the study. In addition, they were asked whether the treatment had been beneficial and were asked to grade their improvement on an ordinal scale.

Results.—The 2 groups were well matched. Five patients in the placebo group and 8 patients in the oxybutynin group withdrew, 3 of the latter because of esophageal reflux. The bladder charts showed that oxybutynin was superior to placebo in reducing daytime urinary frequency, but there were no differences in nocturia. After 1 month, 86% of the patients in the oxybutynin group reported a benefit compared with 55% of the placebo group. By 1½ months, however, this difference was no longer significant. The ordinal rankings showed a similar pattern. Although the oxybutynin dose could be adjusted upward, the median dose remained at 2.5 mg given twice daily at the end of the study.

Conclusions.—Oxybutynin appears ineffective in reducing incontinence in community-dwelling frail elderly individuals with detrusor instability. Subjective ratings suggest that oxybutynin is better than placebo at 1 month but not thereafter. Studies of treatment for detrusor instability should assess the response in terms of reduction in micturition frequency, because these patients will avoid incontinence by urinating more often.

▶ There are relatively few well-controlled trials of drug therapy for urinary incontinence. This is one such study, and it is the first to add subjective outcomes to the usual outcome measure of the number of incontinent episodes. It adds to our understanding of the use of oxybutynin in urge incontinence. Note that the benefit of using oxybutynin to reduce *daytime* incontinent episodes was modest and not significant. However, the patients given oxybutynin thought they were better at one month but not at two. Note also that the side effect profile was similar when an average dose of oxybutynin of 2.5 mg given twice daily was compared with placebo.

Although these data are discouraging with reference to the value of oxybutynin in reducing daytime urge incontinence, many experts believe this drug is particularly helpful when taken in the evening, when nocturnal incontinence is a problem. This would be a good follow-up study.

J.R. Burton, M.D.

The Use of Urinary Catheters Among Elderly Patients Admitted to an Acute Medical Ward
Marcus E-L, Ligomsky H, Ben-Yehuda A, et al (Sarah Herzog Mem Hosp, Jerusalem; Hadassah Univ, Jerusalem)
Aging Clin Exp Res 7:242–244, 1995   2–7

Objective.—Urinary catheterization is a major risk factor for nosocomial urinary tract infections. Given the little information regarding its use in acute hospitals, a study was conducted to evaluate the prevalence, rationale, and natural history of urinary catheterization in elderly patients admitted to an acute medical ward from the emergency room.

Setting.—During a 5-month period, 283 elderly patients (60 years of age or older) were admitted to the ward from the emergency room. Those admitted with a urinary catheter were followed up prospectively on the seventh day postadmission, on discharge, and 1 month postdischarge.

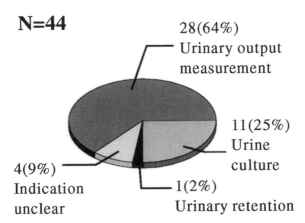

FIGURE 1.—Reasons for urinary catheterization in the emergency room. (Courtesy of Marcus E-L, Ligomsky H, Ben-Yehuda A, et al: The use of urinary catheters among elderly patients admitted to an acute medical ward. *Aging Clin Exp Res* 7:242–244, 1995.)

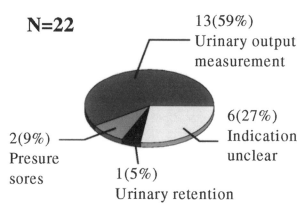

N=22

13(59%)
Urinary output
measurement

6(27%)
Indication
unclear

2(9%)
Presure
sores

1(5%)
Urinary retention

FIGURE 2.—Reasons for urinary catheterization on the seventh day postadmission. (Courtesy of Marcus E-L, Ligomsky H, Ben-Yehuda A, et al: The use of urinary catheters among elderly patients admitted to an acute medical ward. *Aging Clin Exp Res* 7:242–244, 1995.)

Findings.—Eighteen men and 31 women (mean age, 80 years) were admitted with a urinary catheter. The prevalence of urinary catheters was 18%, similar to that reported by Sullivan in an acute hospital but less than that reported by Siers (35%). Principal diagnoses at admission were urinary tract infection in 30%, pneumonia in 22%, uncharacterized fever in 12%, myocardial infarction in 12%, and congestive heart failure in 8%. Most catheters were inserted in the emergency room to measure urinary output (Fig 1). Interestingly, 25% of the catheters were inserted to obtain a urine culture in incontinent or uncooperative patients, and yet these catheters were not removed after urine collection. Furthermore, half of the patients remained catheterized 1 week postadmission, mainly to monitor urine output and for unclear indications (Fig 2). The in-hospital mortality among the 50 patients admitted with a catheter was 38%, which was significantly higher than the 4% mortality rate for those not catheterized.

Conclusions.— Inpatient geriatric assessment should include evaluation of the appropriateness of urinary catheterization. The risk-benefit ratio before and after catheter insertion should be carefully considered. The criteria previously published by Hartstein may be a reasonable approach to the appropriate duration of urinary catheterization after an acute event.

▶ In every acute care hospital in which I have worked or visited, it seems that the placement of a urinary catheter is almost the rite of passage for older patients admitted via an emergency room. In fact, challenging the presence of a urinary catheter is one of the most frequent teaching points of geriatricians while attending or consulting on such patients.

I have selected this paper because of the very high rate and often inappropriate placement of urinary catheters in emergency rooms. In this study, there was a relatively low incidence of only 18% of catheter placement over 5 months among older individuals admitted to the hospital via the emergency room. This level is far lower than I would expect. Perhaps a Hawthorn effect occurred. However, even with this relatively low (but, still, too high) incidence, there are lessons to be learned. Often, the catheter was inserted and the need for the catheter was not reassessed. This is clearly shown in Figures 1 and 2. Twenty-five percent of patients had a catheter placed for a culture, and 9% had them placed for no clear indication. Notice also that at 7 days, 27% of the individuals with catheters no longer had a clear indication for their use. Also at 7 days, nearly 60% of individuals had a urinary catheter remaining for the measurement of urinary output. Quite frankly, I wonder how critical this measurement really was in most patients, particularly 7 days after admission.

Let us all work to stop the inappropriate placement of urinary catheters and to reassess, on a daily basis, their need when they have been placed. Without more conservative use of catheters, there will certainly be inappropriate sequelae, particularly that of infection.

J.R. Burton, M.D.

Geriatric Assessment

The Sepulveda GEU Study Revisited: Long-Term Outcomes, Use of Services, and Costs
Rubenstein LZ, Josephson KR, Harker JO, et al (Univ of California, Los Angeles)
Aging Clin Exp Res 7:212–217, 1995   2–8

Background.—Hospital geriatric evaluation and management units seek to reduce the risks associated with hospitalization in selected, at-risk elderly patients. A previous cost and survival analysis found that 1-year costs were significantly lower for patients managed in the geriatric evaluation unit (GEU), who obtained many other benefits as well. However, the cost-effectiveness of the GEU could not be determined; lifetime costs might actually be higher for patients in the GEU. Functional outcomes were assessed after 2 years, and survival, health care utilization, and direct health costs after 3 years in elderly patients assigned to a GEU or to standard care.

Methods.—The previously reported randomized study included 123 elderly hospitalized patients. All were at least 65 years old and had persistent medical, functional, and psychosocial problems, but none were in obvious need of nursing home placement. The patients assigned to the experimental group received a comprehensive geriatric assessment, treatment, and rehabilitation from an interdisciplinary geriatric team, along with follow-up in the geriatric outpatient clinic. Those assigned to the control group received the usual hospital discharge planning and follow-up services. The outcome measures included a composite, simplified functional score; death; health services utilization; and living location. Total costs were adjusted for survival, and actual costs were based on the number of days at each level of care. Institutional health care costs for the last year of life were evaluated in terms of bed days.

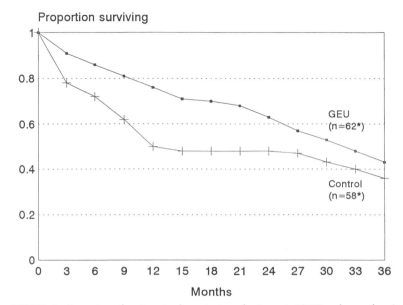

FIGURE 1.—Proportion of patients in the geriatric evaluation unit (*GEU*) and control patients surviving each quarter to 3 years. Based on 62 patients in the GEU and 58 control group individuals with 3-year survival data. *Asterisk* indicates 1 GEU patient and 2 control individuals' survival status was unknown at 3 years. (Courtesy of Rubenstein LZ, Josephson KR, Harker JO, et al: The Sepulveda GEU study revisited: Long-term outcomes, use of services, and costs. *Aging Clin Exp Res* 7:212–217, 1995.)

Results.—Assignment to the GEU had a significant effect on survival through the second year (Fig 1). Including survivors and patients who died, the mean survival at 3 years' follow-up was 2.03 years in the GEU group vs. 1.57 years in the control group. Survivors in both groups represented the full range of functional ability at long-term follow-up. There were no indications that the increased survival time in the GEU group was spent at a reduced level of function. In fact, the patients in the GEU spent significantly more time at the moderate functional level during the second year than the patients in the control group did (Fig 2). There were no significant differences between the groups in mean total institutional costs, though costs were slightly higher for GEU survivors after 1 year and 3 years.

Conclusions.—The benefits of comprehensive geriatric assessment, treatment, and rehabilitation in a GEU for hospitalized elderly patients persist for at least 2 years. The increased length of survival of patients in the GEU does not result in reduced function, nor does it inflate care costs. The GEU approach appears to be cost-effective over the long term.

▶ This abstracted study presents an extended follow-up—now to 3 years—of the well-known Sepulveda randomized GEU trial published in 1984.[1] Recall the dramatic findings among patients in the GEU at the 1-year

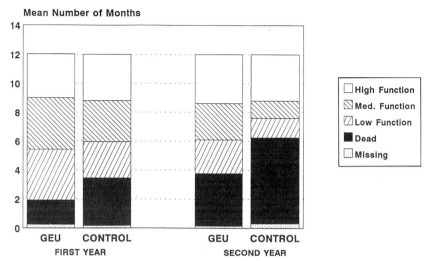

FIGURE 2.—Time spent (mean months per subject) at different levels of function during the first and second year of follow-up of patients in the geriatric evaluation unit (*GEU*) and control group subjects. (Courtesy of Rubenstein LZ, Josephson KR, Harker JO, et al: The Sepulveda GEU study revisited: Long-term outcomes, use of services, and costs. *Aging Clin Exp Res* 7:212–217, 1995.)

follow-up of that landmark study: They had lower mortality, went less frequently to a nursing home, spent less time in a nursing home, had a lower overall cost, and had higher function. Although the study remains difficult to generalize because it is a Veterans Affairs (VA) program, it has provided a powerful incentive to other institutions, including non–VA-based institutions, to properly assess elderly patients in hospitals with the goal of decreasing functional losses and improving survival.

In this report, the positive benefits of the GEU and after-care were evident 2 years after randomization, as shown in Figure 1. The benefit is no longer significant in year 3. Importantly, GEU patients had a higher functional level at year 2 than did controls, as shown in Figure 2. Also, there was no significant cost difference between groups over 3 years with or without adjustment for survival.

Elements of the positive effects of GEU have been replicated in several forms and settings.[2] If health policy experts and insurance programs are to encourage and pay for such assessments, continued studies of the GEU and the more generic comprehensive geriatric assessment that precisely define the target population and link cost savings to improved outcomes are necessary.

J.R. Burton, M.D.

References

1. Rubenstein LZ, Josephson KR, Wieland GD, et al: Effectiveness of a geriatric evaluation unit: A randomized clinical trial. *N Engl J Med* 311:1664–1670, 1984.

2. Stuck AE, Siu AL, Wieland D, et al: Comprehensive geriatric assessment: A meta-analysis of controlled trials. *Lancet* 342:1032–1036, 1993.

Computerized Geriatric Assessment for Geriatric Care Management

De Vore PA (Georgetown Univ, Washington, DC)
Aging Clin Exp Res 7:194–196, 1995   2–9

Introduction.—Geriatric care management requires multidisciplinary collection and analysis of information about elderly patients. Although the care manager may be any of a number of different professionals, the physician is usually the one who must approve the proposed management options. A computer-based approach to the assessment of elderly patients for geriatric care management was described.

Computerized Approach to Geriatric Assessment.—The new approach uses a software program that streamlines the functional assessment of elderly patients. It requires minimal additional staff, so it is cost-effective. The patient is evaluated in a computer-prompted interview, which takes about 1½ hours to perform. With a laptop computer, a caregiver can conduct the interview in the patient's home. Before the physical examination is performed, the software program generates a 10- to 12-page report, including a summary sheet listing positive findings and recommendations for follow-up (Fig 1). The software asks that patients perform certain tasks to assess functional abilities, and it permits individual components of the complete geriatric assessment to be performed without the need to repeat the entire protocol. The program has been shown to improve accuracy in diagnosing new problems, predicting the later need for changes in living status, and facilitating serial testing to track changes in functional capacity.

Discussion.—This software program, whether used by a primary care physician or a nonphysician geriatric care manager, offers many benefits to elderly patients and their families. It also has potential applications for training and outcomes research.

▶ I expect these next few years of medical practice to be characterized in part by the emergence of computer software designed to assist the clinician in data collection and arrangement. This article presents an example of such software developed in a clinician's office and focused on the assessment of older patients. It is menu-driven and can be used in an office or home setting. I believe that we clinicians, even those of us from the precomputer age, will come to recognize the enormous benefit of using computers to assist us in evaluating and managing complicated patients. For example, Figure 1 shows a summary sheet from an assessment and is generated by the computer after the assessment data are entered into the program. A good source of information is available from the American College of Physicians: *Computers in Clinical Practice*, edited by Jerome A. Osheroff, M.D.; Product #33 0300240; Phone: (800) 523-1546, ext. 2600.

J.R. Burton, M.D.

	Risk Factor	Suggested Intervention
A.	Physical	
	Good Nutrition	
*	Underweight	Check serum albumen level
	Vision Adequate	
*	Expiratory Peak Flow below normal	Further evaluation indicated
*	Uses 4 or more prescription drugs	Medication review with primary care physician
*	Possible olfactory dysfunction	1. Sometimes associated with cognitive dysfunction
		2. Install smoke detector
	Low probability of hearing impairment	
*	Medium fall risk for balance maneuvers	1. Transfer training
		2. Balance exercises
		3. Environmental manipulations
	Overall low risk of falling	
B.	Mental	
	No depression based on self-evaluation	
	No depression based on physician's evaluation	
*	Possible cognitive dysfunction	Repeat evaluation in 3-6 months
C.	Functional	
	High probability of being able to function adequately in the community	
*	Physical testing indicated the following functional disabilities:	Physical therapy evaluation
	Dressing self	
	Holding things	
D.	Socioeconomic/Daily Living	
*	Environmental hazards found in the home	Environmental manipulations (e.g., grab bars, handrails)
*	Client has not talked to any friends or relative by phone during the last week	May indicate a functional disability

FIGURE 1.—Assessment summary for a typical patient. (Courtesy of De Vore PA: Computerized geriatric assessment for geriatric care management. *Aging Clin Exp Res* 7:194–196, 1995.)

The Timed Test of Money Counting: A Simple Method of Recognizing Geriatric Patients at Risk for Increased Health Care

Nikolaus T, Bach M, Oster P, et al (Klinikum der Universität Heidelberg, Germany)
Aging Clin Exp Res 7:179–183, 1995   2–10

Objective.—In the functional assessment of elderly individuals, tests simulating everyday activities may offer more objective information than self- or proxy-reports. The development and validation of a simple test to identify elderly patients at risk for increased health care needs, the Timed Test of Money Counting (TTMC), were described.

Methods.—In the TTMC, the patient is asked to open a purse and then remove and count a standardized amount of money. The time required to perform these tasks is measured in seconds. The use of the TTMC was studied in 2 groups of elderly patients: 78 consecutively admitted hospital patients who could be discharged home and 105 community-dwelling patients aged 70 years or older. The patients also underwent a comprehensive geriatric assessment. Health care utilization was assessed 3 weeks after hospital discharge. Eighteen months later, the patients, their caregivers, and their family physicians were asked again about health care utilization and the need for assistance. Receiver operating characteristic analysis was performed to identify the TTMC cutoff points that best identified patients with increased health care needs.

Results.—The reliability of the TTMC was established at baseline in a sample of hospitalized patients. The test demonstrated construct and concurrent validity with other measures of physical function. Of the 152 patients who completed 18-month follow-up, 44 had increased health care

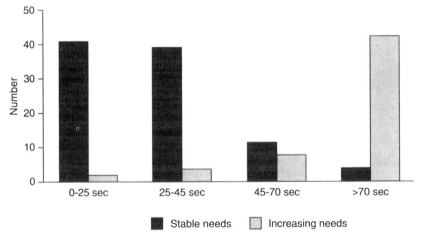

FIGURE 1.—Time score distribution of the Timed Test of Money Counting. (Courtesy of Nikolaus T, Bach M, Oster P, et al: The timed test of money counting: A simple method of recognizing geriatric patients at risk for increased health care. *Aging Clin Exp Res* 7:179–183, 1995.)

needs and 12 had been admitted to a nursing home. The mean time to completion of the TTMC was 31 seconds for patients with stable health care needs vs. 123 seconds for those with increased needs or institutionalization. A cutoff time of less than 45 seconds was established to identify subjects with stable needs, whereas a time of 70 seconds identified those with increasing needs (Fig 1). These cutoff times had a sensitivity of 83%, a specificity of 75%, and positive and negative predictive values of 85% and 75%, respectively.

Conclusions.—The TTMC appears to be a useful test for determining the risk of increasing health care needs among elderly patients. The test is functionally relevant because it includes manual skills, visual acuity, and cognitive capacity. It is quick to perform, requires no special equipment, and can be easily incorporated into routine geriatric assessment.

▶ I am intrigued by simple means of assessing the functional status of older individuals. This study describes such a means—the Timed Test of Money Counting. The test takes just a minute, and it seems to reliably predict whether patients are at risk for increased dependency, up to the 18 months of follow-up in this study.

J.R. Burton, M.D.

Infections

Immunizations in Long-term Care Facilities: Policies and Practice

Nichol KL, Grimm MB, Peterson DC (VA Med Center, Minneapolis; Minnesota Dept of Health, Minneapolis, Minn)
J Am Geriatr Soc 44:349–355, 1996   2–11

Introduction.—The residents of long-term care facilities may be vulnerable to vaccine-preventable diseases, especially influenza, pneumococcal pneumonia, and tetanus. Recognition of the importance of immunization in this population prompted an investigation of the policies and practices regarding resident and employee vaccinations in long-term care institutions.

Methods.—A questionnaire was mailed to all 445 long-term care facilities for adults in Minnesota. Information was requested on immunization policies and programs for the residents and the employees, attitudes toward immunizations, and 12-month vaccination rates for influenza, pneumococcal pneumonia, and tetanus/diphtheria among residents and for influenza, tetanus, and hepatitis B among employees.

Results.—The questionnaire was returned by 90% of the facilities. Among residents, the mean 12-month immunization rates were 84% for influenza vaccination, 11.9% for pneumococcal vaccination, and 2.9% for tetanus/diphtheria vaccination (Table 1). The vaccination rates improved significantly in institutions with formal, written vaccination policies or facility-wide standing orders and in facilities not requiring written consent for immunization. Influenza vaccination was considered very important

TABLE 1.—Long-Term Care Facilities' Immunization Activities
for Residents

	Percent of facilities (n = 399)
Written policies for vaccination	
Influenza	69.3
Pneumococcal	33
Tetanus/diphtheria	16.3
Routine Assessment of Immunization Status	
Influenza	
All residents	94.3
New residents admitted during immunization season	65
Pneumococcal	
Residents ≥65 years	38.9
Residents with chronic cardiopulmonary disease	14.8
Tetanus/diphtheria—primary series	
New residents	6
Tetanus/diphtheria—boosters	
Residents with chronic skin ulceration	2.3
Residents with acute skin trauma	21.4
12-month vaccination rates (spring 1992–spring 1993)	
Influenza	84
Pneumococcal	11.9
Tetanus/diphtheria	2.9
Assessment of vaccination rates included as part of quality assurance/quality improvement activities	
Influenza	40.4
Pneumococcal	7.9
Tetanus/diphtheria	2.6

(Courtesy of Nichol KL, Grimm MB, Peterson DC: Immunizations in long-term care facilities: Policies and practice. *J Am Geriatr Soc* 44(4):349–355, 1996.)

and cost-effective by most of the facilities, whereas the tetanus/diphtheria vaccination was typically considered much less important and cost-effective. Although 86.1% of the facilities had an influenza vaccination program for employees, there was only a 33% 12-month vaccination rate among employees. The other 12-month vaccination rates among employees were 23.2% for hepatitis B and 1.7% for tetanus/diphtheria. Employee vaccination rates were improved in facilities offering onsite vaccination and free vaccination and in facilities providing inservice education regarding immunization.

Conclusions.—Because infectious diseases contribute significantly to the morbidity and mortality of residents of long-term care facilities, the vaccination policies and practices are of vital importance in protecting the health of this vulnerable population. Therefore, long-term care institutions should implement programs to increase immunization rates among both residents and employees.

▶ Residents in nursing homes represent an important target population for vaccinations. Traditionally, such facilities have not had a great rate of immunizing their residents. However, with increased attention to the importance of immunization, vaccination rates have improved considerably in recent years. This study adds to our knowledge of what strategies result in the highest vaccination rates. It is important because it represents a statewide survey that included 399 nursing homes. The greatest immunization rates of patients occurred in those nursing homes when there were written immunization policies, standing orders for vaccine administration, and no requirement for written consent for the administration of a vaccine.

The record on immunization of nursing home staff is not as good as it is for patients. It should be. Health care providers should serve as role models for excellent preventive care, and furthermore, we owe it to our patients to protect them by taking immunization ourselves. In the current study, several strategies improved the vaccination rate among employees. Those strategies were the following: offering the vaccine on site, not charging for administration of the agent, and providing an educational program on the importance and safety of vaccination.

This is an important article to get into the hands of all medical and nursing directors.

J.R. Burton, M.D.

Acute Gastroenteritis in Three Community-Based Nursing Homes
Sims RV, Hauser RJ, Adewale AO, et al (Univ of Pennsylvania, Topton; Lutheran Home, Topton, Pa)
J Gerontol 50A:252M–256M, 1995   2–12

Purpose.—Elderly patients have disproportionately high morbidity and mortality as a result of acute gastroenteritis. Chronic institutionalization is a risk factor for mortality from gastroenteritis; however, few studies have looked at either the risk factors for acute infectious diarrhea in the chronic care setting or the pathogens involved. The epidemiology and pathogenesis of acute, putatively infectious gastroenteritis in the nursing home setting were studied.

Methods.—Patients at 3 community-based nursing homes, which represented a range from intermediate to skilled care, were studied. Five hundred seventy-two long-stay residents were prospectively followed for approximately 8 months for the development of acute gastroenteritis. The study criteria for acute putatively infectious gastroenteritis were diarrhea (i.e., 3 or more loose stools per day, lasting 24 hours or more) plus 1 of the following: diarrhea lasting 48 hours or more, rectal temperature of 100°F or greater, clinical signs of dehydration, hemoccult-positive stool, or part of any outbreak.

Results.—Fifty-three cases of acute gastroenteritis were identified during the study. They made up approximately two thirds of diarrheal illnesses occurring in the 3 nursing homes. There were no associated deaths. The incidence rates ranged from 6.7 to 36.4 cases per 100 patient-years at the 3 nursing homes.

Diarrhea lasting 48 hours or more was present in all cases, new or worsened stool incontinence in 69%, loss of appetite in 47%, and abdominal pain in 22%. Four patients (8%) had behavioral changes, and 16 (32%) had rectal temperatures of 100°F or greater. Forty percent of the stool samples showed fecal leukocytes, suggesting the presence of inflammatory diarrhea. The risk of acute gastroenteritis was more than doubled for patients with an indwelling bladder catheter. Six patients with *Clostridium difficile* were identified, and 1 case was attributed to *Aeromonas/ Pleisomonas* spp. However, submission and testing of stool samples were incomplete, so many potential pathogens most likely went undetected.

Conclusions.—Acute gastroenteritis appears to be a common problem in nursing homes. In most cases, the signs and symptoms are consistent with a relatively mild, self-limited illness. *Clostridium difficile* appears to be an important diarrheal pathogen in the chronic care setting.

▶ This prospective study assessed the epidemiology and pathogenesis of acute gastroenteritis among a cohort of 572 residents of 3 nursing homes over 8 months. Such data are urgently needed to guide clinicians caring for patients in nursing homes. It is of particular note that in almost three fourths of the patients with acute diarrhea, no specific cause was found. About half the episodes of diarrhea had findings consistent with an inflammatory process (fecal leukocytes and/or blood). The article also points out the difficulty in obtaining stool specimens from nursing home patients with diarrhea.

J.R. Burton, M.D.

Nosocomial Transmission of Epidemic Keratoconjunctivitis to Food Handlers in a Nursing Home
Chhabra BK (Univ of Illinois, Chicago)
J Am Geriatr Soc 43:1392–1393, 1995   2–13

Introduction.—Epidemic keratoconjunctivitis (EKC) is usually caused by adenovirus and has an incubation period that is between 5 and 12 days. It is a highly contagious disease that may spread rapidly in an institutional setting because viral shedding may begin from 3 days before to 14 days after symptoms appear, standard disinfectants may not be virucidal, and the virus may contaminate environmental surfaces for up to 1 week. Outbreaks of EKC have been reported in military camps and in the community through contaminated eye solutions and visits to eye clinics. In chronic care facilities, transmission to the staff from residents is known, but transmission of EKC to dietary food handlers who are not involved in direct patient care has not been previously reported.

Setting.—On January 16, 1995, 1 resident and 1 employee in a 7-floor nursing home were found to have conjunctivitis. Despite strict measures for control of infection, 40 of 460 residents and 12 of 350 employees had EKC with unilateral or bilateral erythema, edema, and eye irritation or watery or purulent discharge. The most likely source of infection was an employee who transmitted the infection to residents, and most cases were clustered in the floor for cognitively impaired residents. Of the staff infected, 2 were from the dietary service, where kitchen staff and tray handlers were not all using gloves routinely while handling food trays, either in patient rooms or in the kitchen. These cases were traced to kitchen staff handling food trays from residents subsequently found to have conjunctivitis. Only a few of the bacterial cultures grew pathogenic organisms, and viral cultures were not routinely done because of the high cost of this test.

Recommendations.—This report identifies contaminated trays as a source of transmission of conjunctivitis to food handlers. In addition to inservice training for nursing and housekeeping staff, food handlers should be trained in the use of appropriate precautions. Hand washing alone may not be sufficient to remove adenovirus from contaminated fingers.

▶ This short report delineates an experience with EKC in 1 nursing home. This infection is common and is caused by a highly contagious virus. In this single nursing home experience over a 2½-month period, almost 9% of the nursing home residents and 3.5% of the staff were infected in spite of a vigorous attempt by the nursing home staff to contain the infection. One especially important point emerges from this experience: Use of Gloves—as opposed to hand washing alone—is necessary when anyone, including dietary staff, are in an infected patient's room. Note also that the epidemic emanated from a staff member who should not have come to work with an eye infection.

J.R. Burton, M.D.

The Risk of Midline Catheterization in Hospitalized Patients: A Prospective Study
Mermel LA, Parenteau S, Tow SM (Brown Univ, Providence, RI)
Ann Intern Med 123:841–844, 1995   2–14

Background.—Midline catheters, 3- to 6-inch peripheral intravascular catheters inserted into antecubital veins, are used in both home health care and hospital settings. Although more than 500,000 have been sold, no studies have been published regarding culture of these catheters upon removal or patient follow-up for noninfectious complications. These issues were addressed prospectively to assess the risk associated with use of midline catheters in hospitalized patients.

Methods.—Enrolled in the study were 238 patients, admitted to a university-affiliated hospital between February 1993 and June 1994, who were likely to require at least 7 days of intravascular catheterization. In 251 instances, Landmark (Menlo Care, Inc., Menlo Park, California) midline catheters were inserted into these patients. Adverse reactions were monitored through use of catheter segment, insertion site, hub, blood, and infusate cultures.

Results.—The mean duration of catheterization was 9 days for the 130 patients who remained hospitalized for the duration of catheterization. Catheter cultures were obtained in 140 instances; the incidence of catheter colonization was 5.0 per 1,000 catheter days, and the incidence of catheter-related bloodstream infection was 0.8 per 1,000 catheter days. Significant growth occurred on 3% of hubs and 0.7% of infusate specimens. The per-patient risk of catheter colonization did not differ significantly based on duration of catheterization. Use of the Landmark midline catheters may have been associated with 2 severe, unexpected adverse reactions (53 similar reactions associated with use of Landmark midline catheters had been reported to the Food and Drug Administration as of June 1994).

Discussion.—Midline catheters confer a low risk of infection. No significant difference exists between the risk of bloodstream infection from central venous, as opposed to midline, catheterization. Considering that the incidence density of midline catheter infection decreases with more prolonged dwell time, catheters may not need to be changed on a regular basis in all patients. Midline catheters serve an important function in the care of acute and chronically ill patients, but enthusiasm for use of the Landmark midline catheter has been tempered by published and unpublished reports of life-threatening adverse reactions.

▶ Midline catheters may well serve a special niche in elderly patients who require IV solution for several days or weeks. Midline catheters are peripheral catheters most frequently used in the patient's home but which could easily be more widely used in hospitals and nursing homes. They are called midline because they are inserted into the antecubital veins or the veins of the upper arm.

This study shows that the risk of infection is quite low, although 2 severe systemic reactions occurred that may have been associated with insertions of 251 Landmark catheters. A second study device, the Teflon peripheral catheter, was associated with no such reactions. Midline catheters have several advantages over central venous catheters: reduced costs by a lower per unit cost and by the elimination of the need for chest x-ray; simpler insertion, usually done by nurses; and decreased infection rates. These catheters may be used for prolonged periods (1–3 weeks), which is well beyond that possible with the traditional small distal peripheral catheters.

In spite of advantages that they have, these catheters should be monitored carefully. Approximately 20% of such catheters may have to be removed prematurely because of phlebitis or thrombosis. The Landmark catheter—the midline catheter associated with severe systemic reactions— probably should be avoided pending clarification of the problems. A valuable review of catheter use is provided in an editorial accompanying this paper.[1]

J.R. Burton, M.D.

Reference

1. Maki D: Reactions associated with midline catheters for intravenous access. *Ann Intern Med* 123:884–886, 1995.

Ethics and Advance Directives

The Inaccessibility of Advance Directives on Transfer From Ambulatory to Acute Care Settings

Morrison RS, Olson E, Mertz KR, et al (Mount Sinai Med Ctr, New York; Jewish Home and Hosp for Aged of New York)
JAMA 274:478–482, 1995   2–15

Purpose.—To be effective, advance directives such as living wills, proxy appointments, and durable powers of attorney for health care must not only be completed by the patient but must also be available, recognized, and honored in the clinical setting. The accessibility of patients' previously executed advance directives during acute hospitalization was retrospectively examined for a geriatric patient population.

Methods.—The medical records of 114 geriatric patients who had previously executed advance directives were examined. The patients came from 3 ambulatory care sites for admission to a large teaching hospital in New York City during a 3-year period (185 admissions). The communication of advance directive status on transfer from the outpatient to the inpatient setting was evaluated. The previous outpatient sites of inpatients with previously executed advance directives were retrospectively investigated to determine whether the directives were known to the hospital care providers. It was also noted whether these directives influenced treatment decisions in situations of diminished mental capacity. Charts were evaluated by a single reviewer, with independent verification of some charts done by a second independent observer. An advance directive was considered invoked only if a series of specific criteria were met.

Results.— Concordance between principal and secondary chart review was nearly 100%. The ambulatory physician was involved in the patients' hospital care with 55 admissions. Twenty-nine percent of the patients lacked sufficient mental capacity to make decisions at the time of hospitalization. Directives were recognized during hospitalization for only 26% of patients with previously executed advance directives. With 39% of admissions, the admitting clerk incorrectly documented a lack of an advance directive. For 19% of those admissions in which the patient had an advance directive, the only documentation thereof was a physician's chart notation. The advance directive was recognized in only 14 of the 53 admissions in which patients lacked the capacity to make decisions. When recognized, advance directives influenced treatment for 12 of these 14 patients. Documentation of advance directives was positively associated with white race, elective admission, and involvement of the ambulatory care physician.

Discussion.— Failure of advance directives to be available, recognized, and honored when patients lack cognitive capacity is a significant barrier to their implementation. Responsibility for this lack of recognition rests with admitting clerks, patients and families, nursing homes, and physicians. Copies of advance directives must be transferred along with other medical information from nursing homes to the admitting hospitals. Physicians should document advance directives in patient medical records. This study is the first after passage of the Patient Self-Determination Act to directly assess the accessibility of advance directives on transfer to an acute care setting.

▶ Establishing advance directives regarding one's wishes for health care is important; however, the vast majority of individuals do not establish such directives, and even those who *do* often do not have them recognized, as this study shows. The acute hospital records of 114 elderly patients with previously executed advance directives were analyzed. Of the group of patients judged not to have decision-making capacity who also had a previously developed advance directive, only 26% had their directives recognized. Where available, the directive seemed to influence treatment decisions in 86% of cases.

We need research that shows how to make advance directives simple to develop and use. To get to that point, however, we need to understand the problems with ensuring their use, and one of these is shown in this paper.

J.R. Burton, M.D.

Measuring Capacity to Complete an Advance Directive
Molloy DW, Silberfeld M, Darzins P, et al (McMaster Univ, Hamilton, Ont, Canada; Baycrest Centre for Geriatric Care, North York, Canada; Univ of Toronto)
J Am Geriatr Soc 44:660–664, 1996   2–16

Background.—Advanced directives are increasingly being used. Deciding who is able to complete a directive is difficult. Authorities disagree on criteria for determining this ability as well as who should make the assessment. Two reference standards for ability to complete an advance direction were compared: a multidisciplinary panel, and a team of geriatricians. Two new screening instruments and the Standardized Mini-Mental Status Examination (SMMSE) were compared with reference standards.

Methods.—Elderly individuals from nursing homes, retirement homes, and homes for the aged, representing a broad range of intellectual ability, were studied. Severely demented individuals who appeared clearly incapable of making their own decisions were excluded. The advance directive used allowed individuals to nominate proxies and specify treatment wishes in the event of life-threatening illness and for resuscitation and feeding. Different choices for reversible and irreversible conditions were available. Irreversible or intolerable conditions were defined in personal statements. Study participants were educated about the directive in a general information meeting, and "Let Me Decide" booklets or cassettes were distributed. In addition, a nurse discussed the directive with each individual. Participants were offered the opportunity to watch the educational video again and talk with the nurse. All participants were assessed by the Competency Clinic, a geriatrician, the SMMSE, and Generic and Specific screening instruments. Participants were then randomly assigned to a second geriatrician assessment or to a second Generic and Specific screening.

Findings.—Ninety-six individuals (mean age, 85.5 years) were included. Ninety-two percent were women. The chance-corrected agreement for the 2 geriatrician assessments was 0.78 and between the geriatricians and Competency Clinic assessments, 0.82. Observer agreement for the Generic and Specific screening instrument assessments was 0.77 and 0.90, respectively. The areas under the receiver operating characteristic curve relating the findings of the 3 screening instruments to the Contemporary Clinic, Generic and Specific instrument assessments, and the SSMSE were 0.82, 0.90, and 0.94, respectively.

Conclusions.—Health care providers can make valid, reproducible assessments of elderly persons' ability to complete advance directives. The SMMSE accurately distinguishes between elderly individuals who can and cannot learn about and complete advance directives.

▶ Clinicians are frequently insecure about assessing the capacity of an individual with cognitive impairment to make advance directive decisions. This study adds importantly to an understanding of capacity to complete an advance directive. A rigorous approach using multiple methods of determining capacity were used. There was agreement in this study suggesting that the use of the SMMSE in thoroughly educated individuals was a valid indicator of capacity for advance directives using the cut-point score of 20. These are important data and will hopefully be reconfirmed in other, larger populations.

J.R. Burton, M.D.

▶ Despite broad support for older persons to complete advanced directives, clinicians are frequently concerned that those for whom they may be most imminently relevant are unable to do so because of cognitive impairment. This study focuses precisely on determining which patients are capable of completing an advanced directive and how this can be assessed through brief measures.

As reference standards, the investigators used 2 methods: a Competency Clinic, which used a multidisciplinary panel to review information obtained by a trained nurse, and geriatricians' judgment using agreed upon criteria. These 2 methods demonstrated a high level of agreement ($\kappa = 0.82$). They subsequently used several screening instruments and found the best performance with a SMMSE, using a cut point of 20.

The chief limitation to the study is the use of the standardized rather than the conventional Mini-mental Status Examination. Although the authors attribute some of the high classification power to the use of the SMMSE, which has better reliability than the conventional Mini-mental Status Examination, the standardized version has not gained widespread clinical acceptance.

D.B. Reuben, M.D.

Enhancement of Proxy Appointment for Older Persons: Physician Counselling in the Ambulatory Setting
Meier DE, Gold G, Mertz K, et al (Mount Sinai School of Medicine, New York; Univ of Tennessee, Knoxville; Albert Einstein College, Bronx, NY; et al)
J Am Geriatr Soc 44:37–43, 1996   2–17

Background.—The living will and health care proxy legislation have received widespread publicity. Research has shown that patients are ready to discuss these issues but wait for their physicians to initiate the process. Only a small percentage of adults have completed the necessary documents. The efficacy of physician-initiated counseling on the rate of health care proxy appointment was investigated.

Methods.—Six hundred eighty-seven patients enrolled in a geriatric clinic between March 1991 and June 1993 were included in the study. Physicians counseled these patients on the New York State Health Care Proxy Law, distributed educational materials and health care proxy forms, and provided reminders to 331 of 466 eligible patients.

Findings.—A health care proxy was appointed for 31.5% of the patients eligible for counseling and for 44% of those receiving the intervention. The proxy appointment rate at baseline was only 2.3%. Eighty-one percent of the patients completing the proxy appointment process did so within 3 clinic return visits after the counseling intervention. Only one fourth of the counseled patients not appointing a proxy explicitly declined (Table 2). The rest had not made a decision by the end of the study. Ethnicity,

TABLE 2.—Reasons for Declining to Complete Proxy Form

Reasons	Number of Patients
No interest	18
No one available to appoint	11
Fear or anxiety	5
Leave decision to family	4
Leave decision to MD	1
Other	6
Total	45

(Courtesy of Meier DE, Gold G, Mertz K, et al: Enhancement of proxy appointment for older persons: Physician counselling in the ambulatory setting. *J Am Geriatr Soc* 44(1):37–43, 1996.)

educational level, and more frequent clinic visits were associated with proxy completion. Ninety-seven percent of those who appointed a proxy had good or fair comprehension of the procedure. Ninety-two percent had discussed the appointment with their proxy designees, and 80% had discussed their wishes for care at the end of their lives. A daughter or son was appointed as a health care proxy by 63% of the patients.

Conclusions.—The interventions resulted in one of the higher rates of health care proxy appointment since advance directive laws were passed. Physician counseling of older outpatients therefore seems to be an effective way to increase health care proxy appointments.

▶ It has always been quite surprising to me that only a few patients have actually completed advance directives. This is true in spite of the Patient Self Determination Act of 1991 and the very significant public educational effort made regarding advance directives. This article focuses on the physician's interaction with patients regarding advance directives. It shows that by counseling patients in an ambulatory care setting, physicians can significantly enhance the completion of advance directives by older patients. Almost half of those patients who received appropriate counseling from physicians (which, on the average, took approximately 11 minutes) had very much better than the low rate at baseline. Interestingly, the vast majority of patients who completed advance directives did so by their third follow-up visit after the counseling intervention. Physicians and other ambulatory care health care providers have a very important role in encouraging and helping patients develop advance directives.

J.R. Burton, M.D.

Choices of Seriously Ill Patients About Cardiopulmonary Resuscitation: Correlates and Outcomes
Phillips RS, Wenger NS, Teno J, et al (Harvard Med School, Boston; Univ of California, Los Angeles; Dartmouth-Hitchcock Med Ctr, Hanover, NH; et al)
Am J Med 100:128–137, 1996   2–18

Introduction.—Patients with serious illnesses often must decide whether they want their health care providers to perform CPR if they have a cardiac arrest. The prevalence of the preference to forgo CPR and clinical correlates of this decision were studied in the national multicenter Study to Understand Prognoses and Preferences for Outcomes and Risks of Treatments (SUPPORT).

Methods.—Chart review was performed to collect data on diagnosis, comorbidity, the acute physiology score (APS), the presence of a do-not-resuscitate (DNR) order, the provision of CPR, and the therapeutic intensity. The participating patients were interviewed between the 3rd and 6th days of hospitalization, using a standard interview, to obtain information on demographics, preferences regarding CPR and other interventions, quality of life, daily living function, and outcome expectations. The patients were followed up for 6 months. Correlations between CPR preferences and the other patient and clinical variables were analyzed.

Results.—A total of 1,650 patients were interviewed. Of these, 28% reported not wanting CPR. This preference was independently associated with older age, hospital site, diagnosis, greater functional impairment, and patient perception of a poor prognosis. Only 29% of the patients had discussed their CPR preferences with their physicians, including only 48% of those wanting to forgo CPR. Only 32% of the patients who wanted to forgo CPR had a DNR order. Of the patients who did not want CPR, CPR was performed in 5 of 8 patients without a DNR order and in none of the 26 patients with a DNR order. The 2-month and 6-month mortality rates were significantly higher among the patients who did not want CPR, although the inhospital mortality rates were similar among patients who did and did not want CPR. The intensity of care was slightly greater for the patients who did not want CPR.

Conclusions.—Cardiopulmonary resuscitation preferences are associated with a number of complex factors but are only rarely discussed with physicians or assigned to DNR orders. Therefore, interventions are needed to improve discussion of patient preferences for treatment among seriously ill patients.

▶ This is an extensive study of CPR in seriously ill patients. The study is a component of SUPPORT. In spite of many scientific papers, the public press, and federal legislation, the impact of advance directives remains minimal. It is remarkable that less than one third of seriously ill, hospitalized patients had discussed their preferences about CPR with their physicians. Note also that among those patients who did not want CPR, there was a minimal decrease in the intensity of care, without any significant difference in survival while in the hospital when compared with those patients who elected CPR, if needed. Even when patients deal with advanced directives, it may not affect outcome very much. Much remains to be learned about these issues. One thing, however, seems to be coming clear. Decisions to forgo CPR may not have a significant impact on health care outcomes or expenditures.

J.R. Burton, M.D.

Attitudes of Michigan Physicians and the Public Toward Legalizing Physician-assisted Suicide and Voluntary Euthanasia
Bachman JG, Alcser KH, Doukas DJ, et al (Univ of Michigan, Ann Arbor; Michigan State Univ, East Lansing)
N Engl J Med 334:303–309, 1996   2–19

Introduction.—Legalized physician-assisted suicide has recently been the focus of referenda and legislative and judicial actions. Fundamental to the controversy is disagreement about whether society should permit any form of assisted suicide. Although supporters point out the benefits of

Legislation or Ban

Wider Range of Choices

Suppose that the Michigan legislature were deciding between just two choices. Which do you think would be the better choice?

Some physicians favor a law like Plan A, allowing physician-assisted suicide, whereas others favor a law prohibiting physician-assisted suicide. And some physicians favor no law at all, preferring instead to leave end-of-life decisions to the doctor–patient relationship or guidelines to be provided by the medical profession. Which of these options would you favor most?

"It should definitely/probably enact Plan A for physician-assisted suicide." 56.6%

38.9% "A law allowing physician-assisted suicide."

"Uncertain, can't say." 7.7%

16.1%
4.8%
16.6%

No Law:
"Leave it to the doctor–patient relationship."
or
"The medical profession should provide regulation/guidelines."

"It should definitely/probably keep all physician-assisted suicide illegal." 35.8%

17.2% "A law prohibiting physician-assisted suicide."

FIGURE 1.—How physicians modified their choices between legalizing and banning assisted suicide when "no law" options were included. The figure is based on the responses of the 1,071 physicians who answered both questions. **Right-hand side** of the figure shows the percentages of physicians who gave the responses shown, but it omits the 4.7% who responded "don't know/not sure" to the second version and the 1.8% who gave answers other than those shown. Percentages thus differ slightly from those cited in the text. Questions shown refer to plan A. Some questionnaires referred to "plan A or B." (Reprinted by permission of *The New England Journal of Medicine.* Bachman JG, Alcser KH, Doukas DJ, et al: Attitudes of Michigan physicians and the public toward legalizing physician-assisted suicide and voluntary euthanasia. *N Engl J Med* 334:303–309, 1996. Copyright 1996, Massachusetts Medical Society.)

relieved suffering and individual autonomy, opponents point out the potential for serious unintended consequences and the profound changes such a policy would make in social values. The question of whether physicians should participate in assisted suicide is also central to the controversy. A series of surveys was undertaken to characterize the attitudes of physicians and the public toward assisted suicide.

Methods.—A survey was mailed to 3 geographically stratified, random samples of Michigan physicians: 500 in the spring of 1994, 500 in the summer of 1994, and 600 in the spring of 1995. Similarly, a survey was mailed to 2 geographically stratified, random samples of Michigan adults: 449 in the spring of 1994 and 899 in the summer of 1994. A variety of questionnaires with different questions and wordings was used, but all had questions about legalizing physician-assisted suicide for terminally ill adult patients in uncontrolled pain.

Results.—Usable questionnaires were returned by 1,119 of the 1,518 eligible physicians and 998 of the 1,348 Michigan adults. In a choice between either legalizing or completely banning physician-assisted suicide, 56% of the physicians and 66% of the public supported legalization, 37% of the physicians and 26% of the public supported banning, and 8% of each group were uncertain. Given more choices, 40% of the physicians preferred legalizing physician-assisted suicide, 17% preferred legally banning it, 37% preferred having no law concerning it, and 5% were uncertain (Fig 1). If physician-assisted suicide or voluntary euthanasia was legalized, 52% of the physicians reported unwillingness to participate, 13% would possibly participate in assisted suicide only, 22% would possibly participate in both practices, 10% were uncertain, and 2% did not answer. In the general public, 48% reported that they would possibly request physician-assisted suicide, 30% probably would not, and 22% were uncertain.

Conclusions.—The majority of both physicians and the public favored legalizing physician-assisted suicide as opposed to banning it. A large number of the physicians preferred no legislation regarding physician-assisted suicide and having the issue be regulated within the doctor-patient relationship and medical ethics. These views of the persons most affected by legislative decisions should be considered by policy makers.

▶ Wherever one stands on the issue of physician-assisted suicide, one must be familiar with the arguments for and against such a practice. This study is a survey of the attitudes of Michigan physicians and the people of Michigan toward legalizing physician-assisted suicide and voluntary euthanasia. Figure 1 shows the response of 1,071 physicians who answered the questions on the survey adequately enough to have their data included. Fewer than one fifth of physicians and one fourth of the lay public preferred a ban on physician-assisted suicide. The arguments offered in favor of physician-assisted suicide include the relief of suffering, individual patient autonomy, the patient's right to be free of the intrusion of the state, and that getting the issue open and under some regulation is better than allowing it to occur secretly and in an unregulated fashion.

The arguments offered in opposition to physician-assisted suicide include that it represents a profound change in social values, that it could well have serious, unintended outcomes, and that any small gains of such a practice would not outweigh the anonymous risks.

Also published in this issue of *The New England Journal of Medicine* [1] is a comparable article. In Oregon, physicians have an even more favorable attitude toward physician-assisted suicide. Nearly 50% of physicians surveyed indicated that they would participate in physician-assisted suicide if it were legal. The article that follows (Abstract 2–20) is a survey of ICU nurses and is equally important in our understanding of these issues.

J.R. Burton, M.D.

Reference

1. Lee MA, Nelson HD, Tilden VP, et al: Legalizing assisted suicide: Views of physicians in Oregon. *N Engl J Med* 334:310-315, 1996.

The Role of Critical Care Nurses in Euthanasia and Assisted Suicide

Asch DA (Univ of Pennsylvania, Philadelphia)
N Engl J Med 334:1374–1379, 1996   2–20

Background.—Both U.S. laws and professional nursing codes prohibit euthanasia, although withholding or withdrawing life-sustaining treatment is typically accepted. However, previous studies have reported that a substantial proportion of nurses would be willing to participate in euthanasia under a physician's order if it were legalized. The actual experiences and practices of critical care nurses regarding euthanasia were investigated with a national survey.

Methods.—A random sample of *Nursing* magazine subscribers were sent an 8-page survey asking about the respondents' experiences with requests for euthanasia and their responses.

Results.—Of the 1,600 nurses, 1,139 (71%) completed the surveys, including 852 critical care nurses. Of the 852 critical care nurses, 17% had been requested to engage in euthanasia or assisted suicide and 16% reported having participated in euthanasia or assisted suicide at least once (Table 2). In 8% of those occasions, the attending physician had no knowledge of the euthanasia. The administration of a lethal dose of an opiate was the most frequent method of euthanasia. Another 342 nurses who had not participated in euthanasia reported wanting to engage in euthanasia.

Conclusions.—A substantial proportion of the study nurses had participated in euthanasia and assisted suicide, often without the knowledge of

TABLE 2.—Instances of Euthanasia or Assisted Suicide Reported by 827 Nurses*

CIRCUMSTANCES	NO. OF NURSES (%)	NO. OF INSTANCES REPORTED*	
		EVER	DURING THE PAST YEAR
All cases	129 (15.6)	553	124
Outside a hospital or other medical setting	5 (0.6)	4	0
At the request of the patient	40 (4.8)	133	19
At the request of a family member or surrogate	72 (8.7)	264	67
At the request of another nurse	10 (1.2)	60	8
At the request of the attending physician	83 (10.0)	371	70
At the request of a physician not the attending physician	25 (3.0)	146	30

Note: Number of nurses differs from 852 because of missing data.

* Data are for 127 nurses. Two of the 129 nurses who reported performing euthanasia or assisted suicide were excluded because they reported more than 100 instances each. Instances may be included in more than 1 category.

physicians, patients, or surrogates. The finding of such widespread practices may have public policy implications.

▶ A startling study! Critical care nurses are daily and on a minute-to-minute basis dealing with patients who are likely to die. Surveying such nurses about their belief and role in euthanasia and assisted suicide seems therefore very germane. The results of such a survey were extraordinary, and comments on the results of this study appeared widely in the media.

Table 2 summarizes these data. Sixteen percent of respondents indicated that they had engaged in an act of euthanasia, some doing so without support of another health professional.

The questionnaire, which was said to require only 10 minutes to complete, was not available for review. Therefore, it is possible that there was confusion about the terminology in the questionnaire, and, because it was so short, one cannot have confidence about its overall validity. Also, there was no validation of the instrument, further creating questions about its accuracy and value.

Clearly euthanasia and assisted suicide are important issues for health care professions and the lay public alike in the United States. My conclusion about the survey is that we all would benefit from more education about the ideal management of patients at the end of life. Most of the scenarios related in the article indicate to me that euthanasia was considered when terminally ill patients did not have ideal care. In fact, the American Board of Internal Medicine in 1996 announced an extensive program concerned with improving the care of terminally ill patients. This was widely disseminated to program directors in Internal Medicine.

J.R. Burton, M.D.

Can Physically Restrained Nursing-Home Residents Be Untied Safely? Intervention and Evaluation Design
Neufeld RR, Libow LS, Foley W, et al (Jewish Home and Hosp for Aged, New York; Mount Sinai School of Medicine, New York; Wayne State Univ, Detroit; et al)
J Am Geriatr Soc 43:1264–1268, 1995   2–21

Introduction.—Physical restraint was used for approximately 40% of nursing home residents in the late 1980s. The practice is considered undesirable because it is unnecessary and sometimes harmful, resulting in increased likelihood of disorientation and dependence in dressing. Physical restraints are presumably used in response to dysfunctional and agitated behavior, but restraints have also been implicated as exacerbating agitated behavior. In 1987, the Omnibus Budget Reconciliation Act included a legislative attempt to reduce the use of physical restraints and to define their appropriate use. A clinical intervention program, funded by the Commonwealth Fund, to decrease the use of physical restraints in nursing homes was described. The interventions used and the outcomes measured were defined; detailed results of the program will be presented in future papers.

Program Methods.—Employees of 16 nursing homes with high rates of use of restraints were targeted for receiving education in the use of creative individualized approaches to restraint-free care. The 2-year intervention program, entitled "Retrain, Don't Restrain," consisted of 5 components: a 4-part educational materials package, a 2-day intensive course, quarterly site visits, telephone consultations, and distribution of a newsletter. A nurse in each nursing home served as clinical coordinator and lead a multidisciplinary team in assessing the use of restraints and developing plans for their removal. The outcomes measured included pre- and post-study aggregate and individual facility rates for use of restraints, family attitudes, incidents and accidents, serious injuries, financial impacts, and employee attitudes and work patterns.

Conclusions.—Education of nursing home staff, supplemented with intensive clinical support, was the focus of this demonstration model of restraint-free care. Development of individual care plans that do not include use of restraints was emphasized. Preliminary data suggest that the intervention plan has been well received and appears effective in the goal of enabling restraint-free care. Further details of outcome will be forthcoming in additional publications.

▶ Use of physical restraints can be reduced. This study describes a program that looks easy to implement and also seems to be effective in a variety of facilities in several states. Such programs are necessary, as many institutions still report high use of restraints.

J.R. Burton, M.D.

Nursing Home Survey Deficiencies for Physical Restraint Use
Graber DR, Sloane PD (Med Univ of South Carolina, Charleston; Univ of North Carolina, Chapel Hill)
Med Care 33:1051–1063, 1995   2–22

Introduction.—For many decades, the use of physical restraints has been prevalent in U.S. nursing homes; in the 1980s, however, accumulated research indicated that physical restraints were associated with many adverse effects, including increased numbers of falls and injuries. The Omnibus Budget Reconciliation Act (OBRA) of 1987 mandated new regulations, implemented in 1990, that severely restricted the conditions when restraints may be used. Surveyors issue "deficiencies" when a facility is negligent in meeting the requirements of the OBRA regulations. The impact of these regulations on nursing homes in North Carolina in 1991 was evaluated.

Process.—The study included all 195 North Carolina nursing homes that received Medicaid skilled nursing and intermediate care payments in 1991. A mean of 32.6% of the patients in these facilities were restrained. Citations for violation of the restraint regulations were delivered to 29.2% of these facilities during the study year. The characteristics of facilities unable to meet the new OBRA requirements were examined. These characteristics were then evaluated for correlation with increased proportion of restrained patients.

Outcomes.—Use of restraints was associated with the facility-level factors of the overall disability level and the ratio of licensed vocational nurse or nursing assistant staff to patients. Restraint violations were associated with facility size, proportion of restrained patients, direct costs per patient per day, use of bladder training in less than 3% of residents, and proportion of residents with organic brain syndrome.

Discussion.—Nearly one third of nursing home residents in North Carolina remained physically restrained in 1991, despite the new regulations. The facilities most likely to benefit from education and clinical assistance in reducing physical restraints can be targeted via those characteristics correlated with restraint use and deficiency citation.

▶ This large and important study was conducted in 1991 just after the October 1990 implementation of the OBRA regulations concerning use of restraints in nursing homes. A careful analysis of continued use of physical restraints is provided. Note that, on average, 33% of North Carolina nursing home patients were restrained, with a range of 1.1% to 71%!

The vigorous effort to educate providers of nursing home health care that the use of restraints should be essentially nil needs to continue. Next, hospital personnel need to be educated about how to minimize the use of restraints.

J.R. Burton, M.D.

Retrain, Don't Restrain: The Educational Intervention of the National Nursing Home Restraint Removal Project
Dunbar JM, Neufeld RR, White HC, et al (Jewish Home and Hosp for Aged, New York; Mount Sinai School of Medicine, New York; Rehabilitation Inst of Michigan, Ann Arbor)
Gerontologist 36:539–542, 1996   2–23

Introduction.—Despite a federal mandate against physical restraint of nursing home residents, approximately 300,000 residents remain physically restrained. It is believed that falls and injuries can be prevented by using restraints, but there is evidence that restraints can actually exacerbate injuries. Physical restraints also can cause discomfort and other problems.

Restraint-Removal Project.—A project was created to develop safe and effective ways to replace physical restraints in nursing homes. The goal was to reduce the use of restraints to 5% within 2 years. Sixteen facilities participated, with a total of 2,075 beds from California, Michigan, New York, and North Carolina. The restraint rates in these facilities were more than 30%, and the aggregate restraint rate was 41%. Within 2 years, the restraint rate had fallen to 4%.

Educational Intervention.—The educational program consisted of a 2-day intensive training workshop, a consultation team that visited each facility quarterly and conducted telephone conferences every other week, site visits by project team members, regional conferences in each of the 4 states, and quarterly newsletters. An educational videotape was produced and designed for families of nursing home residents and nursing home staff. Written materials also were created and aimed at administrators, the nurse responsible for the program, and general staff.

Project Review.—At the end of the 2 years, administrators completed a survey of the project. The 2-day training workshop, the site visits, and the videotape were rated the most helpful components of the project. The 2-day workshop created much enthusiasm; even skeptics became convinced that removing constraints was possible and desirable. Site visits helped maintain the momentum of the project.

Discussion.—Facilities may be able to create their own restraint-reduction programs using the methods of this program. Restraint reduction programs need strong leadership and functioning components. Attending a workshop, observing the process, or visiting a facility that does not use restraints are the best ways of learning about restraint-free care. A year after the program ended, aggregate restraint rates were well under 5% at the participating facilities.

▶ Here is another article identifying strategies that led to a sharp reduction in the use of restraints among nursing home residents. This was a national project among 16 randomly selected nursing homes. The outcome was a reduction by 90% in the use of restraints.

The major intervention was a staff educational program. Before the intervention, the involved nursing homes had more than a 30% rate of restraint use among their nursing home patients. In the educational program, the enormous value of a workshop focused on restraint reduction is emphasized. Each nursing home can, and should, make the decision to move forward with a restraint-reduction program. This and the other articles provide strategies about how that can be accomplished.

J.R. Burton, M.D.

Miscellaneous Nursing Home Issues

Hyponatremia in a Nursing Home Population

Miller M, Morley JE, Rubenstein LZ (Mount Sinai School of Medicine, New York; St Louis Univ, Mo; Univ of California, Los Angeles)
J Am Geriatr Soc 43:1410–1413, 1995   2–24

Background.—Increasing evidence suggests that changes in water regulatory capacity accompany the normal aging process. With advancing age, secretion of antidiuretic hormone (ADH) from the posterior pituitary, as well as basal secretion of plasma vasopressin, may be increased. Various acute and chronic illnesses may be accompanied by hyponatremia, and patients residing in nursing homes have been observed to have hyponatremia. The prevalence of hyponatremia in a nursing home population was assessed, and the clinical factors that increased the risk for development of hyponatremia were identified.

Methods.—In a retrospective and prospective review, the records of 119 residents (age, 60–103 years) in a Veterans Affairs nursing home care unit were analyzed for the most recent serum sodium, creatinine, and blood urea nitrogen determinations, as well as all serum sodium determinations during the preceding 12 months; clinical diagnoses, diet, medications, and significant events at the time of recorded hyponatremic episodes; response to acute water-loading in a subset of patients who had hyponatremia at a time when they were medically stable and had no evidence of acute disease or use of drugs that affect water handling; and the number of deaths in the 12 months after entry into the study. For comparison, data from 60 ambulatory patients, 62–91 years of age, who attended a geriatric medicine outpatient clinic were collected.

Results.—Twenty-one nursing home patients had hyponatremia (serum sodium level of 135 mEq/L or less), for a prevalence of 18%, compared with 8% in a similarly aged ambulatory population. However, when all serum sodium determinations for the previous 12 months were examined, 53% of the nursing home residents had at least 1 episode of hyponatremia. There was a high prevalence of CNS disorders in the nursing home patients (82%), but the incidence of cardiovascular disease, diabetes, or use of diuretics was similar in patients with hyponatremia and those without hyponatremia. Hyponatremia occurred more frequently in older patients with CNS disorders (54%), particularly among those with spinal cord disease (100%). Water load testing in 23 patients with hyponatremia revealed impaired water handling that was consistent with the syndrome of inappropriate secretion of ADH (SIADH) in 18 patients. In a review of the records for concurrent events associated with each episode of hyponatremia, the most common factor was increased fluid intake (78%), either orally or intravenously, with hypotonic saline. Other precipitating factors were a low-sodium diet in 32%, tube feeding in 14%, drugs in 11%, and pneumonia in 14%. The mortality rate was 17% in patients with hyponatremia compared with 21% in normonatremic patients.

Conclusions.—Hyponatremia is common in nursing home residents and may be a consequence of impaired ability to excrete water, similar to that seen with SIADH. Increased fluid intake, whether by the oral or IV route or a low-sodium tube-feeding diet, increases the risk of the development of hyponatremia or the worsening of an already present low serum sodium concentration.

▶ Hyponatremia is common among the elderly population. This study, however, shows this problem to be far more common than most of us have thought. Among Veteran Affairs nursing home patients, the point prevalence of hyponatremia was 18%. More dramatic was the remarkable 12-month incidence of slightly more than 50%. Most of those patients with a history of hyponatremia failed a water-loading test, likely indicating the persisting presence of the SIADH secretion. Nearly 80% of the episodes of hyponatremia were associated with a recent adjustment or initiation of oral or IV fluids or of tube feedings. In my view, herein lies the lesson.

In disabled nursing home residents with neurologic disease, clinicians should be cautious when advising fluid therapy because of the very likely presence of SIADH. In such situations, it is probably appropriate to measure plasma sodium concentration a few days after the therapy and adjust the water intake should the sodium concentration decrease. There is one additional point to be made: One of the patients in this retrospective record review had a serum sodium concentration measured 83 times in 12 months. This level of assessment seems in great excess in any circumstances. The highly selective use of laboratory testing is an important part of good clinical practice.

J.R. Burton, M.D.

An Instrument to Assess the Oral Health Status of Nursing Home Residents
Kayser-Jones J, Bird WF, Paul SM, et al (Univ of California, San Francisco)
Gerontologist 35:814–824, 1995   2–25

Introduction.—The oral health status of nursing home residents continues to be neglected. Untreated dental problems can cause pain and systemic infection and can affect an individual's well-being, self esteem, and quality of life. In 1992, federal regulations mandated that nursing home residents have a dental evaluation within 14 days of admission and annually thereafter. The enforcement of this regulation is moving forward slowly, and implementation is problematic, partly because of lack of a valid and reliable instrument to assess the oral health of nursing home residents. The development and testing of an oral health instrument that could be administered by the nursing staff to assess the oral health status of nursing home residents was described.

Setting.—The Brief Oral Health Status Examination (BOHSE) consisted of 10 items that reflect the status of oral health and function (Fig 2). The final score was the sum of each item rated on a 3-point scale, with 0 indicating the healthy end and 2 the unhealthy end. Registered nurses (RNs), licensed vocational nurses (LVNs), and certified nursing assistants (CNAs) underwent two 2-hour training sessions for administering the BOHSE. Each category of nursing staff examined 100 nursing home residents, and their findings were correlated with those of a dentist who examined the same residents. More than half of the residents were 80 years of age and older, and 86% were moderately to severely impaired cognitively.

Results.—Correlation coefficients indicated positive and significant inter-rater reliability among the 3 categories of nursing personnel and the dentist. The LVNs had a slightly higher correlation with the dentist's scores than did the RNs, whereas the CNAs had the lowest correlation. The rates of each nursing staff were consistent, with the same subjects rated similarly

KAYSER-JONES BRIEF ORAL HEALTH STATUS EXAMINATION

Resident's Name _____
Examiner's Name _____

Date _____
TOTAL SCORE _____

CATEGORY	MEASUREMENT	0	1	2
LYMPH NODES	Observe and feel nodes	No enlargement	Enlarged, not tender	Enlarged and tender*
LIPS	Observe, feel tissue and ask resident, family or staff (e.g. primary caregiver)	Smooth, pink, moist	Dry, chapped, or red at corners*	White or red patch, bleeding or ulcer for 2 weeks*
TONGUE	Observe, feel tissue and ask resident, family or staff (e.g. primary caregiver)	Normal roughness, pink and moist	Coated, smooth, patchy, severely fissured or some redness	Red, smooth, white or red patch; ulcer for 2 weeks*
TISSUE INSIDE CHEEK, FLOOR AND ROOF OF MOUTH	Observe, feel tissue and ask resident, family or staff (e.g. primary caregiver)	Pink and moist	Dry, shiny, rough red, or swollen*	White or red patch, bleeding, hardness; ulcer for 2 weeks*
GUMS BETWEEN TEETH AND/OR UNDER ARTIFICIAL TEETH	Gently press gums with tip of tongue blade	Pink, small indentations; firm, smooth and pink under artificial teeth	Redness at border around 1-6 teeth; one red area or sore spot under artificial teeth*	Swollen or bleeding gums, redness at border around 7 or more teeth, loose teeth; generalized redness or sores under artificial teeth*
SALIVA (EFFECT ON TISSUE)	Touch tongue blade to center of tongue and floor of mouth	Tissues moist, saliva free flowing and watery	Tissues dry and sticky	Tissues parched and red, no saliva*
CONDITION OF NATURAL TEETH	Observe and count number of decayed or broken teeth	No decayed or broken teeth/roots	1-3 decayed or broken teeth/roots*	4 or more decayed or broken teeth/roots; fewer than 4 teeth in either jaw*
CONDITION OF ARTIFICIAL TEETH	Observe and ask patient, family or staff (e.g. primary caregiver)	Unbroken teeth, worn most of the time	1 broken/missing tooth, or worn for eating or cosmetics only	More than 1 broken or missing tooth, or either denture missing or never worn*
PAIRS OF TEETH IN CHEWING POSITION (NATURAL OR ARTIFICIAL)	Observe and count pairs of teeth in chewing position	12 or more pairs of teeth in chewing position	8-11 pairs of teeth in chewing position	0-7 pairs of teeth in chewing position*
ORAL CLEANLINESS	Observe appearance of teeth or dentures	Clean, no food particles/tartar in the mouth or on artificial teeth	Food particles/tartar in one or two places in the mouth or on artificial teeth	Food particles/tartar in most places in the mouth or on artificial teeth

Upper dentures labeled: Yes ___ No ___ None ___ Lower dentures labeled: Yes ___ No ___ None ___
Is your mouth comfortable? Yes ___ No ___ If no, explain: _____
Additional comments: _____

Underlined*·refer to dentist immediately

FIGURE 2.—Kayser-Jones Brief Oral Health Status Examination. (Courtesy of Kayser-Jones J, Bird WF, Paul SM, et al: An instrument to assess the oral health status of nursing home residents. *Gerontologist* 35(6):814-824, 1995. Copyright The Gerontological Society of America.)

on repeated testing. The dentist observed that the members of the nursing staff were very conscientious and thorough. In addition, the nursing staff were able to examine 5 cognitively impaired residents when the dentist was unable to do so.

Conclusions.—The nursing staff can be taught to evaluate the oral health of nursing home residents using a brief oral health assessment as a screening evaluation. The RNs and LVNs can be targeted to perform the oral health examinations, whereas CNAs can be taught to report any abnormal conditions. This small study sample should be replicated in multiple sites.

▶ It is increasingly recognized that the oral health status of nursing home residents is poor and that it is often neglected. Many residents have oral health problems that lead to pain, discomfort, infection, or the loss of a sense of well-being. This problem is compounded by the fact that many dentists will not visit nursing homes. The problem of the oral health of nursing home residents has been thought to be so significant that the Omnibus Budget Reconciliation Act of 1987, implemented in 1992, mandated that nursing home residents have a dental evaluation within 14 days of admission and then annually thereafter.

This study is important in that it demonstrates the effectiveness of an oral health instrument administered by nursing staff. There was reasonable correlation among the examiners and appropriate dental referrals resulted. Of course, this study will need to be reproduced in other nursing homes, but it is a first and important step. We should, in my view, be trying to identify the oral health problems of nursing home residents, especially when many of these problems lend themselves to relatively simple therapies that can improve the comfort of our patients.

J.R. Burton, M.D.

The Impact of the 1987 Federal Regulations on the Use of Psychotropic Drugs in Minnesota Nursing Homes
Garrard J, Chen V, Dowd B (Univ of Minnesota, Minneapolis)
Am J Public Health 85:771–776, 1995   2–26

Background.—The use of antipsychotic drugs in nursing homes is regulated under the provisions of the Omnibus Budget Reconciliation Act of 1987. These regulations hold physicians responsible for using a certain class of drugs for specific diagnoses; provide explicit, patient-based conditions for determining the appropriate use of the drugs; and call for sanctions against the institution, rather than the prescribing physician. Antipsychotics are the psychotropic drugs that tend to be used most frequently in nursing home patients. A few studies have sought to determine the impact of the regulations on the use of antipsychotic drugs in nursing homes, and all have documented reductions. A large sample representing all nursing home residents throughout 1 state was studied to determine the impact of the 1987 Omnibus Budget Reconciliation Act drug regulations.

Methods.—The study included all residents aged 65 years of age or older in all 327 Minnesota nursing homes in the 3 years before implementation of the drug regulations and in the first year afterward. In each year, the number of residents was approximately 33,000. A multiyear period before implementation of the regulations was studied to assess previous trends in antipsychotic drug use. To prevent an overestimation of drug use, data on drug administration were gathered from medication sheets rather than from prescription files.

Results.—Most of the residents were very elderly women who required high-level care. The proportion of residents receiving antipsychotic drugs in 1987–1988 was 23%. This figure decreased by approximately 1% the next year, when the draft guidelines for the regulations were published. The proportion decreased to 19% in 1989–1990, then to 15% in 1990–1991, when the new regulations were implemented. The reduction in antipsychotic drugs used was significant for every year studied, relative to 1987–1988. By comparison, 11% to 12% of residents received anti-anxiety drugs throughout the years studied, and 14% to 16% used antidepressants. The only admission practice variable that was significantly related to the level of antipsychotic drug use was the percentage of residents who were using such drugs when they were admitted. Nursing homes in rural areas used significantly more antipsychotic drugs.

Conclusions.—Implementation of the drug regulations included in the Omnibus Budget Reconciliation Act of 1987 has been associated with a significant decrease in the use of antipsychotic drugs in nursing homes. A trend toward reduced use of antipsychotic drugs was also present in the year before implementation. There has been no apparent shift toward the use of benzodiazepine drugs, as had been hypothesized.

▶ This study adds to our knowledge of the impact of the 1987 Omnibus Budget Reconciliation Act (OBRA) federal regulations implemented in October 1990 on the use of psychotropic drugs in the nursing home. It presents a vast statewide data set, including patients covered by all insurance programs and not just Medicaid, as previously reported.

In 1987, when there was no related federal activity, 23% of all residents received antipsychotic drugs. There was only a 1% decrease in the following year, when regulations were published. There then occurred a decrease to nearly 20% in the use of such drugs in nursing home patients over the next 2 years and, finally, a decrease to 15% in 1990–1991, when the regulations were implemented. There was no concurrent increase in the use of antianxiety drugs, which were not subject to regulations.

It is, of course, disappointing that we clinicians needed federal regulations to decrease the use of psychotic drugs in nursing home patients, even when evidence had been published as early as 1980 suggesting that there was misuse of such drugs in nursing homes.[1]

J.R. Burton, M.D.

Reference

1. Ray WE, Fedespeel CF, Schaffner WA: A study of antipsychotic drug use in nursing homes: Epidemiological evidence suggesting misuse. *Am J Public Health* 70:485–491, 1980.

Intraindividual Reproducibility of Postprandial and Orthostatic Blood Pressure Changes in Older Nursing-Home Patients: Relationship With Chronic Use of Cardiovascular Medications

Jansen RWMM, Kelley-Gagnon MM, Lipsitz LA (Harvard Med School, Boston; Univ Hosp Nijmegen, The Netherlands)
J Am Geriatr Soc 44:383–389, 1996   2–27

Introduction.—Elderly residents of nursing homes frequently exhibit postprandial or orthostatic hypotension, both of which are associated with falls and syncope. Some studies have reported that both postprandial and orthostatic hypotension are frequently present in elderly patients. However, it may be difficult to distinguish between them in clinical practice. These 2 conditions were studied in elderly nursing home residents to determine the reproducibility of the blood pressure findings, the extent of their co-occurrence, and their possible modulation with chronic cardiovascular medication.

Methods.—Blood pressure and heart rate changes were evaluated in 22 elderly nursing home residents before and after a postural change from the supine to the standing position and before and after ingesting a 419-kcal liquid meal. The 2 protocols were performed twice with each resident, with the tests separated by 3 days to 2 weeks.

Results.—The blood pressure and heart rate measurements demonstrated similar change curves related to both the meal and posture changes. After the meal, there was a significant decline in the mean systolic blood pressure (16 mm Hg and 12 mm Hg in the 2 tests) and in the mean diastolic blood pressure (8 mm Hg in both tests). However, there were variable individual changes. The mean intraclass correlations for reproducibility of postprandial changes were 0.88 for the systolic blood pressure and heart rate, 0.78 for the diastolic blood pressure, and 0.81 for the mean arterial pressure. Postural changes induced a mean systolic blood pressure increase of 8 mm Hg at 6 minutes in both tests and a mean heart rate increase of 10 bpm at 1 minute in both tests. The mean intraclass correlations for reproducibility of orthostatic changes were 0.72 for systolic blood pressure, 0.50 for diastolic blood pressure, 0.56 for mean arterial pressure, and 0.69 for heart rate.

Of the 22 subjects, 10 had postprandial hypotension, 6 had orthostatic hypotension, and only 2 had both. The blood pressure changes were not affected by the administration of cardiovascular medications 30 minutes before ingesting the meal.

Conclusions.—Blood pressure and heart rate responses to ingesting a meal or to postural changes are reproducible. Postprandial hypotension and orthostatic hypotension are distinct conditions, infrequently occurring together. Postprandial hypotension is more common than orthostatic hypotension. The chronic treatment with cardiovascular medications does not exacerbate orthostatic or postprandial hypotension.

▶ Postprandial hypotension is an important and common phenomenon affecting approximately one third of nursing home patients. The blood pressure changes are substantial and occur, on average, about 45 minutes after a meal. Other studies have shown that meal content is not an important variable. More uncertain, however, has been the knowledge of the reproducibility of the phenomenon in an individual patient. Also it has been unclear as to how the problem is distinct from orthostatic hypotension and what influence drugs may have on changes in blood pressure. This study helps clarify these issues. A carefully done study of 22 patients is reported by the group that first described the problem.[1] Postprandial hypotension is reproducible in repeated study and therefore, the diagnosis can be made in a single assessment. On the other hand, orthostatic hypotension is less reproducible and requires repeated testing. Postprandial and orthostatic hypotension occur infrequently together. Finally, and indeed somewhat surprisingly, taking medications that might lower blood pressure before the subjects ate or stood up did not seem to significantly modify the drop in their postprandial or orthostatic blood pressures.

J.R. Burton, M.D.

Reference

1. Lipsitz LA, Nyqvist RP, Wei JY, et al: Postprandial reduction in blood pressure in the elderly. *N Engl J Med* 309:81–88, 1983.

Benign Prostatic Hypertrophy

Adverse Effects of Medications on Urinary Symptoms and Flow Rate: A Community-Based Study

Su L, Guess HA, Girman CJ, et al (Univ of North Carolina, Chapel Hill; Merck Research Labs, Blue Bell, Pa; Mayo Clinic, Rochester, Minn; et al)
J Clin Epidemiol 49:483–487, 1996   2–28

Background.—In many elderly men, benign prostatic hyperplasia (BPH) causes symptoms of urinary obstruction, necessitating a high number of physician visits and prostatectomies each year. Certain medications adversely affect urologic function, exacerbating urinary symptoms and reducing urinary flow rates. The association of urinary symptoms and medication use was explored in a community-based, cross-sectional study.

Methods.—The study population included 2,115 men, aged 40–79 years, enrolled in the Olmstead County Study of Urinary Symptoms and Health Status Among Men, designed to determine the age-specific preva-

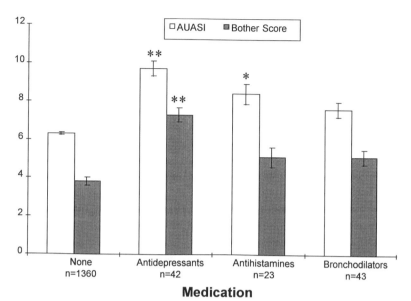

Medication

FIGURE 1.—Age-adjusted mean (±SE) American Urological Association Symptom Index (*AUASI*) and bother scores. *Double asterisk, P < 0.0001; single asterisk, P < 0.05* vs. None category. (Reprinted by permission of the publisher from Su L, Guess HA, Girman CJ, et al: Adverse effects of medications on urinary symptoms and flow rate: A community-based study. *J Clin Epidemiol* 49:483–487. Copyright 1996 by Elsevier Science Inc.)

lence of urinary symptoms. The community-based random sample of white men were followed up and monitored for disease onset and regression.

Findings.—Fifty-one percent of the men said they took 1 or more medications daily. However, only 6% were using medications known to adversely affect urinary function. Forty-three men used bronchodilators; 42, antidepressants; and 23, antihistamines. Men using antidepressants daily had higher age-adjusted American Urological Association Symptom Index (AUASI) scores. This relationship persisted after additional adjustment for the Depression and Anxiety subscales of the General Psychological Well-Being Scale. Men taking antihistamines every day also had higher adjusted AUASI scores. Lower age-adjusted urinary flow rates were associated with the use of antidepressants only (Fig 1).

Conclusions.—The daily use of antidepressants or antihistamines appear to be correlated with AUASI scores 2 or 3 points higher than in men not taking these drugs. These findings are important to clinicians assessing men for causes of voiding dysfunction in accordance with the Agency for Health Care Policy and Research practice guidelines for the diagnosis and management of benign prostatic hyperplasia.

▶ It is well known that many medications affect bladder function. This paper was selected because it quantifies urinary symptoms in a community-based cohort of men who were and were not taking medications. This well-done study shows clearly that those men taking antidepressants or antihistamines daily are likely to manifest urological symptoms significantly higher than men not taking these medications. The bottom line is clear: When evaluating individuals, especially men, with urinary tract symptoms that may be attributable to benign prostatic hyperplasia, the clinician ought to consider medication use, and if present the clinician should see whether modification of medication use is possible before considering other therapies.

J.R. Burton, M.D.

Residual Urine in 75-Year-Old Men and Women: A Normative Population Study
Bonde HV, Sejr T, Erdmann L, et al (Univ of Copenhagen)
Scand J Urol Nephrol 30:89–91, 1996   2–29

Background.—Urologic symptoms such as incomplete bladder emptying are common among the community-dwelling elderly. However, single symptoms have not been reliably correlated with objective findings. Previous studies of the prevalence of incomplete bladder emptying among the elderly have been performed in selected populations; in contrast, this study population consisted of randomly selected, community-dwelling 75-year-old men and women. The prevalence, median, and range of residual urine via nonrepeated sonographic measurements were determined in these patients.

Methods.—As part of a major epidemiologic study (Glostrup) including 154 men and 142 women living in the county of Copenhagen, 116 men and 77 women were examined for residual urine prevalence. Participants voided in private when desired, then immediately (within 10 minutes) underwent transabdominal ultrasonography. Theoretical diuresis produced between voiding and sonography was not subtracted from the residual urine volumes measured. Only those data from the 92 men and 48 women with a prevoid volume of 150 mL or more were included.

TABLE 1.—Prevalence of Residual Urine in 92 Men and 48 Women Aged 75 Years

| Percentiles | Residual Urine Volume (mL) | |
	Men	Women
2.5	13	0
5	15	0
25	49	27
50	90	45
75	135	88
95	297	168
97.5	353	179

(Courtesy of Bonde HV, Sejr T, Erdmann L, et al: Residual urine in 75-year-old men and women: A normative population study. *Scand J Urol Nephrol* 30:89–91, 1996.)

Results.—The median residual urine volume was 90 mL in men and 45 mL in women, whereas the average residual urine volume was 103 mL in men and 59 mL in women. Ninety-one of the 92 men and 44 of the 48 women showed a residual urine volume of more than 10 mL; 1 man had 1,502 mL (Table 1).

Conclusions.—These data from a community-dwelling elderly population do not differ much from data on residual urine prevalence obtained from selected populations. Residual urine may be related to impaired detrussor contractility and/or bladder outlet obstruction, both of which are common in the elderly. Single sonographic measurement of urine volume carries an average error of approximately 50% for true volumes of 50–150 mL and approximately 25% for higher true volumes.

▶ There has been no information from a community-based population of elderly individuals regarding the prevalence of residual urine. This study is important for that reason. An epidemiologic cohort of elderly individuals living in the community was prospectively evaluated. A single graphic measurement of residual volume was obtained. Almost all individuals had a residual urine volume of greater than 10 mL, and many had well over 100 mL. The volumes do not correlate with symptoms. One could debate the validity of a single sonographic residual urine volume determination, because there may be considerable variation of measurements at different times. Nevertheless, these results form a data set, which now can be expanded upon and over time correlated with the development of symptoms. For the clinician, the interpretation of residual volumes must always be individualized.

J.R. Burton, M.D.

Flavoxate Treatment of Micturition Disorders Accompanying Benign Prostatic Hypertrophy: A Double-Blind Placebo-Controlled Multicenter Investigation

Dahm TL, Ostri P, Kristensen JK, et al (Gentofte Hosp, Denmark; Rigshospitalet, Denmark; Aalborg Hosp, Denmark)
Urol Int 55:205–208, 1995   2–30

Background.—Eighty percent of patients with benign prostatic hyperplasia (BPH) experience unstable bladder, characterized by the irritative symptoms of urgency, nocturia, and frequency. Uncontrolled studies have indicated that flavoxate hydrochloride promotes improvement of irritative symptoms in these patients. These findings were challenged with a multicenter, double-blind, placebo-controlled trial.

Methods.—The trial was completed by 65 of the original 70 participants (mean age, 71 years). Treatment in the form of flavoxate, 400 mg given 3 times daily for 12 weeks, was received by 37 patients. Thirty-three patients received placebo. Sufficient statistical power was used in the analyses.

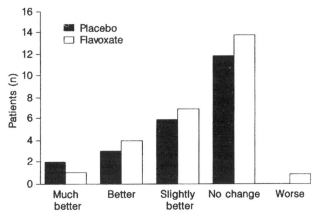

FIGURE 1.—Patient evaluation of treatment (global evaluation). (Courtesy of Dahm TL, Ostri P, Kristensen JK, et al: Flavoxate treatment of micturition disorders accompanying benign prostatic hypertrophy: A double-blind placebo-controlled multicenter investigation. *Urol Int* 55:205–208, 1995, S. Karger AG, Basel.)

Results.—Irritative score decreased significantly in both groups; the difference between groups was not significant. No significant differences in global evaluation were noted between groups at any time during the study (Fig 1). Although statistically significant changes did occur in several variables over time, intergroup differences failed to reach significance. Adverse events were transient and/or mild.

Conclusion.—Although flavoxate has been used extensively to treat urinary tract disorders involving smooth muscle spasm, its use at a dose of 400 mg given 3 times daily for 12 weeks did not prove superior to use of placebo for treatment of symptomatic BPH.

▶ This is a negative study but one that is important because it is a double-blind, placebo-controlled, multisite investigation. It shows that flavoxate is not effective in treating the irritative symptoms of urgency, frequency, and nocturia associated with BPH. The drug is currently available, but it cannot be recommended now that we have this controlled study. These are the kind of studies that are so valuable in guiding clinicians and ideally should be done before a drug is in widespread use.

J.R. Burton, M.D.

Depot Medroxyprogesterone in the Management of Benign Prostatic Hyperplasia
Onu PE (Makurdi Gen Hosp, Nigeria)
Eur Urol 28:229–235, 1995   2–31

Background.—Recognition of benign prostatic hyperplasia (BPH) as an androgen-dependent process has prompted development of medical treatment strategies to decrease bladder outlet obstruction. Recent studies have

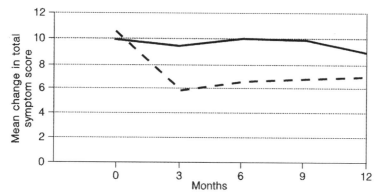

FIGURE 2.—Mean changes in the total symptom score in men with benign prostatic hyperplasia during treatment with depot medroxyprogesterone (*dashed line*) or placebo (*solid line*). Month 0 represents the baseline. (Courtesy of Onu PE: Depot Medroxyprogesterone in the management of benign prostatic hyperplasia. *Eur Urol* 28:229–235, 1995, S. Karger AG, Basel.)

suggested that a progressive decrease in prostatic volume accompanies chronic decrease in intraprostatic dihydrotestosterone. Effective treatment of BPH might therefore be provided by a compound such as medroxyprogesterone acetate, which inhibits luteinizing-hormone release, decreases plasma testosterone synthesis, and inhibits 5-α-reductase. The safety and efficacy of high-dose medroxyprogesterone acetate (depot medroxyprogesterone) for improving symptoms of BPH was examined.

Methods.—Eighty men (mean age, 66 years) with BPH received either depot medroxyprogesterone or placebo in a double-blind, randomized trial. The depot preparation was administered to allow continuous release of the progestational drug for 12 weeks (150 mg in 1 intramuscular injection). Follow-up continued for 12 months; comprehensive clinical examinations and laboratory tests were performed at baseline and at the end of follow-up. Testosterone was measured by radioimmunoassay. The study was completed by 29 patients receiving placebo and 39 patients receiving the treatment.

Results.—After 3 months (the duration of effect of the depot medroxyprogesterone), prostate volume was reduced by 25% among patients receiving the treatment and 3% among patients receiving placebo. Serum testosterone levels reached castration values in treated patients within 3 days; levels in the control group were unchanged. Maximum urinary flow rates among patients receiving the treatment increased by 3.7 mL/sec compared with that of patients receiving placebo. Patients receiving placebo showed no significant decrease in total urinary symptom scores, but scores for patients receiving the treatment decreased by 4.9 points (Fig 2). Irritative symptoms also decreased only in treated patients. After 3 months, reversal occurred in urinary symptoms and urodynamic changes, but status was still significantly improved over baseline. Prostate size returned to pretreatment levels within 18–36 weeks. A significant number of patients receiving the treatment reported impotence, decreased libido, and decreased ejaculate volume, but no hot flashes were reported. Side effects stopped in the fifth or sixth month for all treated patients.

Conclusion.—Depot medroxyprogesterone induces a significant sustained decrease in serum levels of testosterone and a decrease in prostatic volume and urinary symptoms in men with BPH, resulting in increased urinary flow rates. When potency is a secondary consideration, treatment of prostatic obstruction with depot medroxyprogesterone is both safe and effective.

▶ This early placebo-controlled double-blind study of the effects of depot medroxyprogesterone on the symptoms of BPH ties in with Abstract 2–32 very nicely. Medroxyprogesterone is a 5-α reductase inhibitor like finasteride but is also, in contradistinction to finasteride, able to inhibit luteinizing-hormone release and decrease testosterone synthesis. This combination of effects would theoretically lead to a more potent effect on BPH. That seems to be the case. The depot preparation is thought to last about 3 months. The data presented are collected 3 months after a single injection, and it seems to be very effective. Prostatic volume, symptoms, and flow rate all improved. The response was lost as prostate and prostatic volume expanded between 1½ and 3 years after the single injection. Also, and this is no surprise, the administration of methoxyprogesterone resulted in impotence in nearly 65% of men. The cost of the drug for a single injection is $24.60 in Baltimore, midwinter 1996, at a large hospital outpatient pharmacy.

What are needed now are long-term studies.

J.R. Burton, M.D.

Can Finasteride Reverse the Progress of Benign Prostatic Hyperplasia? A Two-Year Placebo-Controlled Study
Andersen JT, Ekman P, Wolf H, et al (Univ of Copenhagen)
Urology 46:631–637, 1995   2–32

Introduction.—Clinical studies with 6–12 months of follow-up have shown finasteride, a potent inhibitor of 5α-reductase, to reduce prostate volume and relieve the obstructive and irritative symptoms of benign prostatic hyperplasia (BPH). In a multicenter study, patients were followed up for 2 years to determine the drug's safety, efficacy, and ability to reverse the progress of BPH.

Patients and Methods.—The double-blind, placebo-controlled trial involved 707 patients enrolled at 59 centers. All patients were in general good health and had moderate symptoms of BPH; the mean age of the group was 65.5 years. After a 1-month, single-blind placebo run-in period, patients were randomized to finasteride (5 mg once daily) or placebo for 24 months. Patients completed a symptom questionnaire at baseline and at scheduled follow-up visits. Urinary flow rates were obtained at these visits for all patients and prostate volume measured in a subset of 416 patients.

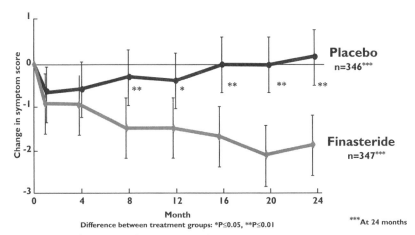

FIGURE 2.—Changes in total symptom score from baseline. Means ± 95% confidence interval. All patients treated analysis. (Reprinted by permission of the publisher from Andersen JT, Ekman P, Wolf H, et al: Can finasteride reverse the progress of benign prostatic hyperplasia? A two-year placebo controlled study. *Urology* 46:631–637, Copyright 1995 by Elsevier Science, Inc.)

Postvoiding residual urine volume and serum prostate-specific antigen were measured in all patients at screening and at 12 and 24 months.

Results.—Placebo-treated patients experienced a small improvement in total symptom score in the first 12 months but returned to baseline scores at 24 months (Fig 2). In contrast, patients in the finasteride group continued to show improvement throughout the treatment period. The difference between the groups was significant at 12 and 24 months. Prostate volume decreased a mean of 19% in the finasteride group and increased a mean of

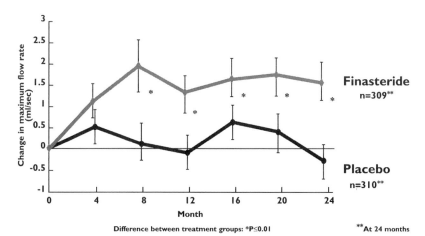

FIGURE 3.—Changes in maximum urinary flow rate (mL/sec) from baseline. Means ± 95% confidence interval. All patients treated analysis. (Reprinted by permission of the publisher from Andersen JT, Ekman P, Wolf H, et al: Can finasteride reverse the progress of benign prostatic hyperplasia? A two-year placebo controlled study. *Urology* 46:631–637, Copyright 1995 by Elsevier Science, Inc.)

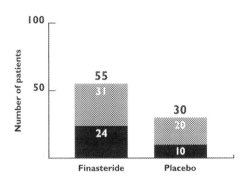

Key: ▓ History of sexual dysfunction (ejaculation disorder, erectile dysfunction, libido decrease, or other)

▒ No history of sexual dysfunction (ejaculation disorder, erectile dysfunction, libido decrease, or other)

FIGURE 7.—Adverse experiences: impotence. (Reprinted by permission of the publisher from Andersen JT, Ekman P, Wolf H, et al: Can finasteride reverse the progress of benign prostatic hyperplasia? A two-year placebo controlled study. *Urology* 46:631–637, Copyright 1995 by Elsevier Science, Inc.)

12% in the placebo group. Maximum urinary flow rate increased significantly in the finasteride group compared to the placebo group (Fig 3). The median percent change from baseline in PSA was +6% with placebo and [min]−52% with finasteride, a significant difference. The 2 groups were similar in proportion of patients who discontinued treatment and who had adverse side effects. However, more patients in the finasteride-treated group had sexual dysfunction vs. those in the placebo group; Figure 7 shows the patients' history of sexual dysfunction at study entry.

Conclusions.—Finasteride was effective and generally well tolerated when used to treat BPH. Patients given placebo reported initial improvement but no long-term benefits, whereas finasteride-treated patients maintained reductions in prostate volume and increases in maximum urinary flow rate over the 2-year study period. Treatment with finasteride can thus reverse the natural progression of BPH.

▶ Here is an excellent multicenter, double-blind, placebo controlled trial of more than 700 patients. The study assesses the effect of finasteride on the progress of BPH. It works! It confirms smaller, shorter, less eloquent studies. Prostate volume is diminished, and symptoms and urinary flow rate are improved. Finasteride is an inhibitor of 5α-reductase, the intracellular enzyme that converts testosterone to dihydrotestosterone, the active form of the male hormone. Prostatic hypertrophy is dihydrotestosterone dependent, so it is logical that this drug is effective.

The drug is well tolerated and adverse effects do not differ extensively from placebo except for impotence, which occurred in 19% of the finasteride group vs. 10% of those taking placebo. Cost is a factor. In Baltimore in the winter of 1996, the cost to the patient for 1 year's supply of the drug at a large hospital outpatient pharmacy was $733.80 ($61.15 per 30 tablets).

Subsequent to this paper, an article comparing terazosin, finasteride, or both in the treatment of BPH has appeared.[1] That study, which also was a placebo-controlled trial, suggests that terazosin was effective whereas finasteride was not. The likely explanation for the difference in the results may relate to the size of the prostate. Walsh has pointed this issue out in an editorial.[2] Finasteride may work only in men with larger glands in which the enlargement causes mechanical obstruction. Finasteride reduces the size of the prostate. Those who do not respond to finasteride may have smooth muscle overgrowth causing obstruction, and this form of BPH may respond to an α1-adrenergic antagonist agent such as terazosin.[2]

J.R. Burton, M.D.

References

1. Lepor H, Williford WO, Barry MJ, et al: The efficacy of terazosin, finasteride or both in BPH. *N Engl J Med* 335:533–539, 1996.
2. Walsh PC: Treatment of benign prostatic hypertrophy. *N Engl J Med* 335:586–587, 1996.

Miscellaneous

Epidemiology of Fecal Incontinence: The Silent Affliction
Johanson JF, Lafferty J (Univ of Illinois, Rockford)
Am J Gastroenterol 91:33–36, 1996 2–33

Background.—The epidemiology of fecal incontinence is still not well documented. Patients were surveyed prospectively during visits to their primary care physician or gastroenterologist to better define the prevalence and demographic distributions of fecal incontinence.

Methods and Findings.—A total of 881 patients aged 18 years or older were studied. The prevalence of fecal incontinence in the whole group was 18.4%. Data were stratified by frequency. Incontinence occurred daily in

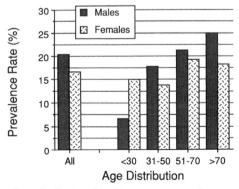

FIGURE 3.—Age and sex distribution of fecal incontinence. Prevalence rates are expressed as the number of affected individuals per 100 (%). (Courtesy of Johanson JF, Lafferty J: Epidemiology of fecal incontinence: The silent affliction. *Am J Gastroenterol* 91(1):33–36, 1996.)

TABLE 2.—Individuals' Attitudes Toward and Treatment of
Fecal Incontinence

	Physician Visits (%)		
	Primary Care	GI	Total
Discussed their incontinence with a physician	20.5	47.9*	33.8
Restricts activity for fear of incontinence	10.5	12.3	11.4
Wears adult diapers or pads	26.0	19.2	22.7
Takes medication to prevent incontinence	6.8	17.8*	12.2

* Statistically significant difference ($P < 0.05$) between patients seen by primary care and gastrointestinal (*GI*) physicians.
(Courtesy of Johanson JF, Lafferty J: Epidemiology of fecal incontinence: The silent affliction. *Am J Gastroenterol* 91(1):33–36, 1996.)

2.7% of the patients, weekly in 4.5%, and monthly or less frequently in 7.1%. The prevalence of incontinence was 12.3% in patients younger than 30 years and 19.4% in those older than 70 years. Incontinence was also 1.3 times more prevalent in men than women (Fig 3). Although the prevalence of fecal incontinence was surprisingly high, very few patients had ever mentioned it to a physician (Table 2).

Conclusions.—The occurrence of fecal incontinence may be more common than previously believed. Only a minority of affected individuals discuss this problem with a physician. Physicians should more actively question their patients about this condition.

▶ These important data on the epidemiology of fecal incontinence are strikingly reminiscent of the data accumulated on urinary incontinence during the past decade or so. Fecal incontinence is far more common than anticipated, and for the most part, it is unrecognized and dealt with inadequately. It has devastating social implications to patients. As with urinary incontinence, symptoms of fecal incontinence should be solicited from older patients. This is especially obvious in Figure 3, which shows the striking age-related increase in prevalence rates.

J.R. Burton, M.D.

Long-Term Outcomes of Patients Receiving Percutaneous Endoscopic Gastrostomy Tubes
Rabeneck L, Wray NP, Petersen NJ (Baylor College of Medicine, Houston)
J Gen Intern Med 11:287–293, 1996   2–34

Background.—Percutaneous endoscopic gastrostomy (PEG), introduced in 1980, is the preferred method for long-term enteral feeding. In 1991, 77,400 PEG tubes were reportedly placed in Medicare recipients. However, there have been no large-scale studies of the long-term outcomes of patients receiving PEG tubes.

TABLE 3.—Complications of Percutaneous Endoscopic Gastrostomy Tube Placement

	No. of Patients*	
Complication	Index (%)	Subsequent (%)
Peritonitis	28 (0.4%)	4 (0.05%)
Cellulitis or abscess of abdominal wall	15 (0.2%)	26 (0.4%)
Puncture or laceration	36 (0.5%)	7 (0.1%)
Hematoma or hemorrhage	75 (1.0%)	18 (0.2%)
Tube malfunction†	121 (1.6%)	134 (1.8%)
Aspiration pneumonia		586 (8.0%)
>1 Complication	17 (0.2%)	23 (0.3%)
Total	292 (3.9%)	798 (10.8%)

* Number of patients with complications during the index and subsequent hospitalizations is reported as a percentage of the full cohort (n = 7,369). Each patient is counted once. The number of patients with aspiration pneumonia after percutaneous endoscopic gastrotomy tube placement could not be determined for the index hospitalization.

† Malfunction includes a tube leaking, dislodging, or migrating.

(Courtesy of Rabeneck L, Wray NP, Petersen NJ: Long-term outcomes of patients receiving percutaneous endoscopic gastrostomy tubes. *J Gen Intern Med* 11:287–293, 1996. Reprinted by permission of Blackwell Science, Inc.)

Methods.—In this retrospective cohort study, data were obtained from 2 computerized databases to determine survival among patients with PEG tubes. A total of 7,369 patients received a PEG tube in fiscal years 1990 through 1992. Their mean age was 68.1 years, and 98.6% of the patients were men.

Findings.—Nineteen percent of the patients receiving PEG tubes had cerebrovascular disease; 28.6%, other organic neurologic disease; and

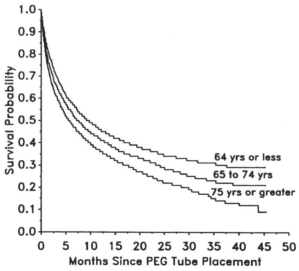

FIGURE 2.—Age-specific survival of 7,369 patients who underwent placement of percutaneous endoscopic gastrostomy (*PEG*) tubes in Department of Veterans Affairs hospitals in fiscal years 1990 through 1992. Differences in survival among the age groups was significant ($P < 0.0001$, log-rank test). (Courtesy of Rabeneck L, Wray NP, Petersen NJ: Long-term outcomes of patients receiving percutaneous endoscopic gastrostomy tubes. *J Gen Intern Med* 11:287-293, 1996. Reprinted by permission of Blackwell Science, Inc.)

15.7%, head and neck cancer. The complication rate associated with the procedure was only 4% (Table 3). However, because of the severity of their underlying illnesses, 23.5% of the patients died in the hospital with PEG tubes in place. Overall, the median survival was 7.5 months (Fig 2).

Conclusions.—The placement of PEG tubes in severely ill patients is widespread. Half of these patients are in the terminal stage of their disease. Future research should focus on whether quality of life and survival are improved by PEG placement.

▶ Approximately 75,000 PEG tubes are placed in the United States each year according to Medicare data. In spite of this widespread use, there are few data on the value and long-term follow-up on this procedure. This study is valuable because it provides 3-year follow-up information for 7,369 patients, almost exclusively men, in the VA system. Table 3 show some of these data. What really is remarkably striking is that nearly 25% of patients who received a PEG tube died during the hospitalization in which the procedure was performed. If this is confirmed in other institutions, it would certainly warrant a global reassessment of the use of this procedure, because it makes no sense whatsoever that it be done in the terminal stages of an illness. These data also provide important information on the complication rate just after placement and subsequently. Ongoing careful analysis of the indications for and outcomes of PEG tubes are desperately needed. In my view, they should not be a ritual of the dying process.

J.R. Burton, M.D.

Telemedicine and Geriatrics: Back to the Future
Williams ME, Ricketts TC, Thompson BG (Univ of North Carolina, Chapel Hill)
J Am Geriatr Soc 43:1047–1051, 1995   2–35

Introduction.—Advances in telecommunications are making possible the provision of universal access to interactive data and communications services from various locations, including the home. Telemedicine systems can provide multiple diagnostic aids, such as, for example, a remote zoom-tilt camera for observing a patient at a remote location. Medical record and laboratory data can also be exchanged via computer, and high-speed data transmission technology enables the simultaneous transmission of multiple types of information (text, images, sound). Such advances in telemedicine must be supported by accommodation of the organizational structure of the health care operation.

Applications in Geriatric Care.—Telemedicine can facilitate more comprehensive evaluation of the health care outcomes of a defined population. Electronic case management via telemedicine technology may be a promising approach to reducing the intimidation wrought by the complicated health care system. The overall goal of electronic case management is to match individuals' needs with health care services received. The key principle of telemedicine is to provide a system that enhances the delivery of health care (especially in rural areas) and is easy to use.

Limitations.—Universal access to health care information may be hampered by nonuniformity between medical information systems. Initial expenses to install telemedicine systems are high. Psychologic barriers may limit full use of advanced technologies; the perception may exist that use of telemedicine threatens the personal nature of the physician/patient relationship.

Conclusions.—The future of telemedicine in geriatric care is not yet clear, but well-designed systems have the potential to reduce patient and provider isolation and to expand educational and research opportunities. The new communications technologies offer potential for enhancing human interaction in geriatric medicine.

▶ This is a very thoughtful essay about telemedicine and geriatrics. In my view, there are enormous opportunities for telemedicine in geriatrics. It seems eminently logical to me that using unobtrusive technologies to link patients who may be acutely ill (located in nursing homes, their own homes, or other facilities) to a central medical resource has enormous potential. Geriatrics generally is an extremely low-technology field, but I believe telemedicine provides an opportunity to improve the care of elderly individuals who do not live near a hospital. The ready transmission of clinical observations such as video camera images, electrocardiograms, x-ray films, vital signs, and historical data by telecommunication systems can only help us provide better care at multiple sites. I encourage clinicians involved in the care of elderly individuals to welcome developments in telemedicine and to work toward making them feasible and appropriate for older patients.

J.R. Burton, M.D.

An Assessment of Surgery for Spinal Stenosis: Time Trends, Geographic Variations, Complications, and Reoperations
Ciol MA, Deyo RA, Howell E, et al (Univ of Washington, Seattle; Seattle Veterans Affairs Med Ctr)
J Am Geriatr Soc 44:285–290, 1996   2–36

Background.—Spinal stenosis is most common in older adults and can cause lower extremity sensory and motor deficits. Its diagnosis has been improved by the ability to obtain axial CT and MR images. To assess the effects of surgical treatment of spinal stenosis, temporal trends and geographic variations in the use of this treatment, the short-term morbidity and mortality of the surgery, and the need for repeated back surgery were investigated.

Methods.—Data were derived from Medicare claims and the National Hospital Discharge Survey (which has data on surgical results between 1979 and 1992). Two cohorts of patients undergoing lumbar spine surgery during 1985 (10,260 patients) and during 1989 (18,655 patients) were

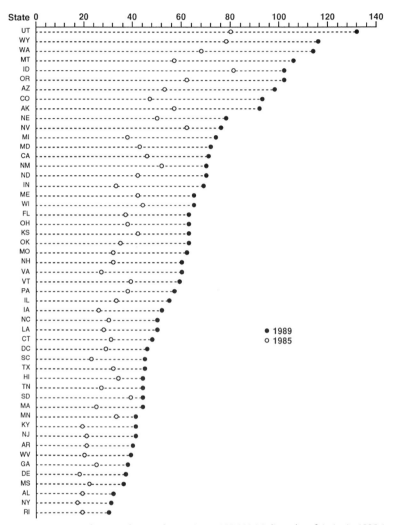

FIGURE 1.—Rates of surgery for spinal stenosis per 100,000 Medicare beneficiaries in 1985 (*open dots*) and 1989 (*filled dots*). (Courtesy of Ciol MA, Deyo RA, Howell E, et al: An assessment of surgery for spinal stenosis: Time trends, geographic variations, complications, and reoperations. *J Am Geriatr Soc* 44(3):285–290, 1996.)

followed up through 1991. Annual surgical rates per 100,000 population were calculated for 1979–1992. Data on postoperative death and complications were analyzed. The time to reoperation was calculated for each cohort.

Results.—The annual rates of surgery to treat spinal stenosis increased eightfold between 1979 and 1992 after adjustment for age and sex (Fig 1), with increases in every state in the United States. There was significant variation between states in the rates of surgical treatment, with the highest rates in both cohorts occurring in the Pacific and Mountain states. Postoperative mortality rates were less than 0.8% for patients younger than 75 years, 1.1% for patients aged 75–79 years, and 2.3% for patients older than 79 years. The likelihood of complications increased in association with age, comorbidity, male sex, and procedures involving spinal fusion. The complication rate was 2.4% in patients without comorbidity and 4.1% in patients with a comorbidity score of at least 3. The probability of reoperation was slightly greater in the 1989 than in the 1985 cohort. However, the 1989 cohort had fewer nonsurgical rehospitalizations for back pain.

Conclusions.—The rate of surgical treatment for spinal stenosis has increased significantly during the past 14 years. However, the complication rate and considerable geographic variations in surgery rates indicate that research is needed to evaluate the relative efficacy of surgical and nonsurgical treatments of spinal stenosis and to clarify indications for surgery.

▶ This extensive survey of spinal stenosis shows a fourfold increase in the rate of spinal surgery among those 65 years of age and older. This rate dwarfs the 40% increased rate for spinal surgery for those younger than age 65 during the 14-year period of this survey. There are, of course, several obvious reasons that could explain this dramatic increase in operations for spinal stenosis in the elderly: increased awareness; improved diagnosis with easier and better imaging; improved surgical and anesthesia techniques; and conceivably, the incidence of spinal stenosis has increased, but that seems unlikely. To me and, I am sure, to health economists, what is so remarkable is the enormous variation among states in spinal surgical rates per 100,000 elders, as shown in Figure 1. It is quite surprising that this remarkable increase in surgical rate has occurred without any published, randomized trials in which surgery was compared with conservative therapy.

The study does not provide any data about the relief of symptoms after surgery, but it does provide a very precise estimate of the risk of complications from spinal surgery. Not surprisingly, this risk increases substantially with increasing age. The reoperation rate in this survey was very substantial, approaching nearly 20%. Clearly a randomized, controlled trial is needed to provide the appropriate guidance to clinicians who are educating their patients about the management of spinal stenosis.

J.R. Burton, M.D.

How Costly Is It to Care for Disabled Elders in a Community Setting?
Harrow BS, Tennstedt SL, McKinlay JB (New England Research Insts, Watertown, Mass)
Gerontologist 35:803–813, 1995   2–37

Purpose.—Quantification of the total costs of community long-term care must include the costs of both the formal care provided by agencies and the informal care provided by family and friends. Estimation of these costs forms a basis for evaluation of current and future trends in providing and financing care for elderly individuals with disabilities. Analyses are described that estimate the total cost of care for a population of community-residing elderly individuals with disabilities. The economic cost of time spent by informal caregivers is considered using a market-value approach.

Design.—The population studied comprised 5,855 adults older than 70 years of age selected for participation in the Massachusetts Elder Health Project (geographically stratified, random sampling). In accordance with the existing sex ratio in the state among those older than 70 years, twice as many women as men were chosen. Baseline data were collected in 1984 and 1985 via extensive interviews conducted with 634 of the 790 respondents who were disabled. Three follow-up interviews were conducted at 15-month intervals beginning in 1988. These interviews included screening of the full study population to identify individuals with change in disability status. Caregiving resources were measured in terms of types and amount of informal and formal services provided in the previous month. These data were collected from the primary caregivers. Hourly wage rates were based on average market value for provision of comparable services.

Results.—Total annual cost of care in the community with mixed formal and informal care was estimated at $9,552, with increased disability resulting in increased cost. Most (76% to 80%) of the costs incurred for community care are for informal assistance, and represent no expenditure of real dollars. The annual cost of all-formal community care was estimated as $13,799; the annual cost of nursing home care in the state is $35,522.

Discussion.—The data from these simulations support the argument that community care costs less than institutional care, even when living expenses are considered and the worst-case scenario substitution of all-formal services is assumed. On an individual basis, however, community care is not always less expensive than nursing home care. Some severely disabled elderly individuals may be cared for less expensively in a nursing home if no informal support is available.

▶ This is a complicated health economics analysis containing important data. Determining the true cost of providing care for disabled elders in various settings is absolutely critical. This study analyzes the cost of formal as well as informal care for community-based elders with various levels of disability. The estimate of the informal cost of providing care at home is likely to become a major concern for HMOs and health economists. If patients and/or their families believe that HMOs are transferring some of their care responsibilities to informal caregivers for the purpose of cutting expenses and increasing profits, a significant backlash will occur. This becomes particularly important as more and more acute care is being provided at home as opposed to in a hospital or nursing facility.

Of course, at some point, for those with especially heavy care needs, the cost of providing that care at home is more than institutional care; this is especially true if housing and food costs are included. Individuals in society will need to have these and similar data if intelligent choices and thoughtful planning are to occur.

J.R. Burton, M.D.

Alternatives to Hospital Care: What Are They and Who Should Decide?
Coast J, Inglis A, Frankel S (Univ of Bristol, England)
BMJ 312:162–166, 1996   2–38

Background.—More information is needed about how patients requiring acute care should best be treated. The potential for changing the balance between primary and secondary care was investigated using a systematic method for identifying alternatives to acute hospital care.

Methods.—A total of 686 hospital admissions were classified into 2 categories: category 1 included patients with no alternative to admission to a hospital with advanced technology, and category 2 included patients who may have received adequate alternative care. Potential alternative forms of care for patients in category 2 were identified. Three panels of physicians participated in the study. Seven general practitioners comprised panel 1, another 7 comprised panel 2, and 6 consultants from general medicine and 1 from geriatrics comprised panel 3.

Findings.—Panels 1 and 2 thought that 51–89 of the hospitalized patients, or 8% to 14%, could have received alternative care. Panel 3 thought that 25–55 patients, or 5.5% to 9%, could have had alternative care. The main alternatives selected by all 3 panels were general practitioner bed and urgent outpatient appointments (Table).

Conclusions.—In this study, 8% to 14% of emergency admissions to general medicine and care of the elderly population may have been man-

---

TABLE.—List of Alternative Forms of Care for the
Assessment Panels

1	Community hospital or general practitioner bed
2	Nursing home—immediate access for short term care
3	Nursing home (elderly mentally infirm)—immedi ate access for short term care
4	Respite care home—immediate access for short term care
5	Residential home—immediate access for short term care
6	Hospice
7	Urgent referral for outpatient treatment or investigation—same day (including X-ray)
8	Urgent referral for outpatient treatment or investigation—next day (including X-ray)
9	Urgent home visit by consultant—within 48 hours
10	Intensive home support—provided within 2 hours
11	Intensive home support—provided within 12 hours
12	Less intensive home support—provided within 12 hours
13	Continuous minor social support in the home—provided within 2 hours
14	Other—to be specified

(Courtesy of Coast J, Inglis A, Frankel S: Alternatives to hospital care: What are they and who should decide? *BMJ* 312:162–166, 1996.)

aged with alternative care, as judged by 2 panels of general practitioners. A panel of hospital consultants estimated that 5.5% to 9% of such admissions could have been managed alternatively.

▶ This article from Britain evaluates whether patients admitted to an acute hospital may have been treated with alternative methods. For a number of reasons this may not be generalizable to the United States. It nevertheless is innovative thinking of the type that, I believe, is also critical in this country. To some extent, the problem in Britain is the reverse of the problem in this country. In Britain there currently is a much greater demand for hospital beds than there are beds. Accordingly, they have worked to create innovative programs of care that might provide acute care without hospitalization. A number of alternatives to hospital care were identified and are listed in the table.

Panels of physicians reviewed the records of patients and made suggestions for care alternatives. A sample of 112 admissions to the hospital were reviewed. A panel of general practitioners believed that between 8% and 14% of all admissions to the hospital could have been properly cared for in alternative situations. On the other hand, consultants believed that only between 5.5% and 9% of such patients could have been cared for in alternative care situations. Such differences in perspective are not surprising.

In the United States, it is time that we look for alternative forms of providing acute "hospital level" care, and this is especially true for elderly individuals. Hospitals are enormously expensive; and, especially in elderly populations, the rate of complications is substantial. Also, many elderly patients find the hospital a threatening and dehumanizing experience. Hospitalization is often associated with the loss of dignity. For these reasons, and not because of a problem of bed capacity, we should begin to evaluate acute care alternatives in this country. From my own experience as an attending physician in an acute hospital, I am certain that a significant portion of patients could be managed quite satisfactorily or even better in an alternative site than the acute hospital. I believe we need to think broadly in this regard.

J.R. Burton, M.D.

Effect of a Prior-Authorization Requirement on the Use of Nonsteroidal Antiinflammatory Drugs by Medicaid Patients
Smalley WE, Griffin MR, Fought RL, et al (Vanderbilt Univ, Nashville, Tenn; Tennessee State Dept of Health, Nashville)
N Engl J Med 332:1612–1617, 1995   2–39

Background.—Drug expenditures in the Medicaid program increased fourfold from 1984 through 1993. To control such expenditures, the Omnibus Budget Reconciliation Act of 1990 established a policy of prior authorization for certain drugs. There is concern, however, that mandatory advance approval may have adverse clinical and economic consequences. The effects of this policy change were examined in a study of nongeneric, nonsteroidal antiinflammatory drugs (NSAIDs) in the Medicaid program in Tennessee.

Methods.—Starting in October 1989, Tennessee Medicaid required prior authorization for all prescriptions for NSAIDs, except those available generically. Spending for NSAIDs made up 11% of the state's Medicaid pharmacy expenditures for 1988. These drugs are widely prescribed, and the more expensive agents can cost 12 times as much as generic ibuprofen. Monthly Medicaid expenditures for NSAIDs were compared for the year before the policy change and the 2 years after its implementation. Also examined were costs for other analgesic or anti-inflammatory drugs, psychotropic drugs, and outpatient services and inpatient admissions for pain or inflammation.

Results.—Enrollment in Tennessee Medicaid increased from 498,821 in the baseline year to 547,403 in the second year after mandatory prior authorization was adopted. An abrupt decrease in the rates of expenditure for NSAIDs occurred with the new policy. For each person-year of enrollment, Medicaid paid $22.41 in the baseline year. After 2 years of prior authorization, this cost was reduced by $11.78 (53%), a change attributed to both an overall reduction in the use of NSAIDs and a shift from nongeneric to generic agents. The estimated savings over the 2-year period after adoption of the prior-authorization policy was $12.8 million. The administrative costs of the prior authorization requirement were approximately $75,000 per year. There was no evidence that the use of other services—including other analgesic and anti-inflammatory drugs, outpatient care, or inpatient admissions—had increased. Those patients who were most affected by the new policy—the regular users of nongeneric NSAIDs—had similar reductions in NSAID use and costs.

Conclusions.—The prior-authorization policy for Medicaid expenditures was successful in reducing payments for NSAIDs in Tennessee. During the first 2 years after the policy was adopted, savings were estimated at $12.8 million. The administrative costs of the program were low, and there was no corresponding increase in the use of other drugs or services.

▶ This important study again points out how regulations—in this case, at the state Medicaid level—powerfully influence, in a positive way, the prescribing patterns of clinicians. Although this study is not limited to the elderly population, it nevertheless is important, because Medicaid is an important insurance program for millions of elders. This Tennessee Medicaid study evaluated the use of NSAIDs by prescription before and after a prior-authorization requirement was implemented. Use decreased dramatically, with enormous cost savings. The study had no way of considering the possibility of worsening patient symptoms or function—a potential outcome of reduction in use of NSAIDs—but it showed no increase in the use of other medications, including prescription analgesics or corticosteroids, which may have been expected if patients' conditions worsened.

I must say, I have long thought that NSAIDs were considerably overprescribed, especially in the elderly population, in whom side effects are often more serious and more common. However, I had no idea that, at least in 1991, NSAIDs amounted to nearly 4% of the prescriptions and were estimated to represent an expenditure of approximately $2.4 billion dollars in the United States.

J.R. Burton, M.D.

3 Geriatric Psychiatry

Introduction

The articles reviewed in this YEAR BOOK include explorations of some of the most intriguing issues in geriatric psychiatry. One important question for clinicians is whether testing for the apolipoprotein 4 allele has reached the stage that clinicians should be using it routinely to confirm a diagnosis of Alzheimer's disease. Several ad hoc groups have convened in the past year, and all conclude that the available data do not support routine testing. All recommend that it be used in research studies. Thus, clinicians are still waiting for a biological test that diagnoses Alzheimer's disease with adequate positive and negative predictive values. The utility of neuropsychological testing for the early detection and staging of Alzheimer's disease is the subject of several articles. In one study of screening for dementia, the memory and initiation/perseveration subscales of the Mattis Dementia Rating Scale had very high sensitivity and specificity in identifying community-residing individuals with dementia. In another study, delayed recall of stories and figures were markedly impaired early in Alzheimer disease whereas naming, fluency, and figure recognition showed a more gradual decline. The authors concluded that the latter tests are better for staging. Parietal asymmetry on positron emission tomography scanning may be an early marker for dementia in individuals who are evaluated for age-related cognitive decline.

In several studies published in the past year, the intriguing question of whether early life education protects against dementia is addressed. Those articles reviewed here continue to support the hypothesis that more education is associated with a lower risk of receiving a diagnosis of dementia. This is such an important issue that continued study is clearly needed. One study even suggests that education may protect against the development of cognitive impairment in younger individuals.

In several of the studies reviewed this year, important points are made about the treatment of depression in the elderly. Hospitalization for major depression is quite infrequent. Selective serotonin reuptake inhibitor antidepressants, although safer than tricyclics in some regards, appear to cause more impairment in body sway and balance (perhaps related to the induction of drug-induced parkinsonism). Recent studies demonstrate that treatments as different as psychotherapy and electroconvulsive therapy are effective in treating late-life depression. Several recent articles review the complex relationship between co-existing medical morbidity and the prevalence and treatment of major depression. Two articles illustrate paradoxes about attitudes toward suicide in late life. Suicidal ideation is quite uncommon in the elderly. Depression is a significant correlate, but other factors contribute to suicidal ideation. A Gallup telephone survey suggests that a perception of failing health and a lack of feeling supported by religious views both correlate with the belief that assisted suicide should be provided.

The challenges presented by cognitive impairment in persons with schizophrenia are addressed in several articles. It is clear that the neuropsychological impairment of persons with schizophrenia is different from those seen with Alzheimer's disease and that patients with chronic schizophrenia and cognitive impairment who come to autopsy are clinically and pathologically different from individuals with Alzheimer's disease. Thus, the neuropathologic basis of the dementia of schizophrenia remains a mystery and evidence of the ability to alter its development and course is lacking.

Several articles highlight important areas in which research is particularly needed. Alcoholism is prevalent but, as a review by the American Medical Association's Council on Scientific Affairs acknowledges, our knowledge base is limited. Post-traumatic stress disorder can occur in elderly veterans of World War II, and cognitive-behavioral treatment is effective in older patients with panic disorder. Findings in the emerging field of outcomes research are reviewed in two articles in this chapter. One study suggests that major depression is better treated in psychiatric units whereas depressed individuals with medical problems might better be treated in general medical units. Some of the same authors demonstrate that prospective payment systems do not significantly lower the length of stay.

Peter V. Rabins, M.D., M.P.H.

Dementia

DETECTION AND STAGING

Statement on Use of Apolipoprotein E Testing for Alzheimer Disease
Farrer L, and the American College of Med Genetics/American Society of Human Genetics Working Group on ApoE and Alzheimer Disease (Boston Univ)
JAMA 274:1627–1629, 1995   3–1

Background.—There is great interest in the possibility of performing DNA tests for the diagnosis and prediction of Alzheimer's disease (AD). Several centers have begun to offer the apolipoprotein E genotype (APOE) polymerase chain reaction assay as a "genetic test" for AD. Although having such a genetic test might improve the diagnosis of AD, a number of key questions would have to be considered before widespread APOE testing could be recommended. Published data on the link between APOE and AD were reviewed for the purpose of making recommendations regarding the use of genetic testing to diagnose or predict AD.

Methods.—The review was performed by a working group of the joint American College of Medical Genetics and the American Society of Human Genetics Test and Technology Transfer Committee. Input from the American Academy of Neurology and the American Psychiatric Association was obtained as well to ensure that the clinicians involved in working with patients with AD and their families were included. A consensus draft was produced and endorsed by the scientific and executive committees of all of the organizations involved, as well as by the National Institutes of Health–Department of Education Working Group on Ethical, Legal, and Social Implications of Human Genome Research.

Recommendations.—The available data showed a strong relationship between the APOE ϵ4 allele and AD, and they suggested that the presence of APOE ϵ4 may constitute an important risk factor for AD. However, there is insufficient evidence to warrant recommending that APOE testing be used for routine clinical diagnosis or for predictive testing. On its own, APOE genotyping is not sensitive or specific enough to be used for diagnosis. Neither should it be used for predictive purposes, because AD can develop in persons without the APOE ϵ4 allele and because many individuals with this allele never get AD. It may also be argued that predictive testing is of value only if some preventive intervention is available. Questions remain regarding how APOE allele associations are affected by race and about possible interactions between APOE and other risk factors.

Conclusions.—The available evidence does not support the use of APOE testing for the diagnosis or prediction of AD, except in carefully designed research protocols. Many of the unanswered questions about the link between APOE genotype and AD may be answered in an ongoing collaborative study. The next few years should tell whether APOE genotyping has other roles in the management of AD.

▶ An ad hoc committee met to review data on the association between APOE and the development of AD. Based on available information, the group concluded that the presence of APOE ϵ4 cannot be used for either predictive testing or clinical diagnosis, because APOE genotype does not provide adequate sensitivity or specificity. They note that further study is needed. The association between APOE ϵ4 and other causes of dementia, the variability among ethnic groups, and the lack of benefit for early recognition are cited as reasons for expressing their conclusions.

Although this article suggests that scientific data for supporting the clinical use of APOE cannot be advocated, it does not discuss such ethical issues as an individual's right to know his or her risk status or the psychological risks and benefits of having negative or positive test results. These challenging issues, which go beyond testing for AD, will confront physicians with increasing frequency in the next decade. Scientific data on APOE is being added at a furious pace, and the value of the test is likely to change in the near future. It will be important to determine not only sensitivity and specificity, but also positive and negative predictive values. The latter are influenced by the prevalence of disorder in the community whereas sensitivity and specificity are not. Because the APOE ε4 allele is relatively new and AD is highly prevalent in late life, predictive values without other data, such as the number of family members affected or the presence of other risk factors, will probably never be useful.

P.V. Rabins, M.D., M.P.H.

Is Senile Dementia "Age-Related" or "Ageing-Related"?: Evidence From Meta-Analysis of Dementia Prevalence in the Oldest Old
Ritchie K, Kildea D (INSERM Equipe "Vieillissement Cognitif," Montpellier, France; Royal Melbourne Inst of Technology, Australia)
Lancet 346:931–934, 1995   3–2

Objective.—Some authors have suggested that the group of disorders comprising the senile dementias represents the end point of the normal cerebral aging process. This hypothesis—which implies that senile dementia will develop in any person who lives long enough—is supported by the exponential increase in the prevalence of senile dementia after 60 years of age. It is possible that the prevalence rate levels off in very old individuals, but there are no data with which to address this issue, which has important scientific and public health implications. A meta-analysis of epidemiologic studies including individuals 80 years of age and older was performed to examine hypotheses regarding the prevalence of senile dementia in the very elderly population.

Methods.—The analysis included 9 epidemiologic studies of senile dementia that provided age-specific prevalence data on subjects older than 80 years. All studies had adequate sampling procedures and used the *Diagnostic and Statistical Manual of Mental Disorders, Third Edition* criteria for senile dementia. Logistic and modified logistic models were used to

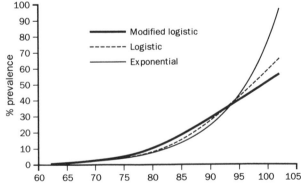

FIGURE.—The relationship, expressed in 3 ways, between age and the prevalence of dementia in meta-analysis of 9 studies. (Courtesy of Ritchie K, Kildea D: Is senile dementia "age-related" or "ageing-related"?: Evidence from meta-analysis of dementia prevalence in the oldest old. *Lancet* 346:931–934, 1995. Copyright by The Lancet Ltd.)

assess whether the prevalence of senile dementia levels off after age 85 years.

Results.—The data suggested that the rate of increase in the prevalence of dementia leveled off with age (Figure). The rate of increase decreased in the age range of 80–84 years. In the oldest age group studied, those aged 95–99 years, the upper end of the 95% confidence interval was only a little greater than 50%. The observed prevalence of senile dementia in that age group was approximately 40%.

Conclusion.—The exponential increase in the prevalence of senile dementia with age decreases beginning in the age range of 80–84 years, before flattening out to zero at age 95 years. Thus, senile dementia appears to occur within a specific age range rather than being caused by the aging process per se. The risk of dementia may decrease for individuals who reach very old age, and this could have important implications for public health policy. The findings suggest that published estimates of the future number of demented elderly individuals may be too high and that etiologic factors other than those involved in normal aging should be sought.

▶ This meta-analysis of 9 epidemiologic studies reviews data on the incidence rates of dementia in individuals older than 80 years of age. The authors demonstrate that the data best reflect a logistic function rather than an exponential pattern of growth (see Figure), and they conclude that the incidence rates level off at age 95 years. Because of the small amount of data and the small number of subjects 90 years of age and older, these conclusions are tentative at best. Nevertheless, they support the hypothesis that dementia is not an inevitable and intrinsic aspect of the chronological aging process. This is most compatible with the hypothesis that dementia is "age-related" rather than "caused by aging." That is, dementia is not an intrinsic and unavoidable component of chronological aging. The debate on this intriguing issue continues. Further data are sorely needed.

P.V. Rabins, M.D., M.P.H.

Intelligence and Education as Predictors of Cognitive State in Late Life: A 50-Year Follow-Up
Plassman BL, Welsh KA, Helms M, et al (Duke Univ, Durham, NC; Johns Hopkins Univ, Baltimore, Md)
Neurology 45:1446–1450, 1995   3–3

Background.—The Army General Classification Test (AGCT) was administered to U.S. military service inductees in the early 1940s as a "test of general learning ability." Scores from this test and a cognitive status test administered later in life provide an opportunity to investigate the relation of intelligence in early adult life and late-life cognitive status. The relation between education and intelligence in early adult life and cognitive function was examined in elderly male twins.

Study Design.—Between 1990 and 1992, 50 years after the administration of the AGCT, 930 men were examined using the modified Telephone Interview for Cognitive States (TICS-m) as part of a study of dementia in twins. The TICS-m scores in later life were correlated with AGCT scores in early life and with years of education. Analysis of heritability was limited to 300 monozygotic and 304 dizygotic twin pairs.

Findings.—Both intelligence and years of education contributed significantly to cognitive status as measured by the TICS-m, with AGCT scores accounting for 20.6% and education accounting for 16.7% of the variance in cognitive status. A multivariable model using AGCT scores, education, and the interaction of the 2 variables as predictors of the TICS-m score explained 24.8% of the variance of the TICS-m. It appeared that these variables may represent a common underlying cofactor although both variables also contained significant individual predictive power. Among the 604 pairs of twins who took the AGCT, heritability for intelligence as estimated by the AGCT score was 0.503, indicating that about one half of the variation observed in the AGCT scores could be attributed to genetic influences.

Summary.—This is the first study to use a direct measure of intelligence, obtained in early adult life, to predict basic cognitive abilities in late life. It appears that those with more education and higher intelligence in early adulthood perform better on tests of cognitive status in late life. This correlation may be helpful when interpreting scores on mental status tests in the elderly or when evaluating risk factors for cognitive decline in late life.

▶ The relationship between early-life cognitive capacity and performance on cognitive tests in late life is controversial. The issue is important because a number of studies have demonstrated that lower education is a risk factor for development of dementia. This study shows that both performance on a cognitive test administered early in life and number of years of education are correlated with current performance on a cognitive screening test. Together, however, these 2 variables explain only 24.8% of the variance. Thus, almost 75% of the variance is unexplained by education and cognitive capacity as measured by a standardized test.

Even though this study does not settle the debate, its results are compatible with the "cognitive reserve" hypothesis. This hypothesis states that individuals with greater cognitive capacity must decline to a greater degree than individuals with less innate capacity before cognitive impairment becomes clinically recognizable. The finding that 75% of the variance in cognitive performance is not explained by early life performance or education suggests 2 possibilities; it is either attributable to the development of cognitive impairment later in life in some subjects or to a continued gain in cognitive capacities throughout adulthood in some subjects. Most plausible, both explanations are true.

P.V. Rabins, M.D., M.P.H.

Education and Change in Cognitive Function: The Epidemiologic Catchment Area Study
Farmer ME, Kittner SJ, Rae DS, et al (NIH, Rockville, Md; Univ of Maryland, Baltimore)
Ann Epidemiol 5:1–7, 1995   3–4

Background.—Several authors have studied the relationship between age and change in cognitive function over time. However, few have studied the correlation between change in cognitive function over time and low educational attainment.

Methods.—The association between educational attainment and decline in cognitive function during 1 year was investigated in 14,883 adults enrolled in the National Institute of Mental Health Epidemiologic Catchment Area Study. Cognitive function was determined by the Mini-Mental State Examination (MMSE).

Findings.—Education significantly predicted cognitive decline among younger as well as elderly adults whose baseline MMSE score exceeded 23 (Table 4). Educational level did not significantly predict cognitive decline among adults with baseline MMSE scores of 23 or less.

TABLE 4.—Estimated Odds Ratio by Age Group for Declining 3 or More Points on the Mini-Mental State Examination (*MMSE*) Over a 1-Year Period Among Participants With Baseline MMSE Score Above 23*

Variable	Baseline MMSE > 23	
	< 65 y	≥ 65 y
Age (y)†	1.1 (1.05,1.2)	2.0 (1.7,2.4)
Education (y)‡	0.5 (0.4,0.6)	0.3 (0.2,0.4)
Ethnicity		
Black	1.4 (1.2,1.7)	2.4 (1.9,3.1)
Hispanic	2.3 (1.9,2.8)	2.0 (1.2,3.4)
White and other	1.0 (reference)	1.0 (reference)
Residence		
Nursing home	3.6 (1.9,6.7)	3.0 (1.9,4.7)
Jail	2.6 (2.0,3.4)	
Mental institution	9.5 (6.0,14.9)	
Household	1.0 (reference)	1.0 (reference)
Substance abuse (lifetime diagnosis)		
Yes	1.1 (0.9,1.2)	1.6 (1.1,2.3)
No	1.0 (reference)	1.0 (reference)
Baseline MMSE score§	0.9 (0.9,0.98)	0.8 (0.8,0.89)
Sex		
Male	1.2 (1.05,1.4)	1.0 (0.8,1.2)
Female	1.0 (reference)	1.0 (reference)

* From the National Institute of Mental Health (NIMH) Epidemiologic Catchment Area Study; note that 95% confidence intervals are in parentheses.
† Associated with an increment of 10 years.
‡ Associated with an increment of 8 years of education.
§ Associated with an increment of 1 MMSE error.
(Reprinted by permission of the publisher from Education and change in cognitive function: The Epidemiologic Catchment Area Study. Farmer ME, Kittner SJ, Rae DS, et al: *Ann Epidemiol* 5:1–7. Copyright 1995 by Elsevier Science Inc.)

Conclusions.—Education appears to protect against cognitive decline even in adults younger than 65 years, in whom the prevalence and incidence of dementia are very low. Thus education or its correlates may protect against processes other than dementia that cause declines in test performance in young adults.

▶ Educational background is one of the issues that clinicians must consider in diagnosing early dementia. Several lines of data now suggest that higher early-life education prevents or delays the development of dementia or, alternatively, makes it more difficult to identify early dementia. This study adds fuel to this debate by showing that even in individuals at very low risk for developing dementia because they are young, cognitive decline is more likely in those with low education. This article has a very useful and readable discussion of this controversial issue. It is an even-handed review and discusses the most important research findings in the area. The authors make the important point that longitudinal studies such as this one are less affected by the confound of early-life education because the individual's education is the same at each measurement point.

This study is intriguing because it demonstrated that among those with better cognition at baseline, lower education predicted greater cognitive decline in both old and young individuals. The implication of this is that the increased risk of cognitive decline associated with low education does not solely operate by leading to dementia, because dementia is rare among the young. Older age, nonwhite race, residence in a nursing home, and prior substance abuse are also risk factors for decline in cognition among this group. There is now widespread interest in the relationship between early-life education and the development of late-life dementia. It will likely be explained by a mixture of brain development and social environment.

P.V. Rabins, M.D., M.P.H.

Clinical Validity of the Mattis Dementia Rating Scale in Detecting Dementia of the Alzheimer Type: A Double Cross-Validation and Application to a Community-Dwelling Sample
Monsch AU, Bondi MW, Salmon DP, et al (Univ of California, San Diego)
Arch Neurol 52:899–904, 1995   3–5

Introduction.—The Dementia Rating Scale (DRS), a psychometric instrument devised to assess the nature and severity of dementia, is relatively brief, is considered reliable, and has clear advantages over other commonly used mental status examinations. It consists of 5 subscales, each of which contributes differently to the total DRS score. Despite widespread use of the DRS, few studies have addressed its clinical validity in detecting Alzheimer-type dementia (DAT). Clinical validation of the DRS was attempted via a study incorporating large sample sizes, consideration of demographic variables, and evaluation of the relative importances of the 5 subscales.

Methods.—Participants included 105 healthy elderly individuals and 254 outpatients with DAT. Multiple regressions of demographic variables were performed on the DRS and its subscales. Optimal DRS cutoff scores were derived using receiver operating characteristic curves. Stepwise logistic regression was used to perform double cross-validation and the results were applied to a community-dwelling population. DRS scores were computed and adjusted for age and education.

Results.—A sensitivity of 98% and a specificity of 97% were calculated for the determined optimal cutoff score for DAT of 129 or less. A combination of the memory and initiation/perseveration subscales correctly classified 98% of all participants, 100% of the 51 participants with DAT confirmed via autopsy, and 92% of a sample (76 patients) of participants with mild DAT. When a community-dwelling population of 238 healthy elderly people and 44 patients with DAT were evaluated based on the derived equation, correct classification occurred for 91% of patients and 93% of normal participants.

Conclusions.—This is the first investigation to comprehensively document the clinical validity of the DRS. The diagnostic accuracy of an abbreviated version of the DRS comprising only the memory and initiation/perseveration subscales seems approximately equal to that of the complete test. However, the original 5-subscale weighting scheme derived by Mattis has been revised for this purpose.

▶ The Mattis DRS is a widely used scale that is longer than the Mini-Mental State Examination but shorter than a typical neuropsychological battery. The results of this study, that a cutoff score of 129 has a sensitivity of 98% and a specificity of 97%, and the demonstration in another sample that 91% of individuals with dementia and 93% of normal subjects were correctly identified by this cutoff score, suggest that the Mattis rating scale can have significant utility for studying individuals with dementia. Although clinical diagnosis remains the "gold standard" in diagnosing dementia, the statistics reported in this paper suggest that the Mattis scale is a valid indicator of the presence or absence of dementia and offers a desirable balance between a test that is both practical and thorough.

P.V. Rabins, M.D., M.P.H.

Cognitive Test Performance in Detecting, Staging, and Tracking Alzheimer's Disease
Locascio JJ, Growdon JH, Corkin S (Massachusetts Inst of Technology, Cambridge)
Arch Neurol 52:1087–1099, 1995   3–6

Purpose.—Behavioral research in Alzheimer's disease (AD) seeks to identify 3 types of tests: tests for detecting AD (i.e., for distinguishing patients with AD from age- and education-matched controls), tests for staging AD (i.e., for measuring differences in the severity of dementia), and tests for tracking the progression of disease. Previous studies have suggested that impairment on tests of delayed recall of verbal material is an early change in AD. A large sample of patients with AD was studied to identify the best cognitive tests for detecting, staging, and tracking AD.

Methods.—The analysis included 123 outpatients with AD, representing a wide range of dementia severity, and 60 normal controls. The 2 groups were similar in age, education, and sex distribution. The subjects in both groups were assessed on 10 different cognitive tests of memory, language, visuospatial ability, and reasoning. Other measures included the Information, Memory and Concentration (IMC) subtest of the Blessed Dementia Scale and an activities of daily living questionnaire. For the patients with AD, the test battery was repeated every 6–24 months over as long as 5½ years' follow-up. In addition to assessing cognitive change over time, the analysis used various techniques to model complex changes in cognitive performance.

Results.—All cognitive scores were significantly lower in the patients with AD than in the normal controls, and the scores of patients with AD grew worse over time. The patients with AD showed rapid declines in delayed recall of stories and figures, and performance on these tests soon bottomed out. As in previous studies, tests of delayed recall were good at identifying patients who had early AD but were not useful for staging purposes. Better tests for staging—i.e., those showing a steady decline over time in the patients with AD—were tests of confrontation naming, semantic fluency, and immediate recognition of geometric figures. The patients' scores on the IMC test increased by approximately 3 points per year for the first 2 years, then by 2 or 3 points per year in the third and fourth years. Scores on the activities of daily living scale increased by approximately 10% per year.

Conclusion.—Some cognitive tests are best for early identification of patients with AD, whereas others are better suited for staging severity of dementia. These findings suggest that atrophy of the cholinergic ventral forebrain neurons and partial deafferentation of the hippocampus—both of which are early changes in AD—might be the underlying cause of impairments in delayed recall. The later, progressive changes in language and visuospatial ability more likely arise from the loss of neocortical neurons and their connections. Tests that are useful in charting the course of AD include the IMC test, tests of activities of daily living, the Boston Naming Test, the Verbal Fluency Test, and the Benton Visual Recognition Test.

▶ Early diagnosis of AD is likely to be important in the future, when preventive treatments become available, because, for most diseases, early recognition leads to better treatment response (this is sometimes called secondary prevention). This study demonstrates that delayed recall of stories and figures decreases early and rapidly and, thus, shows sensitivity to early AD. Other cognitive abnormalities—such as naming, fluency, and figure recognition—show a slower steady decline. The authors conclude that the latter will, therefore, be more useful in the staging of dementia.

Delayed recall is a well-known early sign of memory impairment. The reported dissociation between recall on the one hand and measures of language and visuospatial function on the other supports the Sjögren staging schema of AD. This 3-stage descriptive schema describes memory decline as the predominant symptom for the first 2 or 3 years of AD and indicates that aphasia, apraxia, and agnosia are prominent during the second 3-year phase of the illness.

P.V. Rabins, M.D., M.P.H.

Predictors of Cognitive Change in Middle-Aged and Older Adults With Memory Loss
Small GW, La Rue A, Komo S, et al (Univ of California, Los Angeles; VA Med Ctr, West Los Angeles; Univ of California, Irvine; et al)
Am J Psychiatry 152:1757–1764, 1995   3–7

Background.—According to data from clinical memory tests, age-associated memory impairment occurs in more than 40% of individuals in their fifties and in more than 50% of individuals in their sixties. More severe forms of cognitive impairment occur in 5% to 10% of those older than 65 years of age and in 50% of those older than 85 years. It would be helpful to identify symptoms of the onset of dementia and to predict the rate of cognitive change in older adults. The association between normal cognitive changes associated with aging and changes associated with early dementia is not well understood. The predictors of cognitive change in older adults were tested.

Methods.—Baseline assessments were made in 42 adults between 43 and 81 years of age who had mild memory complaints. The subjects underwent psychiatric and neurologic examinations, MRI and positron emission tomography scans, laboratory tests, and verbal and visual-spatial memory tests. The subjects also completed the Memory Functioning Questionnaire. Follow-up examinations were performed at a mean of 3 years.

Results.—Significant predictors of change in visual-spatial memory were parietal asymmetry, sex, and visual-spatial memory score at baseline. Predictors of change in verbal memory were level of education and verbal memory score at baseline. The following were not significant predictors of cognitive change: other neocortical asymmetry scores, age, family history of Alzheimer's disease, cerebral atrophy, and self-ratings of mnemonic use.

Discussion.—Variables from different domains were included in the analyses, and several of them significantly predicted cognitive change. Parietal symmetry associated with questionable dementia that progresses to Alzheimer's disease may be present in early, age-related cognitive decline. The baseline predictors of change will vary depending on the outcome measure.

▶ This is a potentially important study in the search for the early identification of dementia. Small and colleagues used positron emission tomography scans to determine brain blood flow and performance in patients with decline in visual memory over 3 years. Parietal asymmetry, poor baseline visuospatial memory, and sex predicted rate of change in visuospatial memory, and older age and family history of Alzheimer's disease almost reached statistical significance. The early identification of dementia is a controversial topic because it currently provides no benefit to the subject. In this study, all individuals evaluated had complaints about memory loss. If an accurate test were devised, it would be possible to reassure individuals with memory complaints and no evidence of early dementia that they are not at risk for significant cognitive decline. However, without evidence that pharmacologic or psychosocial benefits can accrue to individuals who have early dementia, such tests cannot be justified. These data are not powerful enough to allow predictions in individual cases; they only show that prognosis can be predicted in groups of individuals. Therefore, the clinical relevance of these studies is yet to be demonstrated.

P.V. Rabins, M.D., M.P.H.

Associations of Status and Change Measures of Neuropsychological Function With Pathologic Changes in Elderly, Originally Nondemented Subjects
Crystal HA, Dickson D, Sliwinski M, et al (Albert Einstein College of Medicine, Bronx, NY; Burke Rehabilitation Inst, White Plains, NY)
Arch Neurol 53:82–87, 1996   3–8

Introduction.—The Bronx Aging Study is a longitudinal study of 488 initially nondemented, community-residing volunteers aged 78 and 85 years at enrollment who were followed up until death. Twenty-nine subjects who had quantitative neuropathologic examinations and at least 2 years of neuropsychological testing were examined to describe the association between status and change of neuropsychological function with pathologic changes.

Methods.—Initial summary neuropsychological score and rate of change score in 29 originally nondemented elderly patients were correlated with postmortem neuropathologic findings of Alzheimer's disease (AD) in 8 subjects, vascular dementia (VaD) in 7, normal aging (NA) in 9, and pathologic aging (PA) in 5.

Findings.—Summary neuropsychological scores at baseline in elderly individuals who subsequently had pathologically confirmed AD or VaD were 0.8 z units lower than those in the NA or PA subgroups. Subjects with AD demonstrated significantly higher rates of change than the NA or PA groups; the AD group declined 3.7 times more readily than the NA group. Baseline scores or rate of change did not differ significantly between the NA and PA groups. Education was strongly associated with initial neuropsychological scores, but not change scores. Initial neuropsychological score and age were the best predictors of change scores.

Summary.—Among initially, nondemented elderly individuals, those who subsequently have AD or VaD develop have lower neuropsychological scores at initial evaluation than normal individuals or those with pathologic aging. In addition, a substantial decline on neuropsychological tests is a predictor of AD. The level of education is strongly associated with initial neuropsychological scores, but not change scores, providing support to the notion that the association of dementia with a low level of education may result from lower levels of "brain reserve" in the less educated.

▶ This is another study that supports the hypothesis that "brain reserve" might explain the finding that individuals with lower education are more likely to suffer from dementia. Among community-residing individuals first examined because they were presumably normal, individuals who eventually had AD or VaD develop had poorer performance on cognitive measures at the time of entry into the study than those who did not become demented. Not surprisingly, individuals who had dementia develop had more rapid declines in cognitive scores than individuals who were not demented. This is compatible with the contention that early dementia is more difficult to detect in individuals with higher education. However, this study does not end the debate on this intriguing and important question. Nevertheless, it is one of the stronger pieces of evidence against the theory that cognitive capacity protects against the development of dementia.

P.V. Rabins, M.D., M.P.H.

Long-Term Stability and Intercorrelations of Cognitive Abilities in Older Persons
Ivnik RJ, Smith GE, Malec JF, et al (Mayo Clinic and Found, Rochester, Minn)
Psychol Assessment 7:155–161, 1995   3–9

Introduction.—Little research has been done on the extent of normal variability in the performance of individuals on multiple tests of different cognitive abilities. It has been assumed that, for a given individual, functioning is similar across cognitive domains and that, in the absence of pathologic conditions, cognitive ability is stable over time. To examine the stability of mental abilities over time, a large group of independently functioning cognitively normal older individuals was tested in 1988 on the Wechsler Adult Intelligence Scale-Revised, Wechsler Memory Scale Revised, and the Auditory Verbal Learning Test. This group was retested in 1992 to examine the long-term stability of multiple tests of cognitive function.

Study Design.—The study group consisted of normal older individuals who participated in the Mayo Older Americans Normative Studies. Of the original 397 participants, 300 were retested. An additional 105 normal older individuals were recruited to be tested for the first time.

Results.—For the 300 participants who underwent retesting, the average interval between testings was 4 years. Of these 300, 52 were excluded from the study either because they had been reexposed to these same tests in other studies or because they were no longer considered cognitively normal. Among the remaining 248 participants, long-term stability coeficients were 0.86 for Verbal IQ, 0.79 for Performance IQ, and 0.61 to 0.78 for Memory/Concentration. Despite this variable performance stability, the average performance of the group on each index was constant. This was because of the age-corrected nature of the scoring on these tests, which masks changes occuring within individuals

Conclusions.—The results challenge the assumption that cognitive abilities are stable over long periods in the absence of pathologic conditions. None of the cognitive abilities measured in this study were truly stable, and the amount of stability was dependent on the type of cognitive ability being assessed. Finally, performance in 1 cognitive domain could not necessarily be used to predict performance in a different cognitive domain. Those who develop and use tests of cognitive performance will have to incorporate these findings into their interpretations of the results.

▶ This study, which presents longitudinal data from the Mayo Older Americans Normative Studies, has made important contributions by providing age-related norms on a number of cognitive tests. Data were reported on 300 individuals who were tested twice (several years apart) and a larger sample of individuals cross-sectionally examined to assess correlations among neuropsychological testings. The results demonstrate a significant degree of variability among tests. The implication of this finding is that variability in performance tests does not necessarily indicate dementia or cognitive impairment.

The study also demonstrates that tests vary in their rates of change. Verbal intellectual skills are most stable, whereas delayed free recall or retention of newly learned information is least stable. Because delayed free recall may be one of the most sensitive tests for dementia (see Abstract 3–6), it will be important to assess longer term follow-up data, as some of the variability within individuals might be evidence of early cognitive decline that did not show up on this 2-year follow-up study.

P.V. Rabins, M.D., M.P.H.

NONCOGNITIVE SYMPTOMS

The Behavior Rating Scale for Dementia of the Consortium to Establish a Registry for Alzheimer's Disease
Tariot PN, Mack JL, Patterson MB, et al (Univ of Rochester, New York; Case Western Reserve Univ, Cleveland, Ohio; Univ of Washington, Seattle; et al)
Am J Psychiatry 152:1349–1357, 1995   3–10

Background.—There is a wide range of psychopathologic signs and symptoms associated with dementia, and up to 90% of patients with dementia exhibit some of these signs during their illness. Psychopathology in these patients is significant in that patients' violent behavior may endanger others or themselves and can result in use of psychotropic medications, institutionalization, or restraint. The Consortium to Establish a Registry for Alzheimer's Disease (CERAD) developed the Behavior Rating Scale for Dementia, a comprehensive scale for describing psychopathology in patients with dementia that can be used by interviewers without extensive training in psychiatry. A pilot study was conducted.

Methods.—The subjects were 303 patients with probable Alzheimer's disease who underwent neurologic and neuropsychological evaluations done by the Consortium. The Behavior Rating Scale for Dementia was administered to each subject within 6 months of evaluation.

Results.—All subjects had at least 1 item that was present during the previous month; the average number of items present per subject was 15. The nature of disturbances varied significantly. The agreement between interviewers was high. There were 8 factors that mapped onto 10 rational domains: depressive features, psychotic features, defective self-regulation, irritability and agitation, vegetative features, apathy, aggression, and affective lability.

Discussion.—This instrument provides a comprehensive, reliable assessment of dementia. It was slightly modified after this study and translated into several languages. The primary goal was not to establish the validity of the instrument. Validation should be done after it has been modified and evaluated across a wider range of psychopathologic disorders.

▶ In recent years, many scales to quantitate the presence of specific symptoms have been developed. This study provides data on the CERAD behavior rating scale, a 51-item structured examination that provides data on a wide variety of symptoms. Factor analysis demonstrates 8 factors, which explain 38.5% of the variance. This article establishes and documents the psychometric properties of the CERAD scale. Similar data are not available on most other scales that seek to measure similar domains. One limitation of this instrument is its length, which will probably prevent its adoption in clinical settings. The next several years will determine which rating scales are adopted by researchers. Studies comparing instruments are sorely needed. It seems likely that longer instruments, such as this one, will be predominantly used in research studies, whereas shorter instruments will be used in drug studies in clinical settings.

P.V. Rabins, M.D., M.P.H.

Assessing Response to Tacrine Using the Factor Analytic Structure of the Alzheimer's Disease Assessment Scale (ADAS): Cognitive Subscale
Olin JT, Schneider LS (Univ of Southern California, Los Angeles)
Int J Geriatr Psychiatry 10:753–756, 1995   3–11

Objective.—The Alzheimer's Disease Assessment Scale-Cognitive subscale (ADASc) is the most commonly used measure of cognitive change in most clinical trials of drugs for Alzheimer's disease. In a multicenter clinical trial of the cholinesterase inhibitor tacrine, factor analysis of the ADASc was used to test whether each factor was sensitive to cognitive decline and whether factors represented distinct areas of cognition that differentially respond to treatment. With factor analysis, items on a test were aggregated on the basis of their relationship to the test's underlying structure.

Study Design.—In a multicenter, 30-week, double-blind, placebo-controlled, randomized trial, patients who met criteria for Alzheimer's disease based on the National Institute of Neurological and Communicative Disorders and Stroke-Alzheimer's Disease and Related Association were assigned to receive placebo or the cholinesterase inhibitor tacrine. Factor analysis was performed on 174 patients who completed the ADASc at both screening and 30 weeks.

Findings.—The factor analysis identified several distinct aspects of cognition, including language functioning, memory, and praxis. These 3 factors accounted for 64.5% of the variance in the ADASc. After 30 weeks, patients who received the placebo showed worsening on each factor score, whereas patients who took tacrine improved, with significant between-group treatment effects. Each ADASc factor score was sensitive to both the cognitive decline in Alzheimer's disease and the clinical effects of tacrine, indicating that tacrine had broad effects on cognition. None of the factors was significantly more sensitive to change than another, indicating that the treatment effect by each factor score was similar in magnitude.

Conclusions.—These findings indicate that the ADASc assesses several distinct aspects of cognition—language, memory, and praxis—and these confirm an earlier factor analysis conducted by Kim et al. Longitudinal change on the ADASc, whether the result of progression of Alzheimer's disease or clinical treatment, is meaningful when measured with a total score or with factor scores. The findings also indicate that the cholinesterase inhibitor tacrine has broad effects on cognition.

▶ The cholinesterase inhibitor tacrine is modestly effective in improving cognitive performance in persons with clinically diagnosed Alzheimer's disease. Because cholinesterase inhibitor therapies were developed because the cholinergic theory of memory suggested that increased synaptic acetylcholine levels might improve memory, it would be assumed that the modest improvement seen in some patients with tacrine might be the result of improvement in memory scores only. Using reanalyzed data from a previously reported tacrine trial, this study demonstrates that tacrine leads to improvement in language and praxis as well as in memory. Each of these is a primary impairment seen in Alzheimer's disease. The results of this study are compatible with either or both of the following: tacrine leads to a specific improvement in several different cognitive capacities that are known to be impaired in Alzheimer's disease, or tacrine has a generalized effect on one or more brain systems that underlie a number of cognitive capacities. If the latter is true, then the modest improvement seen with tacrine results from enhanced functioning of one or more widely distributed systems such as those that maintain attention. Whatever the theoretical implications, these results are important because they demonstrate that the multiple cognitive impairments caused by Alzheimer's disease are potentially responsive to pharmacologic treatment.

P.V. Rabins, M.D., M.P.H.

A Study of Visual Hallucinations in Alzheimer's Disease
Holroyd S, Sheldon-Keller A (Univ of Virginia, Charlottesville)
Am J Geriatr Psychiatry 3:198–205, 1995   3–12

Introduction.—The reported incidence of visual hallucinations in patients with Alzheimer's disease (AD) ranges from 12% to 53%. A number of other visual abnormalities may also be present in patients who have AD, and several studies have correlated these abnormalities with the pathologic findings of the visual system in AD. However, the possible associations between visual hallucinations and the visual system in AD have not been studied. Visual hallucinations in AD were correlated with visual disorders, visual function, and other variables.

Methods.—Ninety-eight patients with probable AD were screened for participation in the study. Those with visual hallucinations were matched by cognitive status to controls without visual hallucinations. The 2 groups were then compared for visual acuity, visual agnosia, and other variables. A model for distinguishing patients with AD with and without visual hallucinations was constructed using conditional logistic regression analysis.

Results.—Eighteen patients with visual hallucinations were identified and matched to 36 controls. The patients with visual hallucinations tended to be older, to be women, and to have visual agnosia and decreased visual acuity (Table 1). A "history of a visual disorder" fell short of significance. The 3 variables that best predicted the presence of visual hallucinations were age, acuity in the "best eye," and visual agnosia. A model including these 3 variables was able to correctly classify 91% of patients as being

TABLE 1.—Comparison of Patients With and Without Visual Hallucinations

Variable	With Hallucinations ($n = 18$)		Without Hallucinations ($n = 36$)		Statistical Analysis
	n (%)	Mean ± SD	n (%)	Mean ± SD	
Age, years	—	79.0 ± 6.2	—	73.6 ± 7.1	$t_{[1,52]} = 2.71; P = 0.009$
Female sex	16 (88.9)	—	21 (58.3)	—	OR = 5.714; $P^* = 0.021$
Visual acuity, "best eye," 20/	—	53.9 ± 16.1	—	41.0 ± 32.5	$t_{[1,51]} = 1.95; P^* = 0.028$
Visual agnosia, /6	—	1.1 ± 2.1	—	0.83 ± 0.4	$t_{[1,52]} = 2.105; P^* < 0.05$
History of visual disorder	6 (33.3)	—	4 (11.1)	—	OR = 4.000; $P^* = 0.056$

* Indicates one-tailed.
Abbreviation: OR, odds ratio.
(Courtesy of Holroyd S, Sheldon-Keller A: A study of visual hallucinations in Alzheimer's disease. *J Geriatr Psychiatry* 3:198–205, 1995.)

hallucinators or nonhallucinators. Only one third of the patients with hallucinations were receiving neuroleptic treatment.

Conclusion.—Visual hallucinations may be found in approximately one fifth of patients with probable AD. In AD, as in other disorders, visual hallucinations appear to be related to the visual system, including cortical pathologic conditions of the occipital and temporal lobes. More research is needed to determine the role of female sex in the development of psychotic symptoms in late life.

▶ Visual hallucinations can be a presenting symptom of AD, or they can develop during the course of the illness. In this study, 18.4% of individuals with AD were found to have visual hallucinations in a cross-sectional assessment. Older age, female sex, worse visual acuity, and a greater degree of visual agnosia were more common in hallucinators; a history of visual disorder approached statistical significance. Logistic regression analysis demonstrates that 3 factors correctly identified 91% of individuals: age (adjusted odds ratio, 1.3), poor visual acuity (adjusted odds ratio, 1.2), and visual agnosia score (odds ratio, 3.2). These data add to evidence suggesting that the development of visual hallucinations is multifactorial. The presence and severity of ocular pathology, the presence of a structural brain disease, and the localization of that disease (as suggested by an association with visual agnosia scores) all contribute to the development of hallucinations.

P.V. Rabins, M.D., M.P.H.

Incidence of Clinically Diagnosed Subtypes of Dementia in an Elderly Population: Cambridge Project for Later Life
Brayne C, Gill C, Huppert FA, et al (Univ of Cambridge, England; Medical Research Council, Cambridge, England; Monash Univ, Melbourne, Australia)
Br J Psychiatry 167:255–262, 1995   3–13

Purpose.—Epidemiologic studies of differential dementia diagnoses are rare. This study attempted to provide information on the incidence rates of Alzheimer's disease (AD) and vascular dementia, based on clinical diagnostic criteria incorporated into the Cambridge Examination for Mental Disorders of the Elderly (CAMDEX).

Study Design.—At baseline analysis, 2,616 participants older than 75 years of age were recruited from 7 family practices. They were interviewed at home using the Mini-Mental State Examination. All who scored 23 or less and 23% of those who scored 24 or 25 were reassessed, including a diagnosis of clinical dementia subtype. These 461 participants underwent follow-up analysis after an average of 2.4 years, using the CAMDEX.

Findings.—The most common diagnosis was AD. Most of the dementia was mild. There was an increase of incidence of AD with age for both sexes. The incidence of vascular dementia also increased with age but then decreased in the oldest age groups. The rates of vascular dementia were higher for men.

Conclusions.—In this study, most of the dementia was of the Alzheimer's type. The well-known increase in dementia incidence that occurred with increasing age was mostly attributable to an increase in AD, rather than to vascular dementia.

▶ It is well known that the incidence of dementia and AD rises with age—until at least age 90. This study demonstrates that this is not the case for vascular dementia. This is important for several reasons. First, this is the first study to show that the increasing prevalence of dementia with age can not be accounted for by an increasing incidence rate of vascular dementia. Second, the demonstration that the incidence of AD continues to rise sharply with age and reaches 6.2% in individuals 85 years of age and older confirms the specific linkage between AD and chronological aging. This supports the controversial hypothesis that AD is an intrinsic aspect of aging (although it certainly does not prove it).

A major limitation of this study is that the diagnosis was made from clinical data using the CAMDEX schedule. Although this instrument has good reliability for the diagnosis of dementia, its reliability for delineation of subtypes is weaker.

P.V. Rabins, M.D., M.P.H.

CAREGIVING

Psychiatric and Physical Morbidity Effects of Dementia Caregiving: Prevalence, Correlates, and Causes
Schulz R, O'Brien AT, Bookwala J, et al (Univ of Pittsburgh, Pa)
Gerontologist 35:771–791, 1995   3–14

Background.—Virtually all studies of caregivers of patients with Alzheimer's disease (AD) and related dementia published in the past decade have reported high levels of burden and distress associated with caregiving. However, many important questions remain. The literature on dementia caregiving was reviewed to determine the prevalence and magnitude of psychiatric and physical morbidity among caregivers, to identify individual and contextual correlates of reported health effects and their underlying causes, and to explore the policy relevance of the research findings.

Review.—Virtually all studies on the psychiatric effects of dementia caregiving report increased levels of depressive symptomatology among caregivers. Research including diagnostic interviews shows a greater prevalence of clinical depression and anxiety among caregivers compared with population norms or control groups. Caregivers also have a higher rate of psychotropic drug use than noncaregivers. The physical effects of caregiving are not as clear. Although caregivers' reported health is worse than that of noncaregivers, the evidence is weak and inconsistent. Predictors generally recognized as being risk factors for negative health outcomes are reported. However, there are relatively few associations unique to caregiving. Most patient characteristics and caregiver contextual variables are not related to caregiver health outcomes consistently.

Conclusions.—Research on the effects of providing care for demented individuals has progressed significantly in the past few years, although prospective studies are lacking. Many questions about the health effects of caregiving could be best answered by following a cohort of individuals making the transition from noncaregiving to caregiving roles. Although some questions still remain, existing findings are robust enough to warrant several policy suggestions. Caregiving produces measurable negative health effects that may be prevented or effectively treated. Also, there are a number of caregiver vulnerability factors to help identify who is most likely to experience negative health effects. Finally, because the problem behaviors of patients with AD are a unique source of distress among caregivers, specific interventions that change patient behavior or empower the caregiver should be developed.

▶ High rates of psychiatric morbidity in persons who care for an individual with dementia have been documented for 20 years. This article is a useful and well-balanced summary of the evidence. It confirms that depressive symptomatology is higher in caregivers, as are categorical major depression and anxiety. It challenges the widely held belief that there is a strong relationship between caregiving and poor physical health. It also confirms the widely reported relationship of psychiatric morbidity with income, poorer self-perception of situation, and low sense of mastery. Thus, caregiving is stressful but is not unique in the mechanisms by which it causes emotional distress.

The authors do not review the roles that religious background and belief systems play in adaptation to stress. This is one resource that is often overlooked by both clinicians and researchers. The authors also do not emphasize adequately that almost all the reviewed studies examine self-selected groups of caregivers. Nevertheless, an important clinical implication of this study is that individuals caring for a person with dementia can be helped by interventions that are helpful in other stressful situations.

P.V. Rabins, M.D., M.P.H.

A Comprehensive Support Program: Effect on Depression in Spouse-Caregivers of AD Patient
Mittelman MS, Ferris SH, Shulman E, et al (New York Univ)
Gerontologist 35:792–802, 1995   3–15

Introduction.—An intervention was developed to provide support for spouse-caregivers of patients with Alzheimer's disease (AD). The effect of this intervention on depressive symptomatology was evaluated in a longitudinal, randomized study.

Methods.—A total of 206 spouse-caregivers were studied for at least 1 year or until the death of the patient or caregiver. After recruitment, the caregivers were randomly assigned to either the treatment or control group, with 103 patients in each group. Patients in the treatment group received the intervention, which included mandatory individual and family counseling, continuously available ad hoc counseling, and support group participation from the time of recruitment until the death of the patient. The caregivers were evaluated every 4 months during the first year, every 6 months thereafter until the patient's death, and finally 1 year after the patient's death. The control group received standard assistance, including resource information upon request.

Results.—At baseline, female caregivers had more depressive symptoms than male caregivers and the severity of the patient's dementia was significantly associated with caregiver depression. After adjustment for caregiver sex and patient dementia severity, there were no significant differences in the number of depressive symptoms at baseline. However, over time, the control group had increasing depressive symptoms, whereas the symptoms in the treatment group were stable. The differences between the 2 groups in depressive symptomatology became significant by the eighth month. Multivariate analysis revealed an interaction between treatment and time. Treatment accounted for 23% of the variance in symptoms.

Conclusions.—An intervention that enhances social support can alleviate depressive symptoms in the caregivers of patients with AD. The treatment effect is typically not immediate, increasing over time.

▶ This article follows up on the authors' previous work demonstrating that persons who care for an individual with AD and who enter into a structured treatment program of group education and emotional support were less likely to place their relative into long-term care. In this article, the authors examine the effects of that intervention on mood and find that male and female caregivers in the active treatment group had a greater improvement in mood than caregivers in the available-resources group. One intriguing finding is that this improvement in mood is, in part, explained by an improvement in satisfaction with help received. This has an important clinical implication: Interventions that enable caregivers to use their available resources better can improve the caregiver's mood and delay nursing home placement. This is a nice demonstration of the power of psychosocial interventions.

Another finding of interest is that lessening financial worries and increasing the number of specific social contacts did not lead to mood improvement. This emphasizes a finding reported in many studies of caregivers and other individuals; the subject's or patient's subjective perception of a situation correlates more with distress than does an "objective" measure of situation severity such as financial difficulty. One finding of this study that is not reported by most other studies is a correlation between increasing severity of dementia and worsening mood. The authors are probably correct in suggesting that this lack of consistancy among studies is best explained by noting that the many different instruments used to measure disease severity vary, and that this is the most likely reason for the variability of this finding.

P.V. Rabins, M.D., M.P.H.

Depression

TREATMENT

Hospitalization for Major Depression Among Older Americans
Callahan CM, Wolinsky FD (Indiana Univ, Indianapolis)
J Gerontol 50A:M196–M202, 1995   3–16

Purpose.—Depression is common among elderly individuals. A representative sample of independently living older Americans was evaluated to report the rate and pattern of hospitalization for major depression. Changes in functional and social characteristics were examined to determine how they related to hospitalization for major depression in this group.

Study Design.—The data source was Version 5 of the Longitudinal Study on Aging (LSOA), which is the 6-year follow-up to the Supplement on Aging that was appended to the 1984 National Health Interview Survey. The LSOA includes 7,527 participants who were at least 70 years of age in 1984. All patients who were hospitalized for major depression among this group were identified. The total number of hospitalizations was tabulated per patient, and the hospital type, length of stay, and cost of care were established.

Findings.—Depression was the primary discharge diagnosis in 0.1% of patients. The mean length of hospital stay was 15 days, and the mean hospital charge was $6,742. The hospital type did not affect length of stay or the charge, but both were higher when major depression was the primay diagnosis. Patients who were hosptalized for major depression had more hospitalizations, longer lengths of stay, and more hospital charges over the 7-year study than did patients who were hospitalized for other reasons. Hospitalization for major depression was not associated with race, sex, education, or social support. Hospitalization for major depression was independently associated with a forced residential move, a history of nursing home care, a decrease in activities of daily living, and perception of poor health.

Conclusion.—One older American per thousand was hospitalized each year of the study with a primary diagnosis of major depression. Hospitalization for major depression was associated with loss of the ability to live independently and a perceived loss of health. Whether mechanisms for coping with these changes could be used to prevent hospitalization for major depression among the elderly population remains an unanswered question.

▶ Data from a nationally representative database were used to determine rates of hospitalization resulting from major depression among older Americans. The 1-year incidence rate of hospitalization for primary diagnosis of major depression was 0.1% (1 per 1,000). The authors note that the epidemiologic catchment study suggests that the yearly incidence rate for major depression is 0.9%. They conclude from this that approximately 11% of older individuals with major depression require hospitalization for depression.

The authors also found that hospitalization was more common among those who had a loss of independent living. Living alone and having a lack of social supports were not independently associated with hospitalization for major depression. The authors note that Jarvik[1] has speculated that a disability leads to depression by engendering a sense of loss of control, and they point out that their data are supportive of this hypothesis.

P.V. Rabins, M.D., M.P.H.

Reference

1. Jarvik LF: The impact of immediate life situations on depression: Illnesses and losses, in Breslau LD, Haug MR (eds): *Depression and Aging: Causes, Care, and Consequences.* New York, Springer, 1983.

Double-Blind, Placebo-Controlled Trial of Methylphenidate in Older, Depressed, Medically Ill Patients

Wallace AE, Kofoed LL, West AN (VA Med Ctr, White River Junction, Vt; VA Med Ctr, Sioux Falls, SD; Dartmouth Med School, Hanover, NH; et al)
Am J Psychiatry 152:929–931, 1995

3–17

Objective.—Although the use of amphetamine preparations in depressed patients is not approved by the Food and Drug Administration, some studies report the beneficial results of methylphenidate on depressive symptoms, particularly with older patients, in whom side effects and slow onset of action of antidepressant drugs are sometimes a problem. The results of a placebo-controlled, double-blind, crossover study of the effi-

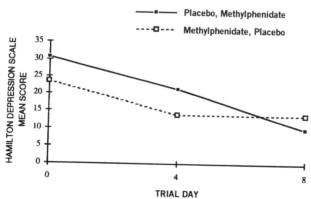

FIGURE 1.—Mean Hamilton Depression Rating Scale scores of 13 patients before and during an 8-day crossover trial of methylphenidate and placebo. (Courtesy of Wallace AE, Kofoed LL, West AN: Double-blind, placebo-controlled trial of methylphenidate in older, depressed, medically ill patients. *Am J Psychiatry* 152:929–931, 1995. Copyright 1995, the American Psychiatric Association. Reprinted by permission.)

cacy of methylphenidate in older, depressed, medically ill patients were presented.

Methods.—Sixteen depressed patients (5 women) with an average age of 72 years and with debilitating medical illnesses were given 5 mg of methylphenidate twice daily for 2 days, 10 mg twice daily for 2 days, and placebo for 4 days. Three patients receiving placebo first were dropped from the study, 1 because of death. Depressive scores were determined at baseline, day 4, day 8 (Fig 1), and 6 weeks after the trial. Four additional patients died during this time.

Results.—Methylphenidate administration improved depressive symptoms significantly more than did placebo. Only those who received methylphenidate before being given placebo had sustained improvement. There were no significant side effects. One patient experienced nervousness that abated after the methylphenidate dose was reduced.

Conclusion.—Methylphenidate is safe and effective in treating older, depressed, medically ill patients in whom rapid resolution of depressive symptoms is desirable to improve care and recovery.

▶ This study reports a small double-blind, placebo-controlled, crossover trial of methylphenidate in elderly, depressed, medically ill individuals. Thirteen subjects completed the trial. Patients receiving methylphenidate had greater improvement than those receiving placebo. Also of note is that improvement was evidenced within several days. This study is limited by small sample size and inclusion of the severity of medical illness; also, the number of individuals remaining in the trial for longer term data assessment was too small to draw adequate conclusions. However, tolerance did not develop in the 5 subjects who continued taking the medication for 6 weeks. Methylphenidate is widely used for the treatment of depression in the medically ill. This study supports its use.

P.V. Rabins, M.D., M.P.H.

Comparative Effects of Sertraline and Nortriptyline on Body Sway in Older Depressed Patients
Laghrissi-Thode F, Pollock BG, Miller M, et al (Univ of Pittsburgh, Pa)
Am J Geriatr Psychiatry 3:217–228, 1995   3–18

Background.—Falls are a major source of morbidity among the elderly population. The use of antidepressants, particularly the tricyclic antidepressants, has been associated with falls among elderly depressed patients. Older depressed patients are now being given selective serotonin reuptake inhibitors (SSRIs) as a safer alternative to tricyclic antidepressants, but their effects on balance in elderly individuals are unknown. The effects of antidepressant drugs on postural stability in older depressed patients was examined using a balance platform.

Methods.—The participants were inpatients of the Geriatric Clinical Research Unit of the Western Psychiatric Institute and Clinic in Pittsburgh.

They had been given a diagnosis of depression and were beginning treatment with either nortriptyline or sertraline. This study group was openly compared with healthy, elderly volunteers who were taking no psychotropic or cardiovascular medication. Body sway was quantified using a balance platform before medication was initiated, 5–7 days after medication was initiated, and 1 week later. All patients were evaluated at the same time of day. All participants were measured in a double leg stance, with feet together, looking straight ahead, focused on an object at a distance of 3 m, and with arms at their sides. They were evaluated both with eyes open and with eyes closed. Blood pressure and pulse were measured before and during each balance assessment.

Results.—The study group consisted of 20 healthy volunteers, 11 patients treated with nortriptyline, and 10 treated with sertraline. The demographic and clinical characteristics of the 3 groups were similar. The sertraline-treated patients had significantly increased postural sway during the first week of drug treatment but were able to compensate and reduce this sway by the second week of treatment. The changes in postural stability occured without hypotension and were clinically observable in 5 patients. Three patients complained of dizziness. There were no falls during the study period. The nortriptyline patients had no significant postural sway changes during the course of this study.

Conclusions.—The use of the SSRI antidepressant sertraline caused significant changes in postural sway in older depressed patients. Therefore, it would seem that to prevent falls, postural stability analysis should be part of the clinical workup for elderly depressed patients receiving SSRI medications.

▶ In this small study, individuals given the SSRI sertraline experienced increased body sway while receiving sertraline but not nortriptyline. Whether this indicates that sertraline specifically, or SSRIs in general, are associated with a high risk of falls remains to be seen. It is now known that SSRIs cause mild parkinsonism in some patients. Therefore, this association has a possible biological mechanism. The results of this study are surprising but should be given careful attention. The assumptions that SSRIs are safer for the elderly population than are tricyclics is challenged by these data, but further studies using larger samples and other SSRIs are needed before any change in practice can be recommended.

P.V. Rabins, M.D., M.P.H.

Long-Term Effects of Cognitive-Behavioural Therapy and Lithium Therapy on Depression in the Elderly

Wilson KCM, Scott M, Abou-Saleh M, et al (Inst of Human Ageing, Liverpool, England)
Br J Psychiatry 167:653–658, 1995   3–19

Background.—Depression has a high relapse rate in the elderly population. Uncontrolled trials have suggested that low doses of lithium can reduce the likelihood of relapse in elderly people with depression. A single study of cognitive-behavior therapy (CBT) in this age group found that it was associated with better maintenance of improvement than insight-oriented therapies. Cognitive-behavioral therapy was studied as an adjuvant to low-dose maintenance lithium therapy for elderly depressed patients in a 1-year follow-up study.

Methods.—Sixty-two consecutive elderly patients with major depressive disorder who were referred to an inner-city psychogeriatric center were studied. Thirty-one patients completed the study. All patients received the usual acute treatment—consisting of antidepressant treatment, major tranquilizers, and/or electroconvulsive therapy—and continuation therapy for depression. In addition, half of the patients received adjuvant CBT. The continuation phase was followed by a 1-year maintenance phase, during which the patients participated in a double-blind, placebo-controlled study of low-dose lithium therapy. This treatment aimed to maintain lithium levels of 0.4–0.8 mmol/L.

Results.—The patients who received adjuvant CBT had significantly lower scores on the Hamilton Rating Scale for Depression during their year of follow-up. However, there were no significant differences in depression scores for patients who took lithium vs. placebo for maintenance therapy.

Conclusions.—In elderly patients with severe depression, CBT can be an effective adjuvant therapy that reduces the severity of depression during follow-up. It can be used on an inpatient or outpatient basis and with patients who are receiving electroconvulsive therapy, antidepressants, and/or major tranquilizers. Further studies are needed to confirm the results. Low-dose lithium maintenance therapy was not effective in this study, most likely because of poor compliance.

▶ Relapse of major depression is common in patients of all ages, including the elderly population. In this small preliminary study, CBT was associated with lower Hamilton Rating Scale for Depression scores at 1-year follow-up than was either lithium carbonate or placebo. Although this finding does not directly address the issue of relapse, it does support the long-term benefit of CBT. A more serious limitation of this study is that it was not performed in a blind fashion. Nor does it appear that subjects were randomized. Therefore, this information should be viewed as preliminary data that document the importance of nonpharmacologic therapy for depression in the elderly population. Furthermore, better-designed studies should follow up on these preliminary data.

P.V. Rabins, M.D., M.P.H.

Comparison of the Efficacy of Titrated, Moderate-Dose and Fixed, High-Dose Right Unilateral ECT in Elderly Patients
McCall WV, Farah BA, Reboussin D, et al (Wake Forest Univ, Winston-Salem, NC)
Am J Geriatr Psychiatry 3:317–324, 1995   3–20

Background.—Electroconvulsive therapy (ECT), an effective treatment for depression among the elderly, is underused. Its underuse may be partly because of concerns about transient memory impairment, a common adverse effect of ECT. The use of right unilateral (RUL) stimulating electrode placement rather than bilateral placement may help mitigate against these memory effects. The efficacy and safety of titrated, moderate-dose RUL ECT were compared with those of fixed, high-dose ECT in elderly depressed patients.

Methods.—Nineteen patients, (mean age, 76 years) were randomly assigned to receive fixed, high-dose RUL ECT or titrated, moderate-dose RUL ECT. The Hamilton Rating Scale for Depression was completed before and after each treatment. The 9 patients receiving titrated, moderate doses had a mean convulsive threshold of 64 mC, with subsequent treatments at a mean dose of 151 mC. The 10 patients in the fixed, high-dose group received all treatments at 403 mC.

Outcomes.—Patients in the fixed, high-dose group responded faster than those in the titrated, moderate-dose group. The mean number of treatments for the 2 groups were 5.7 and 8, respectively. The groups had similar final depression ratings. Memory self-ratings were also comparable between groups.

Conclusions.—When obtaining a fast response or minimizing the total number of treatment sessions is the major concern, fixed, high-dose RUL ECT is superior to titrated RUL ECT. Further research including neuropsychologic tests of memory is needed to verify these findings.

▶ Electroconvulsive therapy has been used for 50 years. Its efficacy in moderate-severe depression and mania is well established. Modifications in technique have developed over the years. Their primary purpose has been to improve safety, although some improvements in efficacy have occurred. Among the most recent and important developments in technique is the work of Sackeim et al.[1] that established methods for determining threshold and dose determination. This study by McCall et al. demonstrates that older individuals improve more quickly with fixed, high-dose treatment even though the final outcomes, measured by depression and self-ratings of memory, were no different. Although economic pressures are mounting to identify treatments that are less costly, this study is too preliminary and the number of patients too small to be the basis of a change in practice. As the authors point out, closer attention to specific neuropsychological testing will be important because the higher-dose treatments could induce delirium more frequently and therefore increase the length of hospitalization. Electroconvulsive therapy is an effective and necessary treatment for severe late-life depression. This study suggests that the methods of delivering ECT can be improved further.

P.V. Rabins, M.D., M.P.H.

Reference

1. Sackeim HA, Prudic J, Devanard DP, et al: Affects of stimulus intensity and electrode placement on the efficacy and cognitive effects of electroconvulsive therapy. *N Engl J Med* 328:839–846, 1993.

Predicting the Course of Depression in the Older Population: Results From a Community-Based Study in The Netherlands
Beekman ATF, Deeg DJH, Smit JH, et al (Free Univ Amsterdam, The Netherlands)
J Affect Disord 34:41–49, 1995   3–21

Objectives.—Data from the Longitudinal Aging Study Amsterdam were analyzed to determine the course of depressive syndrome in a community-based random sample of older individuals and to identify factors predictive of outcome.

Methods.—After the initial interview, follow-up data were collected from 238 individuals, 55–89 years of age, in 5 successive waves covering 1 year. Depression was measured using a self-report rating scale, the Center for Epidemiologic Studies Depression Scale.

Outcome.—Half the elderly individuals experienced a depressive syndrome at some point during the study, 16% suffered an incident depression with half remitting during the study, 8% had depression initially that remitted during the study, 14% were chronically depressed, and 10% had a variable course (Table 3). When simplified to 3 categories, the course of

TABLE 3.—Course of Depression

Course	n	(%)
Never depressed	124	(52.1)
Incident depression with remission	18	(7.6)
Incident depression without remission	20	(8.4)
Remitted depression	19	(8.0)
Chronic depression	34	(14.3)
Variable course	23	(9.7)
Total	238	(100)

(Reprinted from Beekman ATF, Deeg DJH, Smit JH, et al: Predicting the course of depression in the older population: Results from a community-based study in The Netherlands. *J Affect Disord* 34:41–49, 1995, with kind permission of Elsevier Science-NL, Sara Burgerhartstraat 25, 1055 KV Amsterdam, The Netherlands.)

TABLE 4.—Simplified Types of Course of Depression

Course	n	(%)
Never depressed	124	(52.1)
Depressed but not throughout study	80	(33.6)
Chronic depression	34	(14.3)
Total	238	(100)

(Reprinted from Beekman ATF, Deeg DJH, Smit JH, et al: Predicting the course of depression in the older population: Results from a community-based study in The Netherlands. *J Affect Disord* 34:41–49, 1995, with kind permission of Elsevier Science-NL, Sara Burgerhartstraat 25, 1055 KV Amsterdam, The Netherlands.)

the depression indicated increasing duration of depression (Table 4). Of the 60 subjects who were depressed at the start of the study, 32% remitted without a relapse, 25% remitted but relapsed later, and 43% remained chronically depressed. The course of depression was not predicted by age, sex, level of education, or marital status. Health-related variables were predictive of both the onset and the course of depression. Illness episodes before the study, functional impairment (vision and hearing), pain, and subjective health were strongly correlated with the type of course and chronicity. There was a strong linear association between chronicity and contact with physicians, suggesting that treatment could be provided relatively easily.

Summary.—Approximately half of community-based older individuals will experience depression at some point during a 1-year study. Among those who are depressed at the start of the study, a disconcertingly high percentage will be chronically depressed. Indicators of physical health that pertain to global physical functioning are consistently predictive of chronicity.

▶ This study presents data on the development and course of depression during a 1-year period in community-based older individuals. In similar studies in younger individuals, almost 60% of persons identified as depressed either recover fully or recover and then relapse. In this study, 43% of individuals remained chronically depressed. The tables present the findings in more detail. Among the intriguing results are the facts that 16% of individuals in this community cohort developed depression during the course of the study and that only half of these remitted during the period of the study. Of course, some might have remitted after the 1-year period.

The study also examined correlates of chronicity. The presence of physical illness, degree of functional impairment, pain, and self-rated health all correlated with chronic depression, whereas older age was almost statistically significant. The presence of visual and hearing impairments specifically correlated with poor outcome.

These results contradict other epidemiologic studies that suggest that depression becomes uncommon in later life. They demonstrate both that depression is prevalent in old age and that new cases are constantly developing. Treating co-existing mood and physical illness simultaneously is likely to benefit a significant number of older persons.

P.V. Rabins, M.D., M.P.H.

MEDICAL COMORBIDITY

Mental Well-Being in People With Non–Insulin-Dependent Diabetes

Viinamäki H, Niskanen L, Uusitupa M (Kuopio Univ Hosp, Finland; Univ of Kuopio, Finland)

Acta Psychiatr Scand 92:392–397, 1995   3–22

Introduction.—Depression and mental comorbidity are more common in somatically ill individuals than in the general population, but the impact of diabetes on mental well-being is not known. The prevalence of minor mental disorder and depression in elderly patients with non–insulin-dependent (type 2) diabetes mellitus was studied.

Methods.—The study was based on cross-sectional data from the 10-year follow-up of 82 patients with type 2 diabetes with a mean age of 66.9 years and 115 nondiabetic control individuals of the same age; both groups were randomly selected from the general population. Both groups completed self-rating questionnaires, including the General Health Questionnaire (GHQ) for assessment of minor mental disorder and the Zung Self-rating Depression Scale for measuring depressive symptoms.

Findings.—Among elderly individuals with type 2 diabetes, the prevalence of cases of minor mental disorder (GHQ score >2) was 40% and the prevalence of depression (Zung score ≥50) was 11%, and both rates were similar to those of nondiabetic individuals. However, diabetic individuals with mental disorders were more severely affected than controls. The mean scores of GHQ and Zung scores tended to be higher in patients with diabetes than in control individuals. Logistic regression analyses demonstrated that minor mental disorder and depression were most clearly associated with symptomatic neuropathy. Age, sex, degree of obesity, mode of treatment, or levels of cardiovascular risk factors such as lack of exercise, blood pressure levels, smoking, or serum lipids were not related to minor mental disorder and depression.

Implications.—The impact of type 2 diabetes per se on minor mental disorder or depression in elderly individuals is not overwhelming. However, diabetic individuals appear to have markedly impaired well-being, and treatment of its underlying factors may improve overall treatment compliance. In particular, symptomatic neuropathy is significantly associated with minor mental disorder and depression. In some patients, refractory hyperglycemia may respond to antidepressive medication and psychotherapy.

▶ Many studies suggest that medically ill individuals have higher rates of depression than matched individuals without medical illness. This study did not confirm this finding in individuals with non–insulin-dependent diabetes mellitus. It did find, however, that within the group of individuals with diabetes, the presence of neuropathy was significantly correlated with depression. This adds to a growing body of information suggesting that chronic pain can be a cause of depression. The intriguing finding that antidepressant treatments can lessen the pain of neuropathy and also improve mood is reason for optimism and supports the need to recognize and aggressively treat neuropathic pain. The mechanisms leading to the association between chronic neuropathic pain and depression are not known. Cross-sectional studies such as this one do not prove a direction of causality. On the other hand, this study does highlight the importance of identifying neuropathic pain in diabetic patients. It would be intriguing to determine whether earlier recognition of neuropathy could prevent the development of depression or lessen its severity.

P.V. Rabins, M.D., M.P.H.

The Impact of Depression on Functioning in Elderly Patients With Low Vision

Shmuely-Dulitzki Y, Rovner BW, Zisselman P (Jefferson Med College, Philadelphia)

Am J Geriatr Psychiatry 3:325–329, 1995   3–23

Background.—Visual impairment is one of the most common, disabling conditions among elderly individuals. However, there have been no studies directly assessing the effects of depression and low vision on functioning in this population. The impact of depression on elderly patients at a low-vision clinic at 1 urban eye center was investigated.

Methods and Findings.—A geriatric nurse-practitioner interviewed 70 low-vision clinic patients older than 65 years using a structured clinical format to diagnose depression according to *Diagnostic and Statistical Manual of Mental Disorders,* Third Edition, Revised (DSM-III-R) criteria. Criteria for major depression were met by 38.6% of patients. Although depression was not associated with severity of visual impairment, depression was directly correlated with functional impairment. Depression was the factor most strongly associated with functional impairment.

Conclusions.—More than one third of the elderly patients had high levels of depression. Recognizing and treating depression in visually impaired elderly individuals may decrease functional disability and improve quality of life.

▶ Sensory impairments are prevalent in later life and are often hypothesized to be a precipitant of depression. This study examined the inter-relationships among visual impairment, depression, and functional impairment. The finding that visual impairment and depression are unrelated is surprising and unintuitive. On the other hand, the strong relationship between functional impairment and depression is both plausible and understandable. This suggests that it is not the impaired vision per se that leads to demoralization but how this impaired vision impacts on every day functioning that is key in precipitating depression.

This finding offers strong support for the rehabilitation model in which the maximization of function is a primary focus. It would be very interesting to determine whether a rehabilitation program focused on improving function would prevent or relieve depression. The major limitation of this study is that it used a general measure of functional impairment rather than a measure of impaired function resulting from visual impairment. This is problematic because it is possible that impairments other than visual were present and that these other impairments explain the lack of a relationship between the degree of visual impairment and depression.

P.V. Rabins, M.D., M.P.H.

Prevalence and Correlates of Depression in a Population of Nonagenarians

Forsell Y, Jorm AF, von Strauss E, et al (Karolinska Inst, Stockholm; Australian Natl Univ, Canberra)
Br J Psychiatry 167:61–64, 1995   3–24

Objective.—Despite the limited studies, there is evidence that depression is not uncommon in the oldest old. The prevalence of depressive symptoms and syndromes in nonagenarians and the correlates of depression in this age group were assessed.

Methods.—A total of 329 individuals aged 90 and older and registered in a parish of Stockholm, underwent extensive clinical examination by physicians and nurses. Depression was diagnosed using the *Diagnostic and Statistical Manual of Mental Disorders*, Fourth Edition (DSM-IV) and ICD-10 criteria and correlated with physical health, disability in daily life scored on the Katz Activity of Daily Living scale, sex, use of drugs, social circumstances, and cognitive function measured on the Swedish version of the Mini-Mental State Examination.

Findings.—The prevalence of major depressive episodes was 7.9% as defined in DSM-IV and 9.1% as defined in ICD-10 (mild, moderate, and severe depressive episode combined). The prevalence was similar in men and women, but depression was significantly related to the presence of malignant tumors, increased number of drugs taken, increased cognitive dysfunction, and increased disability in daily life. Multiple linear regression analysis identified disability in daily life and use of psychotropic drugs as the only factors that significantly correlated with depressive symptoms and syndromes.

Conclusion.—The prevalence of major depressive episodes in nonagenarians is slightly higher than the 2% to 4% prevalence typically reported in the younger elderly. Depression in the oldest old is associated with disability in daily living and use of psychotropic drugs, similar to that seen in younger adults. It appears that disability, rather than the physical disease per se, is the important risk factor for depression.

▶ We know little about the presence of nondementing psychiatric illness in the very old. This interesting study from a population sample in Stockholm demonstrates the prevalence of major depression is quite high in this very elderly group (7.9%). If a slightly broader definition of depression is used, prevalence increases to more than 9%. This finding demonstrates that depression remains a significant clinical problem in the very old and, indeed, might even be more prevalent in this age group than in the young old.

Perhaps the greatest limitation of this study is that the instruments it used have not been validated in very old individuals. Because no data on this issue are available, the study should not be dismissed because of this, but validity studies are certainly needed. Another finding of the study that must be cautiously interpreted is the finding that severe depression is associated with degree of functional disability. Because this is a cross-sectional study, we have no way of knowing whether the depression caused the disability, the disability caused the depression, or the two are related to some third factor such as poor physical health.

P.V. Rabins, M.D., M.P.H.

Depressive Symptomatology and Hypertension-Associated Morbidity and Mortality in Older Adults

Simonsick EM, Wallace RB, Blazer DG, et al (Natl Inst on Aging, Bethesda, Md; Univ of Iowa, Iowa City; Duke Univ, Durham, NC; et al)
Psychosom Med 57:427–435, 1995   3–25

Background.—Among older adults, there is a high prevalence of hypertension, which is an important risk factor for stroke and mortality. Similarly, depressive symptoms are common among the elderly and are a risk factor for cardiovascular disease. The diminished motivation, energy, and concentration associated with depression may have implications for blood pressure control and may precipitate a general health decline. The prevalence of concurrent depressive symptoms and hypertension in the elderly and the impact of depressive symptomatology on blood pressure control, stroke, and cardiovascular disease mortality were investigated.

Methods.—Data on social, behavioral, and environmental characteristics of elderly individuals and their morbidity and mortality were derived from the Established Populations for Epidemiologic Studies of the Elderly, which gathered data on older adults in 3 communities. Only data for individuals with diagnosed hypertension were used. Depressive symptomatology was assessed using 3 different instruments in the 3 communities, all having items derived from the Center for Epidemiologic Studies–Depression Scale, during years 3 and 6 of the study. Data on morbidity and mortality were collected annually for 6 years.

Results.—High depressive symptomatology was present in 9.4% to 13.5% of the men and 20.6% to 27.1% of the women with diagnosed hypertension. These depressed patients consistently had significantly higher rates of disability, angina, myocardial infarction, stroke, and digitalis treatment. There was a trend toward an association between high depressive symptomatology and poor blood pressure control, but this association did not attain significance. The depressed men and women in

2 communities each had rates of stroke 2.3–2.7 times higher than the nondepressed individuals.

Conclusions.—Hypertensive patients with high levels of depressive symptoms have an increased risk of stroke, which may be partly related to poor blood pressure control. However, the data do not allow conclusions regarding the nature of the association: whether depressive symptoms are a cause or consequence of morbidity. Further study of this relationship is warranted.

▶ This study illustrates many of the complexities that bedevil researchers trying to understand the relationship between depression and medical co-morbidity even when the data are longitudinal. Because the relationship between depressive symptoms and higher blood pressure was present at the beginning of the study, the authors were not able to determine whether depressive symptoms result from hypertension (e.g., caused by hypertension-related brain vascular disease that induces a depression), whether depression interferes with participation in treatment for hypertension and increases the risk of stroke, or whether the symptoms measured by the instruments overlap. Nevertheless, the finding that rates of stroke were between 2.3 and 2.7 times higher in individuals with high depressive symptomatology is extremely important.

The study also illustrates several methodological points. The authors are to be congratulated for comparing findings across the different study sites. No finding was present at all sites in both men and women. The reason for this is not clear. Unfortunately, the 3 sites used different forms of the instrument to measure depression. This weakens the capacity to examine these important questions and suggests that multisite centers should be required to use similar instruments.

Both depression and hypertension are treatable. Good data exist to demonstrate that prompt, effective treatment of each improves health and well-being. Whether there is something unique about the association between depression and hypertension remains to be seen, but the evidence presented here suggests a synergistic relationship. Future studies might establish whether early treatment of depression or hypertension prevents the development of, or improves the outcome of, the other.

P.V. Rabins, M.D., M.P.H.

Depression in a Long-Term Care Facility: Clinical Features and Discordance Between Nursing Assessment and Patient Interviews
Burrows AB, Satlin A, Salzman C, et al (Harvard Med School, Boston)
J Am Geriatr Soc 43:1118–1122, 1995   3–26

Background.—Although depression is common among nursing home residents, it is diagnosed and treated infrequently. Nurses report more symptoms of depression than do doctors, and they may represent a valuable resource for the identification of depressed patients. A group of nursing home patients who were identified by their long-term care nurses as being depressed but who were not being treated for depression were examined.

Study Design.—The study participants were residents of an academic, long-term care facility who did not live in units designed for dementia or behavioral disorders. Each resident had a bimonthly functional assessment that included a rating of depression. Residents rated as depressed by caregivers and not receiving antidepressants were chosen to participate in this study. The participants were examined by semistructured interviews and a modified Cornell Scale for Depression. Both nurse and patient were interviewed by the same person.

Study Group.—Of the 495 residents, 110 were rated as depressed by the primary nurse. Of these 110 patients, 58 were not receiving antidepressant medication. Twenty-one patients were excluded from the study because of Mini-Mental State Examination scores less than 10, inability to communicate, acute mental illness, death, or schizophrenia, leaving 37 patients in the study group. The average age of these patients was 88 years, and the majority were female.

Findings.—When patient interviews were analyzed using *Diagnostic and Statistical Manual of Mental Disorders,* Third Edition, Revised (DSM-III-R) criteria, 9 patients in the study group met the criteria for major depression, 20 met the criteria for nonmajor depression, and 8 had no apparent mood disorder. The correlation between nurse and patient interview Cornell scores was poor, particularly for patients with nonmajor depression.

Conclusions.—Nurses in long-term care facilities often reported depressive symptoms in patients who were not given a diagnosis of depression. These nurse-derived patient ratings did not correlate well with ratings derived from patient interviews. The authors of this study did not attempt to determine whether patient interviews or nurse ratings were more accurate in the diagnosis of patient depression. However, these findings do suggest that caregivers have access to different information than physicians and that this may provide a valuable resource in the care of the depressed elderly nursing home resident.

▶ This study documents the well-known fact that nurses' and residents' ratings of depressive symptoms in nursing home residents are often discordant. In general, nurses report more symptoms. A substantial body of studies demonstrates that the ascertained rates of depression in the elderly population depend significantly on the source of the information. What remains to be demonstrated is the validity of such a diagnosis; i.e., we do not know who is more accurate: residents, staff, or family.

The predictive validity of diagnosis has been shown in studies that demonstrate that individuals with staff- and instrument-rated depression have poorer outcomes (i.e., nursing home placement, rapidity of cognitive decline, and short-term death rates) than do nondepressed individuals. Similar studies that use these outcomes to compare prediction among different raters would be an important step in deciding the best source of ratings.

Even more convincing would be data demonstrating response to pharmacologic and behavioral treatments for depression. Until we have such data, the reliance on external informants used by Alexopoulos in developing the Cornell Scale for Depression is appropriate.

P.V. Rabins, M.D., M.P.H.

Major and Minor Depression in Later Life: A Study of Prevalence and Risk Factors
Beekman ATF, Deeg DJH, van Tilburg T, et al (Free Univ of Amsterdam)
J Affect Disord 36:65–75, 1995   3–27

Background.—Depression is one of the most common psychiatric disorders among elderly persons. It has been associated with declines in well-being and levels of daily functioning and an increased risk of functional impairment, mortality, and use of health services. The prevalence rates of minor and major depression appear to shift in the older age group, with the prevalence of major depression decreasing and that of minor depression increasing among the older elderly. Whether major and minor depression in this age group are determined by different sets of risk factors was investigated.

Methods and Findings.—The study participants were part of the Longitudinal Aging Study Amsterdam, a 10-year longitudinal study of the predictors and consequences of changes in well-being and autonomy among individuals aged 55–85 years. The prevalences of major and minor depression were 2.02% and 12.9%, respectively. Fifteen percent had clinically relevant levels of depressive symptoms. Neither age nor sex substantially affected associations with a comprehensive set of risk factors. However, the distribution of risks for major and minor depression differed markedly. Major depression appeared more often to be an exacerbation of a chronic mood disorder, rooted in long-standing vulnerability factors. Minor depression more often appeared to be a reaction to the stresses commonly experienced in later life.

Conclusions.—If these findings are verified by longitudinal studies, they will have major implications for clinical practice. For elderly individuals with minor depression, treatment would be aimed primarily at the amelioration of the effects of current stresses, such as lack of interpersonal support and impaired daily functioning resulting from physical disease. For those with major depression, treatments found effective in younger adults would be used without delay.

▶ The results of this study are surprising and add to the increasing database supporting the idea that minor and major depression may be distinct conditions. The demonstration that major depression is more likely to reflect a chronic mood disorder and that minor depression is more likely related to precipitating life events does not support the hypothesis that major and minor depression are on a continuum. The authors state that these results imply that the treatments for the 2 conditions should be different. This is certainly a testable hypothesis. However, before treatment studies are initiated it will be important to confirm these results in longitudinal studies. Recall bias is always a potential major source of confound in cross-sectional studies and necessitates confirmation in prospective cohorts. Further research into minor and major depression will need to document similarities or differences in course, treatment response, comorbidity, familial studies, and outcomes. Premature closure on the questions raised by this study would be harmful to the many patients who have these disorders.

P.V. Rabins, M.D., M.P.H.

The Impact of Somatic Morbidity on the Hamilton Depression Rating Scale in the Very Old
Linden M, Borchelt M, Barnow S, et al (Free Univ of Berlin)
Acta Psychiatr Scand 92:150–154, 1995   3–28

Background.—The Hamilton Depression Rating Scale (HDRS) is the most commonly used scale for assessing the depressive syndrome. However, many items on this scale refer to somatic symptoms, which jeopardize the validity of HDRS scores in patients with comorbidity. The validity of the HDRS in patients with depressive illness and somatic diseases was investigated.

Methods.—Five hundred sixteen patients aged 70 years and older were studied. Internists and psychiatrists independently evaluated these patients. The internists then rated each positive HDRS item on the extent to which it reflected somatic illness.

Findings.—More than half of all psychiatrist-rated positive scores on 8 items could be related to somatic disease according to the internists. Patients with corrected HDRS scores had a greater rate of medication use and cardiovascular diagnoses. The interpretation of items rated by psychiatrists as being more severe was less ambiguous.

Conclusions.—Multimorbidity can impair the validity of the HDRS total and individual scores. The strong emphasis on psychomotor and somatic symptoms, which commonly occur in elderly persons, casts doubt on the validity of the HDRS.

▶ This study examines one of the major challenges of clinical practice: How does one distinguish between somatic complaints secondary to depression and somatic complaints that reflect physiologic disease? One of the strengths of this study is that it comes from a representative community sample of older individuals. A second strength is that it used the HDRS, the most commonly used instrument to rate depression. Its central finding is that several symptoms identified by psychiatrists as positive on the HDRS have a significant probability of being rated by internists as being caused by physical illness. Apparently, all patients in the study were evaluated in person by both a psychiatrist and an internist.

Unfortunately, this study has a central flaw, which demonstrates the difficulty of doing research on this subject. In fact, this difficulty is the same one faced by the clinician: How does one validate whether depression is present and whether a specific somatic symptom is caused by depression or a physical illness? In this study, the internist's opinion was used as the "gold standard" to categorize a specific symptom as possibly or very probably caused by a somatic rather than a psychiatric cause, but no data are presented to demonstrate that the internist is any more reliable or valid at making this distinction than a psychiatrist. Clinical experience suggests that the distinction is a difficult one and that no one profession is better than the other at making the differentiation. Before accepting this study as having any utility, it would be important to determine the reliability of the observations among internists and psychiatrists. Follow-up medical and psychiatric evaluations, course of illness, and response to treatment could provide data by validating the diagnosis. Exploratory analyses might identify other markers that can improve accuracy.

The HDRS remains widely used. The Yesavage Geriatric Depression Scale was specifically developed to avoid reliance on somatic items. However, no convincing data exist that allow the clinician or researcher to decide whether the HDRS or Geriatric Depression Scale is better for a specific purpose. Follow-up studies would be helpful in addressing the important questions raised by this study. Unfortunately, the data presented in this study do not help advance our understanding of this difficult issue.

P.V. Rabins, M.D., M.P.H.

SUICIDE

Attitudes of Older People Toward Suicide and Assisted Suicide: An Analysis of Gallup Poll Findings
Seidlitz L, Duberstein PR, Cox C, et al (Univ of Rochester, New York)
J Am Geriatr Soc 43:993–998, 1995   3–29

Introduction.—In November 1992, the Gallup Organization surveyed a large group of independently living older Americans to determine their attitudes toward suicide and assisted suicide. The demographic and psychosocial correlates of these attitudes were also investigated.

Study Group.—The sample included 541 women and 261 men selected on the basis of randomly generated telephone numbers. Participants had to be at least 60 years of age and living independently.

Study Design.—The telephone interview was conducted by trained Gallup employees and focused on 5 items assessing attitudes toward suicide. Each attitude was examined as it related to the age, sex, race, marital status, income, religious feelings, health, and family relationships of the respondent.

Findings.—The majority of respondents did not view suicide favorably, although opinion was about evenly divided in cases of incurable disease with severe suffering. Univariate analysis indicated that age, sex, race, marital status, income, and religious feeling all influenced attitudes toward suicide. The best univariate predictor was religiousness. Logistic regression indicated that race and religiousness predicted agreement with assisted suicide; religiousness and income predicted agreement with a society that respects suicidal wishes; sex and family relationships were associated with the attitude that suicide is personal; and age and marital status did not independently predict attitudes toward suicide.

Conclusions.—This Gallup telephone survey of older Americans provides a glimpse of the view of the elderly toward suicide and assisted suicide at this time. Nonreligious white men with strained family relationships and a perception of failing health had the most lenient attitude toward suicide. These factors are known risk factors for completed suicide. Health care providers need to understand the attitudes of their older patients toward end-of-life decisions and to determine whether these attitudes are linked to known risk factors for attempted suicide.

▶ Forty-one percent of participants in a 1992 Gallup Organization survey of 802 individuals who were 60 years of age and older believed that physician-assisted suicide should be legalized. Respondents who were male; white; separated or divorced; and reported that religion played a minor, little, or no role in their life were more likely to support physician-assisted suicide. As the authors note, these are risk factors for suicide.

Because these data are cross-sectional, conclusions must be very tentative. For example, several recent studies have demonstrated a significant degree of variability and advanced-directives over time. It may well be that attitudes toward suicide will change over time. Experience teaches us that attitudes about illness and death often change when the issue becomes an actual possibility rather than an abstract possibility. The recent report of an increase in suicide among the very old[1] and the apparent change in attitude towards the ethics of suicide and physician-assisted suicide reported in this study require that these contentious issues be discussed and debated further.

P.V. Rabins, M.D., M.P.H.

Reference

1. Suicide among older persons—United States, 1980–1992. *MMWR Morb Mortal Wkly Rep* 45:3–6, 1996.

Factors Associated With the Wish to Die in Elderly People
Jorm AF, Henderson AS, Scott R, et al (Australian Natl Univ, Canberra; Mental Health Research Inst of Victoria, Australia)
Age Ageing 24:389–392, 1995   3–30

Objective.—Data from an Australian epidemiologic study of individuals aged 70 years or older were analyzed to determine the prevalence of the wish to die in elderly individuals and to investigate the factors associated with it.

Methods.—The participants were interviewed using the Canberra Interview for the Elderly, a standardized psychiatric interview for use by lay interviewers covering dementia, depression, and related disorders. The participants were asked whether, in the past 2 weeks, they had felt that they wanted to die and, if so, if they had such thoughts repeatedly. Three classes of possible risk factors were investigated, including sociodemographic factors (age, sex, and marital status), mental health factors (depression, cognitive impairment), and physical health (poor self-rated health, disability, pain, sensory impairment, and living in a nursing home or hostel).

Results.—Response rate was 69%. Only 21 (2.3%) elderly persons reported repeatedly having had a wish to die during the previous 2 weeks. Depression was an important risk factor for wishing to die, but a small minority of patients had no evidence of depressed mood. After adjustment for depressive symptoms, multiple logistic regressions identified unmarried status, poor self-rated health, disability, pain, hearing impairment, visual impairment, and residential care as statistically associated with the wish to die. The strongest association was with being in residential care.

Summary.—The wish to die has a strikingly low prevalence in elderly individuals. Although the wish to die in the elderly may be associated with depressed mood, depression is not invariably present. Other factors are independently linked to the wish to die, and further studies should evaluate whether treatment of these factors can restore the desire to live.

▶ It is widely believed that depression is common in older individuals and that the wish for life to end is also likewise common. This study has 2 strengths in addressing these issues. It is an epidemiologic study and collected enough data to examine a number of hypotheses. The finding that only 2.3% of individuals aged 70 years or older studied in this Australian sample reported having had the wish to die during the 2 weeks before the study is unexpectedly low. Furthermore, most individuals who express this wish are depressed. There is also a relationship between the wish to die and a number of social and demographic variables. It is more likely in those who are single, and who live in a nursing or a group home. It is also related to physical health variables: poor self-rated health, pain, and hearing and visual impairment. These relationships suggest the wish to die is multifactorial.

The strong association with depression suggests that individuals who express a wish to die should be assessed carefully for the presence of depression. Clinical experience suggests that, when depression is present and responds to treatment, the wish to die usually abates. However, for individuals who are not depressed or who are depressed but give reasons unrelated to their depression, the appropriate course for the clinician is less established. Referral for help with social problems, supportive listening, and explorations of the meaning of death are appropriate clinical options.

P.V. Rabins, M.D., M.P.H.

The Long-Term Effects of Later Life Spousal and Parental Bereavement on Personal Functioning

Arbuckle NW, de Vries B (Univ of British Columbia, Vancouver, Canada)
Gerontologist 35:637–647, 1995

3–31

Background.—Investigators have found the death of a spouse or a child to be the most disruptive and stressful of familial losses. The long-term effects of bereavement on personal functioning were examined in older adults 2–15 years after the death of a spouse or adult child, with particular attention to the significance of sex and of the type of bereavement.

Methods.—Data were obtained from the large national survey, *Americans' Changing Lives: Wave 1, 1986.* Three study samples of adults older than 55 years of age were identified: 41 parents (19 men and 22 women) who had lost an adult child, 143 widowed adults (31 men and 112 women), and 407 nonbereaved adults (164 men and 243 women). The deaths had occurred 2–15 years previously (average, 6.4 years for parents and 7.5 years for spouses). Personal functioning was assessed with measures of perceived health, self-efficacy, depression, life satisfaction, fatalism, vulnerability, future planning, and the ability to complete plans. The effects of age, education, income, race, unexpectedness of loss, duration of bereavement, type of bereavement, and sex on the measures of personal functioning were examined in multiple regression analyses.

Results.—Perceived health was significantly predicted only by education and income. These factors were also important predictors of self-efficacy, as were sex and the type of bereavement. Sex, age, education, and the duration of bereavement had significant effects on the depression index. Life satisfaction was largely dependent on income and the duration of bereavement, but there were no differences in the effects of the type of bereavement. Sex was a significant predictor of fatalism and vulnerability, but not future planning. There was a significant interaction effect between sex and spousal bereavement as the ability to complete plans was predicted. Education, income, age, race, and the duration of bereavement also had significant effects in the prediction of these measures of future orientation. The sex effects always predicted lower levels of personal functioning among women.

Conclusions.—The variations in personal functioning variables were only modestly explained by differences in sex and the type of bereavement, which suggests that long-term adaptation to bereavement is a complex process that encompasses both psychological and physiological variables considered within both familial and sociohistorical contexts.

▶ Bereavement is a universal human experience that also occurs in animals. Previous studies of bereavement have fallen into 3 categories: descriptive studies, which demonstrate that usual grief follows a predictable course in most individuals; studies that examine the relationship between depression and grief after the bereavement; and long-term studies; which suggest that the bereaved are at higher risk for adverse physical health. In general, these previous studies have examined small groups of individuals who were not randomly ascertained.

A major strength of the Arbuckle and de Vries study is that it used a national probability sample. Several findings are intriguing. First, adverse effects of bereavement such as lower life satisfaction can persist for a number of years. Second, widowed adults reported higher self-efficacy than a long-term married comparison group. These findings suggest that bereavement may have long-term adverse effects, but that positive benefits can also be identified.

However, the limitations of the study are significant and undermine confidence that these relationships are true. The findings are based on cross-sectional comparisons; individuals were not identified before their bereavement and followed over time, but rather the data were collected at one time. Also, there is no measure or discussion of the quality of relationships between the bereaved and the deceased person. Finally, because this study is cross-sectional, it could not examine which bereavement had adverse effects on physical health.

P.V. Rabins, M.D., M.P.H.

Schizophrenia

Cognitive Impairment in Elderly Schizophrenia: A Dementia (Still) Lacking Distinctive Histopathology
Arnold SE, Trojanowski JQ (Philadelphia)
Schizophr Bull 22:5–9, 1996   3–32

Introduction.—Since the first descriptions of schizophrenia, there has been controversy regarding the nature of cognitive impairment in the disease; some investigators emphasize the general disorder of thought processes without cognitive deterioration while other investigators emphasize the progressive cognitive deterioration.

Longitudinal Studies.—There have been few longitudinal studies of schizophrenia that examine cognitive performance. Most have found significant heterogeneity in the patients studied, with a subgroup experiencing declining orientation, memory, and other cognitive functions. This heterogeneity may reflect differing pathological processes in schizophrenia or treatment differences that have modified the disease course.

Cross-Sectional Studies.—Cross-sectional studies of schizophrenia have generally found increasing cognitive impairment and negative symptoms as well as decreasing positive symptoms with increasing age. One study showed no correlations between cognitive performance and neuroleptic use or somatic treatments such as electroconvulsive therapy, insulin coma, and leukotomy. In this same study, a subgroup of patients retested after 1–2 years had no significant cognitive deterioration.

Autopsy Studies.—Postmortem studies have not revealed recognizable neuropathologic abnormalities such as neurofibrillary tangle, senile plaque formation, excess protein abnormalities, or apolipoprotein E genotype distribution that explain severe dementia in schizophrenic patients. However, some studies have found more Alzheimer's disease (AD) lesions in schizophrenic patients, particularly those treated with antipsychotic medication. This raises the possibility that neuroleptic treatment may induce neurofibrillary tangle formation. These conflicting findings may be related to misdiagnosis, which has been found to occur frequently.

Conclusions.—Better-designed studies are needed. These should use standard diagnostic and assessment instruments to study both community and institutionalized patients and psychiatric control groups with longitudinal follow-up. The possibility of both AD-specific markers and less specific markers (such as neuron loss, astrogliosis, microglia proliferation, synapse-related proteins, metabolic markers, neurochemical markers, and programmed cell death markers) should be evaluated. Because cytoarchitectural, morphometric, synaptic, and neuroreceptor abnormalities have been found in schizophrenic patients, particularly in the hippocampal region, the possibility that these abnormalities may enhance the significance of subtle neurodegenerative pathology should be explored.

▶ When Emil Kraepelin first described the disease we now call schizophrenia, he chose the label "dementia praecox" because he recognized that the disease caused social deterioration. This article provides a useful reminder that schizophrenia is sometimes associated with a dementia in late life and that neuropathologic studies are not yet able to explain this. As reviewed in this article, more recent studies tend to find little neuropathology even in severely incapacitated individuals whereas studies that rely on autopsy material collected in the past find higher rates of AD pathology. This review reminds us that it is important to pay attention to details such as how samples were collected and to review whether appropriate diagnostic standards were used. Using currently available neuropathologic, neurochemical, and molecular biological approaches, researchers should be able to unravel the mystery.

P.V. Rabins, M.D., M.P.H.

Clinical and Neuropsychological Characteristics of Patients With Late-Onset Schizophrenia
Jeste DV, Harris MJ, Krull A, et al (San Diego VA Med Ctr, Calif; Univ of California, San Diego)
Am J Psychiatry 152:722–730, 1995   3–33

Purpose.—The definition of late-onset schizophrenia remains controversial. The goal of this research was to examine the clinical and neuropsychological characteristics of patients who had clearly defined late-onset schizophrenia.

Study Design.—Patients were recruited from a Veterans Administration Medical Center, a university Medical Center, county mental health services, and private physicians in the San Diego area. Over 3 years, 74 patients were referred for psychotic symptoms that had developed after the age of 45 years. Some participants were excluded because of a failure to comply, substance abuse, dementia, earlier onset of symptoms, or diagnosis of other psychotic syndromes. Exclusion of these participants permitted the selection of 25 patients, who met the *Diagnostic and Statistical Manual of Mental Disorders,* Third Edition, Revised (DSM-111-R) criteria for late-onset schizophrenia as the study group. This group was compared with 39 participants with early-onset schizophrenia and 35 normal participants. All participants were assessed by a structured neurologic and medical history and underwent a complete physical examination.

Findings.—All 3 groups had similar levels of education, but the normal group was significantly older. The late-onset and normal groups had more women than did the early-onset group. There was a significantly higher proportion of patients with the paranoid subtype of schizophrenia in the late-onset group than in the early-onset group. The late-onset and early-onset group were similar to each other, but different from the normal group on psychopathology tests. Most of the late-onset group had chronic illness. None of the normal group had a family history of schizophrenia, while the same proportion of both late- and early-onset patients did have a family history of schizophrenia. The early-onset patients had occupational difficulties since early adulthood and had frequently not been married. The late-onset group had had jobs or raised families until middle age. At the time of the study, the proportion of currently married patients was the same in both the early- and late-onset groups. Both schizophrenic groups were similar in psychosocial history variables, including childhood variables, and were significantly different from the normal group. The schizophrenic participants were significantly worse than the normal participants on measures of executive functions, learning, motor skills and verbal ability, but were similar to the normal group in delayed recall, perceptual motor skills, and sensory abilities.

Conclusions.—Patients with late-onset schizophrenia, after the age of 45, were quite similar to early-onset schizophrenics in ratings of psychopathology and neuropsychological impairment and quite different from normal volunteers. These findings support the DSM-IV assertion that late-onset schizophrenia is similar to early-onset schizophrenia. The late-onset group had better premorbid functioning in adolescence and early adulthood and was more likely to have the paranoid subtype of schizophrenia. It will be necesssary to study larger groups to determine whether late-onset schizophrenia is a distinct schizophrenia subtype.

▶ In this study, 25 individuals who met the criteria for schizophrenia developing after 35 years of age were compared with 39 individuals in whom schizophrenia developed before age 45 years and 35 normal individuals. The 2 groups of individuals with schizophrenia were similar in psychopathology, family history, childhood social adjustment, and patterns of neuropsychological impairment. This study adds to data supporting the contention that schizophrenia-like illnesses that develop after age 45 years are part of the schizophrenic spectrum. The demonstration of high rates of childhood social maladjustment in the late-onset group suggests that individuals with the late-onset condition may have been predisposed to development of the disorder early in life but were protected by an as-yet-unidentified factor.

P.V. Rabins, M.D., M.P.H.

Memory Functions in Geriatric Chronic Schizophrenic Patients: A Neuropsychological Study

Harvey PD, Powchik P, Mohs RC, et al (Mount Sinai School of Medicine, New York)

J Neuropsychiatry Clin Neurosci 7:207–212, 1995   3–34

Background.—Studies on memory functions in schizophrenia have demonstrated deficits in acquisition and short-term retention of information, but not in remembering information that was successfully learned. These findings suggest that anatomical circuits responsible for memory functioning are impaired in schizophrenia and that these memory deficits reflect a neuropsychological deficit that may be localized to these regions. However, nearly all these studies of memory function in schizophrenia have examined young patients, most of them younger than 45.

Methods.—In 49 geriatric, chronically institutionalized schizophrenia patients, memory functions were examined with a battery of tests sensitive to neuropsychological impairments in either temporal or frontal regions, including tests on spatial delayed response and spatial delayed alternation; verbal recall and recognition; digit span; and supraspan digit learning. All patients met *Diagnostic and Statistical Manual of Mental Disorders,* Third Edition, criteria for schizophrenia and all had global Clinical Dementia Rating (CDR) scores of 2 (moderate) or lower and had not received leukotomy.

Results.—On the basis of the CDR scores, 24 patients were considered cognitively impaired and 25 were less impaired. Except for the correct recall of the first supraspan digit string, cognitively impaired patients demonstrated significantly more impairment in memory measures than the less cognitively impaired. Principal component analysis showed that performance on tests sensitive to frontal and temporal lobe memory functions had a statistical factor structure consistent with their putative localization. Furthermore, discriminant factor analysis indicated that both factors contributed independently to the differentiation of cognitively impaired and less impaired cases.

Summary.—These findings suggest that, in elderly patients with schizophrenia, clinically rated cognitive impairments are associated with deficits in memory functions that are hypothetically localized in both the frontal and temporal regions of the cerebral cortex, and the patterns of impairments are not consistent with a generalized deficit.

▶ This is a preliminary study of cognitive performance in elderly individuals with life-long schizophrenia. The results confirm what Emil Kraepelin reported 100 years ago: Individuals with the disease we now call schizophrenia can suffer from a generalized decline in cognitive performance, which manifests itself in impaired social and interpersonal performance. The more interesting finding of this study is the fact that the impairments were not generalized and therefore are different from those found in Alzheimer's disease. The results suggest that impairments are primarily in "frontal" and "temporal" cognitive functions. However, this interpretation must be interpreted with caution because the authors do not report scores on tests that measure performance in other cognitive realms. Presumably those data will be published in the future. The study also found significant variability in cognitive impairments among individuals. This suggests that there is not one single pattern of brain involvement in chronic schizophrenia.

Neuropathologic studies are now being published on this sample from New York state as well as from other samples.[1] They also support the conclusion that the dementia seen in elderly individuals with schizophrenia is neither Alzheimer's disease nor any other pathologically recognizable dementing illness. The causes of these neuropathologic changes and their linkage to the decline in social and cognitive function in schizophrenia is unknown. The answer to this question might lead to better treatments and perhaps even prevention of decline.

P.V. Rabins, M.D., M.P.H.

Reference

1. Bogerts B, Hantsch J, Herzer M: A morphometric study of the dopamine-containing cell groups in the mesencephalon of normals, Parkinson patients and schizophrenics. *Biol Psychiatry* 18:951–969, 1983.

Miscellaneous

Alcoholism in the Elderly
Council on Scientific Affairs, AMA (AMA, Chicago)
JAMA 275:797–801, 1996   3–35

Introduction.—Alcoholism is an increasing problem among elderly patients. However, alcoholism is a treatable disease. Physicians should increase their efforts in the prevention, diagnosis, and treatment of alcoholism in the elderly.

Epidemiology.—Community studies have reported a prevalence of 2% to 10% for alcoholism, alcohol abuse, or problem drinking in the elderly population. In elderly patients, there are 2 types of alcoholism: that which occurs earlier in life and that which occurs late in life. Situational factors appear to be more strongly related to late-onset alcoholism, whereas family history or genetic influences play a greater role in the etiology of early-onset alcoholism. Alcoholism is more likely to occur in elderly patients who are affluent, have higher formal education, and are isolated.

Effects of Alcohol Use Related to Age.—Elderly patients may have higher blood alcohol concentrations than younger patients ingesting the same quantity of alcohol. This effect is probably related to the lower water volume in older patients. Heavy drinking can affect nutritional status by interfering with food intake and by increasing the need for particular nutrients. Chronic heavy drinking is associated with numerous diseases: liver disease, ulcers, respiratory disease, stroke, myocardial infarction, and cancers of the mouth, larynx, and esophagus. Bone fractures are more common, possibly related to a greater decrease in bone density in elderly alcoholic patients. Many of the commonly prescribed drugs for elderly patients interact with alcohol. Even moderate alcohol use can cause abrupt onset organic brain syndrome. There is conflicting evidence of an effect of alcohol on cognitive deterioration. However, heavy drinking is associated with dementia and other psychiatric disorders, particularly depression, in the elderly.

Diagnosis.—A thorough physical examination, including laboratory tests and mental status evaluation, are necessary. Obtaining a thorough history is essential, with particular attention to the pattern and extent of current alcohol use. Self-administered screening instruments are often useful. Alcoholism should be suspected in patients with frequent falls, bruises, and emergency department visits, as well as in patients with medical problems associated with alcohol use, such as hyperuricemia, gastrointestinal disturbances, hypertension, insomnia, malnutrition, and unstable diabetes. It may be necessary to differentiate between alcoholism and other psychiatric disorders.

Treatment.—Because withdrawal from alcohol can be potentially life-threatening, detoxification should ideally occur in a hospital, with careful monitoring of benzodiazepine therapy, hydration needs, and thiamine therapy. After detoxification, a long-term treatment plan should be developed with the patient and family, which should include appropriate referrals. The physician may be essential in secondary prevention, with attention to early warning signs and prompt intervention.

Conclusions.—New guidelines should be developed and disseminated concerning the prevention, diagnosis, and treatment of alcoholism in elderly patients. In addition, more instruction on alcoholism and aging is needed in the medical curriculum, more research on alcoholism in the elderly is needed, and public education about alcoholism should be developed for the elderly population.

▶ This is a useful compendium of current knowledge and current opinions about alcohol abuse in the elderly. It combines a thorough review of the literature with the opinions of a number of national experts. Although the report highlights differences between early- and late-onset alcoholism, it notes that some individuals categorized as having late-onset alcoholism are likely to have had onset in early life but were undetected or undiagnosed until a life event such as retirement caused the alcoholism to be noticed by others. The paper offers no data to support this hypothesis, however. In my clinical experience, retirement or death of a spouse does lead to increased use of alcohol in some individuals whose use previously had been moderate, but dramatic changes in drinking habits late in life seem rare.

This report also highlights that certain settings increase the likelihood that alcohol abuse will be identified. Emergency departments, acute hospital medical units, and acute psychiatric units are 3 such settings. The article points out that the phenomenon of higher blood alcohol concentrations for a given quantity of alcohol, which is common in the elderly, is most likely explained by a lower total body water volume in which the alcohol is distributed. The report also highlights the lower recognition rates among physicians for identifying alcoholism in the elderly.

Treatment is organized into 4 categories: attending to emergency situations, detoxification, working with patients and their families, and developing a long-term treatment plan. Treatment programs that emphasize social relationships work better with older individuals than those that rely on confrontation. This review does not note the difficulty in treating older alcohol abusers who have few social supports and no longer are employed, two of the factors that clinicians attempt to modify to increase the likelihood of treatment compliance.

P.V. Rabins, M.D., M.P.H.

Convergent Validity of Measures of PTSD in an Elderly Population of Former Prisoners of War
Neal LA, Hill N, Hughes J, et al (RAF Hosp Wroughton, Swindon, Wiltshire, England)
Int J Geriatr Psychiatry 10:617–622, 1995   3–36

Objective.—Several instruments are available for assessment of symptoms of posttraumatic stress disorders (PTSD) in the general adult population, but their validity or reliability in the elderly has yet to be defined. The spectrum of current symptoms of PTSD in elderly former World War II Far East prisoners of war was examined, and the validity of 3 self-report PTSD scales as continuous and dichotomous measures of PTSD in this population was assessed.

Methods.—Thirty World War II Far East prisoners of war were examined. The participants were aged 70–85 years, and all were Caucasian. One woman was included. They were administered a structured clinical interview for PTSD based on *Diagnostic and Statistical Manual of Mental Disorders*, Third Edition, Revised (DSM-III-R) criteria—the Clinician Administered PTSD Scale (CAPS-1)—and 3 self-report psychometric instruments—impact of event scale (IES), the Minnesota Multiphasic Personality Inventory-Posttraumatic stress disorder subscale (MMPI-PTSD subscale), and the Mississippi scale for combat stress disorders. The CAPS-1 was the "gold standard" against which all 3 psychometric instruments were validated.

Results.—At 46 years after their release as prisoners of war, 30% of participants met the DSM-III-R diagnosis of PTSD and 90% complained of at least 1 symptom of intrusion or avoidance related to their captivity. Two scales correlated highly with the total score of the CAPS-1. The Mississippi scale was the most accurate measure of PTSD severity. At a

Moving?

I'd like to receive my *Year Book of Geriatrics & Gerontology* without interruption.
Please note the following change of address, effective:

Name: _____

New Address: _____

_____

City: _____ State: _____ Zip: _____

Old Address: _____

_____

City: _____ State: _____ Zip: _____

Reservation Card

Yes, I would like my own copy of *Year Book of Geriatrics & Gerontology*. Please begin my
subscription with the current edition according to the terms described below.* I understand that I
will have 30 days to examine each annual edition. If satisfied, I will pay just $66.95 plus sales tax,
postage and handling (price subject to change without notice).

Name: _____

Address: _____

City: _____ State: _____ Zip: _____

Method of Payment
O Visa   O Mastercard   O AmEx   O Bill me   O Check (in US dollars, payable to Mosby, Inc.)

Card number: _____ Exp date: _____

Signature: _____

LS-0908

*Your *Year Book* Service Guarantee:

When you subscribe to the *Year Book*, we'll send you an advance notice of future volumes
about two months before they publish. This automatic notice system is designed to take up as
little of your time as possible. If you do not want the *Year Book*, the advance notice makes it
quick and easy for you to let us know your decision, and you will always have at least 20 days
to decide. If we don't hear from you, we'll send you the new volume as soon as it's available.
And, of course, the *Year Book* is yours to examine free of charge for 30 days (postage, handling
and applicable sales tax are added to each shipment.).

BUSINESS REPLY MAIL

FIRST CLASS MAIL   PERMIT No. 762   CHICAGO, IL

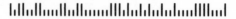

POSTAGE WILL BE PAID BY ADDRESSEE

Chris Hughes
Mosby-Year Book, Inc.
161 N. Clark Street
Suite 1900
Chicago, IL 60601-9981

NO POSTAGE
NECESSARY
IF MAILED
IN THE
UNITED STATES

BUSINESS REPLY MAIL

FIRST CLASS MAIL   PERMIT No. 762   CHICAGO, IL

POSTAGE WILL BE PAID BY ADDRESSEE

Chris Hughes
Mosby-Year Book, Inc.
161 N. Clark Street
Suite 1900
Chicago, IL 60601-9981

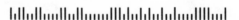

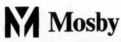 **Mosby**

Dedicated to publishing excellence

cutoff score of 81, the Mississippi scale had a sensitivity of 0.78 and a specificity of 0.57. The MMPI-PTSD subscale was the most efficient dichotomous measure of PTSD, with a sensitivity of 0.89 and specificity of 0.62 at a recommended cutoff score of 17. The IES avoidance subscale failed to discriminate avoidant symptoms from those of intrusion. The positive predictive values of the scales were uniformly low when the cutoff scores were adjusted downward for screening.

Conclusions.—These findings indicate that self-report scales for chronic PTSD should be interpreted with caution when used in the elderly. These measures require further evaluation of their validity.

▶ This study examines the validity of several instruments that have been devised to identify PTSD in combat veterans. Because individuals who fought in World War II are now at least in their 70s, the subjects of the study are of interest to individuals treating the elderly. This study does not strongly support the validity of the instruments it studied. However, a more notable result is the finding that some symptoms of PTSD can persist for more than 50 years. The demonstration that 30% of individuals fulfilled criteria for PTSD and that almost all individuals had at least 1 intrusive or avoidant symptom associated with PTSD has significant clinical relevance and strongly suggests that all individuals with a history of combat experience should be asked about the symptoms of PTSD. The study has several limitations, however, to its applicability to all veterans. All subjects were prisoners of war and were ascertained because they had visited a Royal Air Force hospital in England. Thus, the sample is neither representative of former prisoners of war nor combat veterans in general. In addition, the study offers no evidence on the treatability of these symptoms. Nevertheless, the findings deserve clinical attention because these symptoms can cause significant distress and can theoretically respond to treatment even after 50 years.

P.V. Rabins, M.D., M.P.H.

Cognitive-Behavioral Therapy in Older Panic Disorder Patients
Swales PJ, Solfvin JF, Sheikh JI (Stanford Univ, Calif)
Am J Geriatr Psychiatry 4:46–60, 1996   3–37

Background.—Several studies have reported the efficacy of cognitive-behavioral treatment for panic disorder in younger patients. The results of a pilot study of cognitive-behavioral therapy for panic disorder among elderly patients were reported.

Methods.—Twenty self-referred patients, aged 55–80 years, began the study. All lived in the community and met *Diagnostic and Statistical Manual of Mental Disorders*, Third Edition, Revised (DSM-III-R) criteria for panic disorder. Fifteen patients completed the 12-week study of 10 treatment sessions, which consisted of cognitive, behavioral, and relaxation strategies. Self-report measures were used to assess cognitive, behavioral, physiologic, affective, and global domains.

Findings.—Significant improvements in panic-associated cognitions, physiologic symptoms, and avoidance behaviors were noted on posttreatment compared with pretreatment measures. The posttreatment improvements persisted for the 3 months of follow-up.

Conclusions.—Although this pilot study is inherently limited, the significant differences between pretreatment and posttreatment measures, along with findings from previous research, seem to indicate true treatment effects. The current protocol of cognitive, behavioral, and relaxation interventions appears to effectively ameliorate panic-associated cognitions, physiologic symptoms, and avoidance behaviors in elderly patients with panic disorder.

▶ Cognitive-behavioral therapy is effective in treating panic disorder in the nongeriatric population. This small, uncontrolled trial supports the efficacy of this approach in a sample of self-referred individuals with a mean age of 63.2 years. However, well-designed, controlled, double-blind studies—including comparisons between psychotherapy and pharmacotherapy—are needed. This study is a reminder that older individuals can respond to the same psychotherapy-based treatments as younger individuals.

P.V. Rabins, M.D., M.P.H.

Occult Caffeine as a Source of Sleep Problems in an Older Population
Brown SL, Salive ME, Pahor M, et al (Natl Inst on Aging, Bethesda, Md; Universita Cattolica del Sacro Cuore, Rome; Univ of Iowa, Iowa City)
J Am Geriatr Soc 43:860–864, 1995   3–38

Background.—Many medications contain caffeine, which can interfere with sleep. A dosage of 2 tablets of a typical over-the-counter analgesic given 4 times daily contains the equivalent of 4 weak cups of coffee. The effect of caffeine on sleep can be more profound in older adults, and sleep problems may be associated with higher mortality and nursing home placement. Approximately 25% of older adults report sleep problems, and caffeine may contribute to this. The effect of caffeine in medications on the sleeping patterns of older adults was investigated.

Methods.—At the third annual follow-up to the Iowa 65+ Rural Health Study, 2,885 participants between 67 and 105 years of age completed a survey that included questions about sleep problems, use of medications, and caffeine intake. Responses were analyzed after adjustment for factors that could obscure the relation between caffeine and sleep.

Results.—The reported use of medications containing caffeine was 5.4%. Individuals who used medication with caffeine had more trouble falling asleep. No other significant risk of sleep problems was associated with this type of medication. After controlling for other factors that could interfere with sleep, the use of medications with caffeine was still associated with a significant risk of sleep problems. Those who took over-the-counter medications without caffeine did not have the same risk of sleep problems.

Conclusions.—The caffeine in various medications may contribute to sleep problems in older adults. Patients should be advised by their health care providers about the potential problems in falling asleep associated with the use of caffeine, especially in over-the-counter analgesics. Older patients should be advised to read labels and avoid medications that contain caffeine.

▶ Complaints of sleep disorder are common in the elderly population. This study documents that the use of caffeine-containing medications is associated with sleep problems. Although sleep disorder and sleep complaints have many determinants, the clinician is most interested in those that can be modified. Thus, clinicians evaluating patients who complain of poor sleep should question them about the use of caffeine-containing medications and foods and should attempt to remove them from patients' diets. It is important to note that this is a cross-sectional descriptive study and, therefore, does not prove that sleep would improve if the use of caffeine-containing analgesics were discontinued. Nevertheless, physicians should ask about the use of caffeine-containing analgesics when evaluating patients for sleep disorders.

P.V. Rabins, M.D., M.P.H.

Quality of Care for Depressed Elderly Patients Hospitalized in the Specialty Psychiatric Units or General Medical Wards
Norquist G, Wells KB, Rogers WH, et al (Natl Inst of Mental Health, Rockville, Md; Univ of California, Los Angeles; RAND, Santa Monica, Calif)
Arch Gen Psychiatry 52:695–701, 1995   3–39

Background.—The assessment of the quality of care of individuals with mental disorders is important for research and for developing policy. It is important to know whether these patients receive better care in mental health units or in general medical wards. The results of studies addressing this issue have been inadequate for a variety of reasons. The quality of care of elderly inpatients with depression in psychiatric units was compared with that in general medical wards of hospitals in 5 states.

Methods.—The medical records of 2,746 patients older than 65 years of age who had depression were examined retrospectively. Quality of care was determined by measures of clinical assessment, services provided, and outcomes.

Results.—Of the 2,746 patients studied, 1,295 were in psychiatric units and 1,451 were in general medical wards. In the psychiatric units, more admissions were considered appropriate, the overall psychological evaluation was better, patients were more likely to receive psychological assessment and services, there were more general medical complications, and implicit measures of clinical status at discharge were better. Patients in general medical wards were more likely to receive traditional general medical services.

Conclusions.—These patients may have received better psychological care in psychiatric units than in general medical wards of hospitals. The quality of care for patients with depression in general medical wards can improve, as can the quality of care for general medical complications in psychiatric units. Postgraduate training for general medical providers should be improved, and practice guidelines for treating depression, with emphasis on the elderly population, should be developed.

▶ Studies of the quality of medical care and the outcome of treatment have taken on added importance in an era of attempts to diminish the cost of care and improve its efficiency of delivery. The strengths of this study included examination of the records of 3,626 hospitalized patients in Medicare databases of 5 states and comparison of persons treated for major depression in psychiatric units and general medical units. One serious limitation is that 24% of patients who had a serious medical condition were excluded. As is usual with outcome studies, a clinician panel rated severity of illness at the time of admission, quality of care during the admission, and outcome.

Although this is a limit in that no a priori standard was measured, this is the standard in the field. The findings are that patients in psychiatric units were more likely to be considered appropriate admissions, to have had better quality clinical assessments, to receive better psychological care, and to be rated as having more improvement. Individuals hospitalized in medical units received better general medical services and had fewer medical complications.

The authors concluded that the overall quality of psychiatric care was better in the psychiatric units but that the quality of medical care was better in the medical units. This is an important result. As the authors discuss, one implication of this finding is that medical care needs must be better met in psychiatric units and that psychiatric needs must be better met in medical units. However, the exclusion of a significant number of individuals with severe medical complications limits the applicability of the findings to many older individuals who have both major depression and serious medical co-morbidity.

P.V. Rabins, M.D., M.P.H.

Precipitating Factors for Delirium in Hospitalized Elderly Persons: Predictive Model and Interrelationship With Baseline Vulnerability
Inouye SK, Charpentier PA (Yale Univ, New Haven, Conn)
JAMA 275:852–857, 1996   3–40

Background.—Delirium is a common, serious problem among hospitalized elderly patients. A predictive model for delirium based on precipitating factors during hospitalization was developed and validated prospectively.

Methods.—Two prospective cohort studies were conducted, one for model development and one for validation. The participants were 196 and 312 patients, respectively, aged 70 years and older, with no delirium at baseline.

Findings.—Thirty-five patients (18%) in the first cohort became delirious during hospitalization. Independent precipitating factors included the use of physical restraints, malnutrition, more than 3 medications added, the use of a bladder catheter, and any iatrogenic event. Each of these factors preceded the onset of delirium by more than 24 hours. A system of risk stratification was developed by adding 1 point for each factor. Three percent of patients with no points became delirious, compared with 20% of those with 1 or 2 points and 59% with 3 or more points. In the validation cohort, delirium developed in 47 patients (15%). The corresponding rates of delirium for low-, intermediate-, and high-risk groups were 4%, 20%, and 35%, respectively. Baseline and precipitating factors independently, significantly contributed to the onset of delirium.

Conclusions.—This simple predictive model can be used to identify elderly hospitalized patients at high risk for delirium. Precipitating and baseline vulnerability variables contribute significantly to the development of delirium in this population.

▶ Dr. Inouye's important work regarding delirium continues to improve our understanding of this common source of medical and psychiatric morbidity in inpatient settings. This study identified 5 factors associated with the incidence (i.e., the new development) of delirium in hospitalized patients. These findings were confirmed in a second cohort; using these 5 factors to identify high-risk individuals, approximately one third of individuals were identified at risk for having delirium develop. Of most interest, perhaps, is the finding that vulnerability (i.e., pre-existing) and precipitating factors act both independently and in concert. Although this is not surprising, it does illustrate the difficulties faced by clinicians and researchers in developing ways to prevent delirium, to improve early recognition, and to shorten its course. It is always possible that factors such as use of restraints, which was the factor with the highest likelihood of association (relative risk, 4.4 times), indicate the subtle presence of early delirium. This may also be a marker for other risk factors such as dementia.

P.V. Rabins, M.D., M.P.H.

Effects of Medicare's Prospective Payment System on Service Use by Depressed Elderly Inpatients

Davis LM, Wells KB, Rogers WH, et al (Rand Corp, Santa Monica, Calif; New England Med Ctr, Boston; Natl Inst of Mental Health, Rockville, Md; et al)
Psychiatric Serv 46:1178–1184, 1995   3–41

Objective.—Implementation of Medicare's prospective payment system (PPS) for inpatient care has resulted in reductions in resources for many medical and surgical services by reducing length of stay and intensity of services. However, these effects are less clear in inpatient psychiatric care. The effects of Medicare's PPS on hospital care received by elderly depressed patients in acute care general medical hospitals was examined.

Study Design.—Medical records of 2,746 depressed Medicare patients aged 65 and older, who were admitted to a general hospital in 5 states, were examined. For both the medical and psychiatric portions of hospital stay, length of stay and intensity of clinical services before the implementation of PPS (1981–1982) and after its implementation (1985–1986) were compared. Care provided on units exempt from PPS was compared with care provided in nonexempt units. Multiple regression analysis was employed, with each analysis controlled for the level of sickness at admission.

Findings.—The average length of stay fell by up to 3 days after PPS implementation in each type of treatment setting, particularly in hospitals without a psychiatric unit. However, this reduction was partially offset by proportionately more admissions to psychiatric units, which had longer lengths of stay. Thus, overall length of stay among elderly depressed Medicare patients did not significantly decrease over time. The intensity of services, particularly doctor and other therapist visits, increased after PPS implementation. In particular, the increase in intensity of services in nonexempt psychiatric units had matched that of the exempt units by the post-PPS period.

Summary.—Implementation of Medicare's PPS is not associated with an overall reduction in length of stay among elderly depressed patients admitted to general hospitals, although the intensity of a few specific therapeutic services in nonexempt psychiatric units has increased post-PPS.

▶ This is an important study that assessed the impact of prospective payment on the hospital care of elderly individuals with depression. By comparing individuals treated in units under the prospective payment system to individuals on units exempt from this system, the authors were able to determine the effects of prospective payment. The results strongly suggest that prospective payment does not diminish the cost of care for elderly depressed individuals and in fact may cause an increase in intensity of service use. These findings suggest that the inpatient treatment of depression is not subject to inappropriate physician or health care provider behavior. Rather, it is most compatible with the conclusion that the treatments patients are now receiving are appropriate and that financial incentives for hospitals to decrease this care do not change physician behavior. In an era in which cost containment and allegations of overuse of services abound, it is reassuring to know that practitioners will not bow to financial incentives in every instance. These results also suggest that the added burdens that will accrue to clinical care over the next several years as Medicare becomes an integral part of managed care might not lead to the cost savings hoped for by health planners. Rather, they may only increase the bureaucratic burdens on practitioners.

P.V. Rabins, M.D., M.P.H.

4 Geriatric Neurology

Introduction

As in past years, much of this chapter about geriatric neurology focuses on dementia. In the research area, we are excited about the role of oxidative stress in neurodegenerative diseases. Therapeutic trials of anti-oxidants, including deprenyl, are underway to try to slow progression of Alzheimer's disease (AD).

Apolipoprotein E (APOE) research also continues to command attention. Many studies have confirmed that individuals with the APOE ϵ 4 allele, particularly homozygotes, are more at risk for AD. If this finding improves our understanding of the pathogenesis of AD, it may lead to more effective therapies. In addition, a diagnostic adjunctive test is already available commercially, along with tests of CSF levels of β and τ. My view is that we need to know more about the risks associated with APOE status, based on genetic studies not molecular studies. Once this knowledge is gained we need to make sure that physicians understand the implications of the test for family members and its use in the differential diagnosis of dementia.

This year the Agency for Health Care Policy and Research published long-awaited guidelines for early recognition of dementia, which should assist primary care physicians. I often wonder whether we could increase our detection of dementia if we could persuade every primary care physician to ask their elderly patients to remember three objects and assess their recall two minutes later. Specific mental status testing must be incorporated into patient assessment, and I believe that three-item recall is as good a screen as any single-test item.

As of this writing in November 1996, we expect that a new drug, Aricept, will soon be approved for the treatment of AD. This novel cholinesterase inhibitor is administered only once a day, and it is not associated with the toxicity of tacrine hydrochloride. However, despite our continued excitement about new medications, creative psychosocial interventions also need to be developed. One area that needs considerable investment is the use of information systems, both to educate caregivers and to provide entertainment for patients with dementia.

Dementia continues to pose challenging ethical questions, such as how to obtain informed consent from demented patients. I expect that in the next several years a number of groups will be looking at this issue, including the International Working Group for Harmonization of Dementia Drug Guidelines, in cooperation with Alzheimer's Disease International. We need to continue to encourage individuals to develop advanced directives that address the possibility of dementia. Most important, we need to involve healthy and affected individuals in our deliberations concerning critical ethical issues.

Diagnosis and treatment of vascular dementia received renewed attention this year. There is a complex area of overlap between AD and vascular dementia, as vascular mechanisms may be at work in AD. International collaborative efforts are focusing on developing better criteria and ways of assessing vascular components of dementia. We have greater consensus about diagnostic criteria for AD than we do for vascular dementia. Medications under development may be effective in treating vascular dementia as well as AD.

Management of stroke is undergoing a revolution as we redefine it as brain attack and as thrombolytic therapy becomes more readily available. Moreover, basic science studies are suggesting that mechanisms can be developed to protect the brain from ischemic damage. At the same time, however, we must develop more effective interventions for first strokes. We also need to be more efficient in incorporating consensus developed by governments and academics into physician practice.

Treatment options for Parkinson's disease continue to increase. A number of new medications are likely to be approved in the next few years, including some new dopamine agonists with different profiles of dopamine receptor specificity. Moreover, surgical interventions such as pallidotomy are growing in importance for selected patients. As always, we must recognize that patients with AD are more at risk for Parkinson's disease and vice versa.

The last section of the chapter, general geriatric neurology, includes several articles about the exceedingly important topic of falls. All primary care physicians need to understand the frequency of falls and how they can be prevented. This section also includes a brief summary of preventive health care for the elderly.

Peter J. Whitehouse, M.D., Ph.D.

Dementia

BASIC RESEARCH

Aging, Energy, and Oxidative Stress in Neurodegenerative Diseases
Beal MF (Harvard Med School, Boston)
Ann Neurol 38:357–366, 1995   4–1

Background.—The causes of neuronal death in neurodegenerative diseases are unknown. Cell death appears to involve both excitotoxicity and oxidative damage, and these processes could result from defects in energy metabolism. Current knowledge about the roles played by energy metabolism, excitotoxicity, and oxidative damage in normal aging and in neurodegenerative diseases was reviewed.

Discussion.—Defects in energy metabolism, excitotoxicity, and oxidative damage likely play an interrelated role in the pathogenesis of neurodegenerative diseases. Energy metabolism defects could result in neuronal depolarization, activation of N-methyl-D aspartate excitatory amino acid receptors, and increases in intracellular calcium. These changes are buffered by mitochondria, which seem to play an important role in oxidative damage in neurodegenerative diseases. Mitochondria are the main intracellular source of free radicals, the generation of which is enhanced by increased mitochondrial calcium concentrations. Mitochondrial DNA may be especially vulnerable to oxidative stress, and studies have suggested that normal aging is associated with damage and deterioration of respiratory enzyme activity. These "normal" changes could be part of the reason for the late onset of neurodegenerative diseases; the energy metabolism defect could be dormant until age-related declines in oxidative metabolism occur. The resulting slow excitotoxicity may be followed by increased free radical generation, and this feed-forward cycle would eventually result in neuronal death.

Recent studies have demonstrated increased oxidative damage to macromolecules in several neurodegenerative diseases, i.e., amyotrophic lateral sclerosis, Huntington's disease, Parkinson's disease, and Alzheimer's disease. Several different therapeutic approaches have been proffered, including glutamate release inhibitors, excitatory amino acid antagonists, agents to improve mitochondrial function, free radical scavengers, and neurotrophic factors. These approaches might be made more effective by using combinations of agents at sequential steps in the degenerative process.

Summary.—Recent studies suggest that defects in energy metabolism, excitotoxicity, and oxidative damage could play a pathogenetic role in the neuronal death occurring in neurodegenerative diseases. All of the treatment possibilities mentioned are being pursued in human studies. Once their effectiveness is established, it may be possible to identify and treat patients at risk for neurodegenerative diseases at a presymptomatic stage.

▶ One of the oldest scientific theories of aging relates oxidative stress and damage to the accumulation of free radicals. This excellent review article summarizes the potential role of oxidative stress in a variety of neurodegenerative diseases, including Alzheimer's disease. The article concludes by discussing some of the therapeutic implications of this approach and the efforts that are already under way to develop therapies.

P.J. Whitehouse, M.D., Ph.D.

Apolipoprotein E Genotype and Association Between Smoking and Early Onset Alzheimer's Disease

van Duijn CM, Havekes LM, van Broeckhoven C, et al (Erasmus Univ, Rotterdam, The Netherlands; TNO Inst of Prevention and Health Research, Leiden, The Netherlands; Univ of Antwerp, Belgium)

BMJ 310:627–631, 1995   4–2

Purpose.—There is an inverse association between smoking and Alzheimer's disease, which may be the result of some neuroprotective effect of smoking, or it may be explained by bias resulting from a lower rate of survival among smokers. One report has suggested that the increased risk of early death among smokers could result in a decreased frequency of the apolipoprotein e4 allele, which has been linked to an increased risk of both late- and early-onset Alzheimer's disease. The possible role of the apolipoprotein e4 allele in the association between smoking and early-onset Alzheimer's disease was investigated.

Methods.—A population-based study included 175 Dutch patients with early-onset Alzheimer's disease and 2 independent control groups of 159 and 457 individuals. The patients with Alzheimer's disease and individuals in the control groups were matched for age, sex, and place of residence. The mean age of the patients with Alzheimer's disease was 57 years at the time of diagnosis and 63 years at the time of the study. The frequency of the apolipoprotein e4 allele and the relative risk of early-onset Alzheimer's disease were the main outcome measures. The second control group was added to find out whether subjects with a history of smoking had a lower frequency of the apolipoprotein e4 allele.

Results.—No decrease in the frequency of the apolipoprotein e4 allele was found to explain the inverse association between smoking history and early-onset Alzheimer's disease. In both control groups, the frequency of this allele was significantly greater among subjects with a history of smoking than among those who had never smoked; the difference stemmed mainly from subjects with a family history of dementia. Control subjects who had a family history of dementia and who had smoked 11 pack-years or more had a 27% higher frequency of apolipoprotein e4 allele. Among carriers of this allele who had a family history of dementia, the risk of early-onset Alzheimer's disease was much reduced (odds ratio, 0.10) for those with a history of smoking.

Conclusions.—An increase in mortality among smokers who carry the apolipoprotein e4 allele does not account for the inverse association between smoking history and early-onset Alzheimer's disease. However, the presence of this allele and of a family history of dementia strongly influence the association between smoking and Alzheimer's disease. Treatment with nicotine or nicotine derivatives may be a promising approach to patients with familial Alzheimer's disease who carry the apolipoprotein e4 allele.

▶ A number of neuroepidemiologic studies have shown that smoking diminishes the risk of Alzheimer's disease. Apolipoprotein E status and smoking are also both related to the likelihood of vascular disease, including vascular dementia. This study demonstrates that both apolipoprotein E and smoking history have effects on Alzheimer's disease and that one cannot be explained in terms of the other. Interestingly, it also shows that the association of Alzheimer's disease with smoking is affected by the apolipoprotein E status: Smoking has a stronger protective effect in individuals with the apolipoprotein e4 allele. This relationship is not understood, but it may represent a clue that should be followed up with biological studies to examine the reactions between apolipoprotein E and nicotinic receptors.

P.J. Whitehouse, M.D., Ph.D.

Prevalence of Dementia and Distribution of ApoE Alleles in Japanese Centenarians: An Almost-Complete Survey in Yamanashi Prefecture, Japan
Asada T, Yamagata Z, Kinoshita T, et al (Yamanashi Med Univ, Tamaho, Japan; Yamanashi Univ, Kofu, Japan; New York Hosp, White Plains)
J Am Geriatr Soc 44:151–155, 1996   4–3

Background.—Discrimination between a normal mental state and dementia in very old patients has received considerable attention. However, some researchers have proposed the inevitability of dementia at the extreme limits of the life span. The apolipoprotein E (ApoE) ϵ4 allele has been identified as a genetic risk factor for Alzheimer's disease (AD). However, it has been proposed that this allele is more a predictor of the age at onset than of the ultimate risk of AD, suggesting that its prevalence would decrease with age. To examine this potential association, the prevalence and types of dementia were studied in centenarians.

Methods.—Forty-seven centenarians underwent an examination, which included an interview, physical examination, functional assessment, mental examination, and routine laboratory tests. The diagnosis and severity of dementia were determined using the *Diagnostic and Statistical Manual,* Third Edition, Revised (DSM-III-R) criteria. The diagnosis of probable and/or possible AD was determined using National Institute of Neurological and Communicative Disorders and Stroke–Alzheimer's Disease and Related Disorders Association criteria. Blood samples were obtained from 33 centenarians and 224 other older adults with dementia with onset at an age younger than 90 years; the samples were analyzed for ApoE genotyping. The 6-month mortality rate was determined.

Results.—There was a 70.2% prevalence of dementia in the centenarians, with a mean age of onset of 98 years. Probable or possible AD was diagnosed in 75.8% of the subjects with dementia. There was a 6-month rate of 27% among the subjects with dementia and 0% among the subjects without. Apolipoprotein E ϵ4 alleles were found in 4.6% of the subjects overall and in 5.9% of the subjects with AD. There was a tendency of decreasing ApoE ε4 allele frequency with increasing age at onset.

Conclusions.—Centenarians have a high prevalence of dementia. The development of AD in centenarians is not associated with the ApoE ε4 allele.

▶ Apolipoprotein E is now available commercially to potentially assist in the diagnosis of AD. One of the controversies about its use is that the data available for interpreting this information clinically are based on a limited sample of individuals. Therefore, this study is interesting for 2 reasons: It involved Japanese subjects in whom there were different baseline rates of different ApoE subtypes; and more than 70% of this population of centenarians had dementia, yet ApoE status did not predict whether AD would be present. Thus, both age and ethnic group need to be considered by clinicians considering using ApoE status as an adjunct to diagnosis.

P.J. Whitehouse, M.D., Ph.D.

Apolipoprotein E Type 4 Allele and Cerebral Glucose Metabolism in Relatives at Risk for Familial Alzheimer Disease
Small GW, Mazziotta JC, Collins MT, et al (Univ of California, Los Angeles; Univ of California, Irvine; Duke Univ, Durham, NC; et al)
JAMA 273:942–947, 1995   4–4

Objective.—Positron emission tomography (PET) with fludeoxyglucose F 18 in patients with Alzheimer's disease (AD) has shown a consistent pattern of reduced glucose use that begins in the superior parietal cortex and spreads inferiorly and anteriorly into the inferior parietal, superior temporal, and prefrontal cortices. It is also well known that the apolipoprotein E type 4 allele (APOE e4) is a risk factor for familial AD. The association between APOE e4 and reduced brain function was assessed in relatives of patients with AD with and without APOE e4.

Methods.—Thirty-eight subjects met the inclusion criteria of the study and received APOE genotyping and PET scanning. Twelve subjects were at-risk relatives of patients with AD who had APOE; 19 subjects were at-risk relatives of patients with AD without APOE; and 7 subjects were patients with probable AD. The neuropsychological performance of the subjects was determined by the Mini-Mental State Examination. Magnetic resonance imaging scans were performed to determine the presence and degree of cerebral atrophy and white matter hyperintensity.

Results.—The mean age and neuropsychological performance of the subjects in both at-risk groups did not differ significantly. The group with dementia scored lower than the at-risk groups on the Mini-Mental State Examination. An association of APOE e4 with lower cerebral parietal metabolism was noted. Parietal metabolism was significantly lower in at-risk subjects with APOE e4 than in those without APOE e4. In addition, left-right parietal asymmetry was significantly higher in at-risk subjects with APOE e4 than in those without. The patients with probable AD had significantly lower left and right parietal metabolism than the at-risk group with APOE e4. Atrophy ratings from MRI scan results were not significantly different between the at-risk groups, but were significantly greater in the group with dementia compared with the at-risk group without APOE e4.

Conclusion.—The presence of APOE e4 in nondemented individuals who are at risk for inheriting AD is associated with reduced cerebral parietal metabolism and increased asymmetry. These glucose metabolic measures may provide a means of monitoring experimental treatment during the early phases of AD.

▶ One approach to the diagnosis of AD has been PET. This and other functional neuroimaging techniques have shown differences between patients with AD and controls, usually decreased temporal and parietal metabolism. In this study, subjects at risk for familial AD who did not differ from controls on neuropsychological performance were shown to have lower cerebral glucose metabolism associated with APOE e4 status. It is interesting that changes in brain metabolism occur before pronounced neuropsychological deficits can be detected. Moreover, it raises the possibility that these kinds of neuroimaging studies can be used to monitor the results of experimental therapies. Although not abstracted here because of space restrictions, a number of other recent papers about APOE status are worth reviewing.[1-6]

P.J. Whitehouse, M.D., Ph.D.

References

1. Dal Forno G, Rasmusson X, Brandt J, et al: Apolipoprotein E genotype and rate of decline in probable Alzheimer's diease. *Arch Neurol* 53:345–350, 1996.
2. Duara R, Barker WW, Lopez-Alberola R, et al: Alzheimer's disease: Interaction of apolipoprotein E genotype, family history of dementia, gender, education, ethnicity, and age of onset. *Neurology* 46:1575–1579, 1996.
3. Farrer LA, Cupples LA, van Duijn CM, et al: Apolipoprotein E genotype in patients with Alzheimer's disease: Implications for the risk of dementia among relatives. *Ann Neurol* 38:797–808, 1995.
4. Mak YT, Hiu H, Woo J, et al: Apolipoprotein E genotype and Alzheimer's disease in Hong Kong elderly Chinese. *Neurology* 46:146–149, 1996.
5. Myers RH, Schaefer EJ, Wilson PWF, et al: Apolipoprotein E e4 association with dementia in a population-based study: The Framingham Study. *Neurology* 46:673–677, 1996.
6. Tsuang D, Kukull W, Sheppard L, et al: Impact of sample selection on APOE e4 allele frequency: A comparison of two Alzheimer's disease samples. *J Am Geriatr Soc* 44:704–707, 1996.

Reduction of β-Amyloid Peptide$_{42}$ in the Cerebrospinal Fluid of Patients With Alzheimer's Disease

Motter R, Vigo-Pelfrey C, Kholodenko D, et al (Athena Neurosciences Inc, South San Francisco, Calif; Univ of California, San Diego; Univ of California Los Angeles, Torrance; et al)
Ann Neurol 38:643–648, 1995   4–5

Objectives.—The diagnosis of Alzheimer's disease (AD), the most common form of dementia in the elderly population, is accomplished clinically by exclusion of other dementing illnesses. The utility of measurements of the β-amyloid (AB) protein and the microtubule-associated protein τ in the CSF for the diagnosis of AD was studied prospectively.

Methods.—Thirty-seven patients with diagnosed AD, 32 patients with non-AD neurologic disease (ND), and 20 patients without dementia (NC) were evaluated clinically and neurologically. Apolipoprotein E (APOE) was genotyped, and total AB, AB$_{42}$, and τ levels were determined by enzyme-linked immunoabsorbent assays.

Results.—Total AB levels were not significantly different among the 3 groups of patients, but levels of AB$_{42}$ were significantly lower in the AD group (383 pg/mL) than in the ND (543 pg/mL) and NC (632 pg/mL) groups. The 505-pg/mL level was identified as the cutoff for separating AD patients from ND and NC subjects. In contrast, τ levels were significantly higher in AD patients (407 pg/mL) than in ND (168 pg/mL) and NC (212 pg/mL) controls, and a cutoff of 312 pg/mL was chosen to separate AD patients from ND and NC subjects. Simultaneous measurement of AB$_{42}$ and τ in the same CSF samples revealed that elevated τ and reduced AB$_{42}$ levels predicted AD in 22 of 23 cases, and high AB$_{42}$ and low τ levels were observed only in control subjects. The frequency of the APOE allele was high in the AD group, compared with the control groups, but the frequency of APOE alleles had no effect on τ, AB, or AB$_{42}$ levels.

Conclusion.—Combined measurement of AB$_{42}$ and τ levels in the CSF may aid in the diagnosis of AD.

▶ Improving our ability to diagnose AD continues to be a major challenge. This group from Athena Neurosciences has demonstrated that levels of AB peptide extending to position 42 were lower in the CSF of patients with AD compared with ND and NC controls. As in other studies of CSF and plasma markers, there were overlaps between patients with AD and control subjects.

This group is developing a commercial approach to the diagnosis of AB that combines this test of AB protein with tests of τ levels in CSF, which have been shown to be increased in patients with AD. It remains to be seen, however, what these tests permit in terms of improved diagnostic sensitivity and specificity over standard current practice. These improvements will need to be dramatic, and perhaps tied to therapeutic interventions before the expense of performing CSF examinations in all patients with dementia is warranted. History is still the best diagnostic tool for AD, and even the roles of blood tests and structural neuroimaging, which are currently standard tools, need to be further examined.

P.J. Whitehouse, M.D., Ph.D.

DIAGNOSIS AND STAGING

Linguistic Ability in Early Life and Cognitive Function and Alzheimer's Disease in Late Life: Findings From the Nun Study
Snowdon DA, Kemper SJ, Mortimer JA, et al (Univ of Kentucky, Lexington; Univ of Kansas, Lawrence; Univ of Minnesota, Minneapolis)
JAMA 275:528–532, 1996   4–6

Background.—Low levels of education have been associated with a higher risk of Alzheimer's disease and dementia. A proposed explanation for this association is that individuals with an insufficient cognitive or neurologic reserve capacity may be vulnerable to the development of dementia. It was hypothesized that linguistic ability in early life may be more appropriate than education as an indication of neurocognitive reserve and as a predictor of cognitive ability in late life. The potential association between linguistic ability in early life and cognitive function and neuropathologic evidence of Alzheimer's disease in late life was examined in participants in the Nun Study.

Methods.—A total of 93 American sisters born before 1917 were studied. At an average age of 22 years, all had written autobiographies, which were analyzed for idea density and grammatical complexity. At an age of 75–95 years, the sisters were evaluated for cognitive function with 7 neuropsychological tests. Fourteen participants who died were evaluated neuropathologically with quantitation of senile plaques and neurofibrillary tangles.

Results.—There were significant associations between idea density and grammatical complexity and between idea density and education level. Cognitive function was strongly associated with idea density, and less strongly with grammatical complexity. Of the 14 sisters with neuropathologic evaluations, all of those with low idea density and none of those with high idea density had confirmed Alzheimer's disease.

Conclusions.—Early linguistic ability is strongly correlated with later cognitive function and Alzheimer's disease, suggesting that low linguistic ability in early life is an important marker of the risk of Alzheimer's disease. Because only 1 sister had neuropathologic evidence of Alzheimer's disease without intellectual decline, it is unlikely that the development of dementia is related to the reserve capacity of the brain, rather than to neuropathologic components.

► This widely publicized study of nuns living in the Milwaukee area provides interesting evidence concerning the relationship between cognitive abilities earlier in life and the development of dementia in late life. We must remember that the sample size is small, the population is unique, and the correlations between early idea density and grammatical complexity in autobiographies and later life dementia are unbelievably high. Nevertheless, the study is well done and provocative.

The question is whether their cognitive function 58 years earlier was at that time a function of the environment in which the nuns were educated or of premorbid abilities, present perhaps at birth, and "hard-wired" into the nervous system. Thus, although provocative, the study does not help us resolve the issue of whether one is born with a brain more resistant to Alzheimer's disease, which is also more likely to allow one to write more linguistically complex material, or whether one's early education contributes to a brain that is more resistant to the disease through intellectual activities. The answer is likely that both genes and environment play a role, emphasizing the importance of examining gene–environment interactions. Cases in this study also remind us that plaques and tangles do not equate to dementia. Individual nuns in this particular study either had many plaques and no dementia or severe dementia and no plaques and tangles.

P.J. Whitehouse, M.D., Ph.D.

A Follow-Up Study of Age-Associated Memory Impairment: Neuropsychological Predictors of Dementia
Hänninen T, Hallikainen M, Koivisto K, et al (Univ of Kuopio, Finland)
J Am Geriatr Soc 43:1007–1015, 1995   4–7

Background.—Age-associated memory impairment (AAMI) has been proposed as a diagnostic entity. AAMI is based on subjective memory decline, objective evidence of memory loss, adequate intellectual function, and the absence of dementia or other disease affecting memory occurring in an individual older than 50 years of age. Age-associated memory impairment has been seen as an intermediate state on a continuum between normal aging and dementia. To investigate this theory, the clinical course of AAMI was explored with follow-up of a cohort of patients who were given the diagnosis of AAMI. Also investigated were the dimensions of cognitive functions that could predict progression from AAMI to dementia.

Methods.—Two cohorts of research subjects in 2 age groups, including 592 randomly selected individuals aged 68–78 years and 250 aged 60–67 years, were screened for the prevalence of AAMI. The screening process included a structured interview that rated subjective complaints of memory loss, evaluated objective memory capacity, assessed mental state, and tested memory and frontal executive functions using standard instruments. From the 2 cohorts, AAMI was diagnosed in 229 research subjects, who were invited for a follow-up evaluation an average of 3.6 years after the screening evaluation, again using standard evaluation instruments.

Results.—Follow-up was complete for 176 of the 229 research subjects who originally had a diagnosis of AAMI. Of the 176 patients, AAMI was diagnosed in 104 (59.1%) at follow-up, whereas 16 (9.1%) received a diagnosis of dementia; a mild decline without dementia was noted in 13

(7.4%). Memory had improved in 17 (9.7%). Nine (5.1%) no longer had any subjective complaints about memory. The patients who progressed to dementia had significantly poorer performance in baseline tests, particularly on the Buschke Selective Reminding (testing total recall), Visual Reproduction (testing immediate recall), Verbal Fluency on Category, Benton Visual Retention, Paired Associated Learning, and Verbal Fluency on Letters.

Conclusions.—The incidence of dementia among patients with AAMI is slightly greater than the reported incidence in the general population, although some patients may have improved memory. In the majority of patients, however, AAMI is nonprogressive. Patients who progress to dementia can be predicted with baseline neuropsychological tests.

▶ This article examines the challenging issue of the relationship between normal age-related memory changes and subsequent development of dementia. Specifically, it explores "age-associated memory impairment," a term that was replaced in the *Diagnostic and Statistical Manual of Mental Disorders,* Fourth Edition (DSM-IV) by "age-associated cognitive decline." In their study of Finnish individuals, the authors found that certain neuropsychological tests better predict who is more likely to have Alzheimer's disease develop rather than have nonprogressive memory difficulties. The tests that provided the greatest differentiation were total recall from Buschke Selective Reminding and immediate recall from Visual Reproduction. Also playing a role were fluency tests on categories or letters (e.g., "Name as many foods as possible in one minute").

This work supports other recent studies.[1, 2] Although the 3 studies involved very different patient populations, they all confirm the impression of many clinicians that memory impairment is an early sign of dementia and that recall is harder than recognition. Verbal fluency is perhaps as much a measure of executive function as of memory.

References

1. Masur DM, Sliwinski M, Lipton RB, et al: Neuropsychological prediction of dementia and the absence of dementia in healthy elderly persons. *Neurology* 44:1427–1432, 1994.
2. Newman SK, Warrington EK, Kennedy AM, et al: The earliest cognitive change in a person with familial Alzheimer's disease: Presymptomatic neuropsychological features in a pedigree with familial Alzheimer's disease confirmed at necropsy. *J Neurol Neurosurg Psychiatry* 57:967–972, 1994.

Memory Complaints and Memory Impairment in Older Individuals

Jonker C, Launer LJ, Hooijer C, et al (Free Univ, Amsterdam, The Netherlands; Erasmus Univ, Rotterdam, The Netherlands)
J Am Geriatr Soc 44:44–49, 1996   4–8

Background.—Interpretation of an older patient's complaint of memory loss may be complex. Individuals with dementia are more likely to complain about their memory than are those without dementia, but evidence also exists that individuals may complain about their memory for other reasons, such as depression. Nondemented, nondepressed individuals living in the community are proportionately the largest group at risk for memory impairment. The relationship between complaints about memory and cognitive test performance was evaluated in such a population.

Methods.—Of the 4,051 participants in the Amsterdam Study on the Elderly (65–85 years of age), 2,537 respondents who were neither demented nor depressed were included in the analysis. Answers to questions about the presence or absence of memory complaints and memory-related problems were classified into 4 categories of subjective memory complaints. Cognitive function was assessed by deriving subscales based on questions from the CAMCOG and several other mental status tests.

Results.—Memory complaints and problems were noted for 22.1% of nondemented, nondepressed individuals, compared with 36.7% of depressed individuals and 46.4% of demented individuals. Cognitive subscales correlated negatively with age and positively with premorbid verbal intelligence. Scores were higher for men than for women on most cognitive tests. After adjustment for these associations, individuals with self-reported memory complaints and memory problems, compared with those without memory complaints or problems, showed increased risk of poor performance in recall, factual memory, time and place orientation, and concentration, but there was no increased risk of poor performance at language, verbal abstraction, or copying design.

Discussion.—Individuals living in the community who are neither depressed nor demented and who have complaints about memory perform less well on cognitive tests than do those without memory complaints. Individuals reporting both memory complaints and memory-related problems perform even less well on cognitive tests. Asking questions about memory complaints as well as memory-related problems may identify a wider group at risk. This distinction may be important because older individuals sometimes perceive their memory to be generally impaired, yet specific questioning about activities reveals substantially less impairment. Subjective memory complaints should be considered a potential indicator of memory impairment signaling a need for follow-up.

▶ The Amsterdam Study on the Elderly has been a useful community-based study of elderly individuals. In this portion of the study, the researchers address an important topic for clinicians: the prognostic value of subjective memory complaints. When do such complaints portend that a neurologically significant memory problem will occur in the future? Some of us have been touting the clinical pearl that if the family complains about the patient's memory, the problem is likely to be early dementia, whereas if the patient complains about his or her own memory, the problem is more likely to be depression.

In this study, individuals with depression were not studied and the CAM-COG was used to assess cognition. Although the authors include a number of caveats about their finding, they present the concern that subjective memory complaints can warn of subsequent dementia. For nondepressed individuals, the clinician would do well to consider referral to a neuropsychologist or at least a follow-up visit in 6 months.

P.J. Whitehouse, M.D., Ph.D.

The Natural History of Alzheimer's Disease: A Brain Bank Study
Jost BC, Grossberg GT (Saint Louis Univ, Mo)
J Am Geriatr Soc 43:1248–1255, 1995   4–9

Background and Objective.—Studies of the natural history of Alzheimer's disease are complex because the diagnosis of this disease is based on exclusion and because natural history studies are longitudinal by design. The only way to confirm a diagnosis of Alzheimer's disease is by autopsy. The natural history of Alzheimer's disease has not been formally studied in large numbers of patients in whom the disease was confirmed by autopsy. Persons with Alzheimer's disease who are registered in a brain bank before or at death are ideal subjects for natural history studies. The natural history of Alzheimer's disease and the clinical and demographic characteristics of patients with this disease were described.

Methods.—Data from 100 patients with autopsy-confirmed Alzheimer's disease were collected. Data pertaining to family and clinical history, use of medication, nutrition, clinical testing, behavioral symptoms, and deficits in cognitive function and daily activities were analyzed.

Results.—These results are expressed in mean values. The time between symptom onset and diagnosis was 32.1 months; this interval was longer for patients younger than 65 years of age at time of diagnosis, women, and those with a family history of dementia. Patient age at diagnosis ranged from 52 to 89 years (mean, 74.7 years). A diagnosis was made at an earlier age in men than in women. The time between diagnosis and institutionalization was almost 2 years. Patient age at institutionalization ranged from 60 to 92.5 years (mean, 77.6 years). The time between symptom onset and institutionalization was 56.5 months; this interval was shorter for patients older than 65 years of age at time of diagnosis and those with no family history of the disease. Duration of disease was defined as the time from symptom onset to death. Disease duration was nearly 8.5 years and was longer in patients who were younger at onset, women, and those with a family history of dementia.

Discussion.—Other diseases, consequences of the aging process, and denial on behalf of the primary caregiver can play a role in the sometimes long delays between onset of symptoms and a diagnosis of Alzheimer's disease. Further analysis of these findings will address the role of medical history; education; and functional, behavioral, and cognitive impairment on the duration of disease and other variables.

▶ This article was selected for overtly personal reasons—I reviewed this article and recommended its acceptance in the *Journal of the American Geriatrics Society.* It is a study of 100 cases selected from the autopsy program at St. Louis University School of Medicine. Dr. William Deal and I wrote an editorial commenting on this article from the postmodern perspective.[1] The word "postmodern" engenders strong reactions, as was evidenced from subsequent correspondence in the journal. The major point to be made, which I think bears repeating in this YEAR BOOK, is that physicians need to be more aware of the cultural context in which medicine exists. Science and medicine are losing some of the privileges of their positions in society, which were based on a degree of independence from social and cultural forces. Postmodernism, one of the major cultural trends that is affecting the humanities, literature, architecture, and art, asks us to think more critically about the limitations of the vantage points that we assume as scientists and clinicians in approaching health problems that are emerging in a broader cultural context.

P.J. Whitehouse, M.D., Ph.D.

Reference

1. Whitehouse PJ, Deal WE: Situated beyond modernity: Lessons for Alzheimer's disease research (editorial). *J Am Geriatr Soc* 43:1314–1315, 1995.

Predicting the Onset of Alzheimer's Disease Using Bayes' Theorem
Prince MJ (Inst of Psychiatry, London)
Am J Epidemiol 143:301–308, 1996   4–10

Background.—The apolipoprotein E e4 (apoE e4) allele is known to be strongly associated with Alzheimer's disease. However, on its own, apoE e4 is not specific enough to be used as a screening test for Alzheimer's disease. Bayes' theorem offers a means of evaluating the effect of some new information on the likelihood that a certain outcome will occur—in this case, the effect of a test result on the probability of a disease. When likelihood ratios for separate tests are developed and combined, the joint effects of the tests on disease probability can be assessed. Bayes' theorem was used in an attempt to develop a test battery capable of predicting the onset of Alzheimer's disease.

Methods.—Several tests that were moderately predictive of Alzheimer's disease were combined in an attempt to develop a more effective combination of tests. The tests selected were the Paired Associated Learning Test, the Trailmaking Test, and Raven's Progressive Matrices; these were combined with consideration of patient age and a family history of dementia. Participating in the study were 1,454 elderly individuals from a previous study of hypertension. The cognitive tests were all administered at study entry—between 1983 and 1985—and again 1 month later. None of the subjects had signs of dementia at baseline. The mean age was 70.5 years, and all were hypertensive. The subjects were followed up through 1990–1991, when dementia status was assessed.

Results.—Subjects in whom dementia developed during follow-up performed less well on the cognitive tests at baseline. The combined tests' ability to predict dementia and Alzheimer's disease depended on the false positive rate level considered. At a 9% false positive rate, 52% of cases of Alzheimer's disease were identified. At a false positive rate of 29%, 90% of cases were identified. A split-half reliability exercise suggested that the test performed approximately as well in a test data set as in the development data set, with areas under the receiver operating characteristic curve of 0.82 and 0.78.

Conclusions.—Although the study does not offer a practical test battery for the prediction of Alzheimer's disease, it does suggest that a Bayes' theorem approach could be useful for this purpose. A cognitive test battery could be combined with an apoE e4 test as a likelihood ratio approach for prospective identification of patients at increased risk for Alzheimer's disease. The next step would be ethically sound trials of new treatments for individuals at risk.

▶ Bayes' theorem should not be unknown to clinicians. It describes the effect of new information (e.g., a test result) on the probability of an outcome (e.g., a disease). If multiple tests are performed, their results can be combined so that their joint effect on determining the probability of a disease can be assessed. Bayes' theorem is important to all of medicine but particularly for Alzheimer's disease because there has been a rapid increase in the amount of information that is claimed to assist the diagnostic process.

This study focuses on a combination of simple cognitive tests, age, and family history. However, it alludes to the test for apoE e4 status, which clearly affects the risk for Alzheimer's disease. In the United States, AD-MARK is being marketed, a diagnostic test for Alzheimer's disease that considers apoE e4 status and levels of Aβ and τ in CSF. However, it is not clear to me that we have adequately described the populations for which these tests will be used and analyzed the mathematical probabilities that will allow us to assess whether these biological tests offer a significant increment of diagnostic specificity and sensitivity.

P.J. Whitehouse, M.D., Ph.D.

Reversible Dementia: More Than 10% or Less Than 1%? A Quantitative Review
Weytingh MD, Bossuyt PMM, van Crevel H (Academic Med Ctr, Amsterdam)
J Neurol 242:466–471, 1995   4–11

Objective.—The reported percentages of reversible dementia vary widely. In a systematic, quantitative review of the literature, the factors behind the variation were identified, and a more accurate estimate of the prevalence of reversible dementia was obtained.

Methods.—A literature search of publications on reversible dementia from 1972 through 1994 produced 1,232 studies, of which 16 (with a total of 1,551 patients) met the inclusion criteria. The percentages of reversed dementia varied widely. The average for potentially reversible dementia was 15.2%; for partly reversed dementia, 9.3%; and for fully reversed dementia, 1.5%. Depression and intoxication by drugs were the most frequent causes of reversible dementia. The percentage of partial and full reversal of dementia decreased in the more recently published studies.

Conclusion.—Because reversible dementia is very rare, a full clinical investigation of elderly outpatients with dementia is not likely to detect treatable causes of the dementia.

▶ Clinicians should always try to identify partially or fully reversible causes of dementia (e.g., surgically removable structural lesions or endocrine abnormalities). There has been controversy, however, concerning the prevalence of reversible dementias in different populations. The site of clinical practice has a large effect on the number and causes of reversible forms identified.

This paper, a review of studies conducted between 1972 and 1994, reports depression and drug intoxication to be the most frequent causes of reversible dementia, followed by metabolic and neurosurgical disorders. I suppose the good news is that the percentage of individuals found to have reversible dementia in outpatient settings was less than expected, perhaps as a result of earlier detection by primary care physicians. On the other hand, this finding may reflect the aging population and the greater likelihood that detected dementia is caused by Alzheimer's disease or a disorder that is not reversible. In an age in which new diagnostic approaches are being developed (e.g., apolipoprotein E type and β amyloid in CSF), this paper also reminds us that we know precious little about when to conduct a full clinical evaluation with "routine" blood and imaging studies.

P.J. Whitehouse, M.D., Ph.D.

Epidemiology

Prevalence of Alzheimer's Disease and Dementia in Two Communities: Nigerian Africans and African Americans

Hendrie HC, Osuntokun BO, Hall KS, et al (Indiana Univ, Indianapolis; Univ of Ibadan, Nigeria)
Am J Psychiatry 152:1485–1492, 1995   4–12

Introduction.—It is believed that Alzheimer's disease is caused by a combination of aging along with genetic and environmental factors. However, little is certain regarding nongenetic risk factors other than family history and age. Identification of environmental risk factors would be facilitated by the identification of populations with high and low prevalence of the disease. Therefore, the prevalence of Alzheimer's disease was compared in 2 populations from the same ethnic group: Nigerian Africans living in Ibadan, Nigeria, and African-Americans living in Indianapolis, Indiana.

Methods.—Elderly individuals and a family member were interviewed in the community screening phase in 2,494 households in Ibadan and 2,212 households in Indianapolis. In addition, the African-American residents of 20 nursing homes in Indianapolis were screened for dementia. The screening instrument included literacy-independent items drawn from several standard measures of mental state and memory. A detailed cognitive and medical history report was obtained from a key informant. Individuals with poor cognitive performance during the screening interview were clinically evaluated for Alzheimer's disease or other forms of dementia.

Results.—Dementia was diagnosed in 65 patients in Indianapolis and in 28 patients in Ibadan. There were 49 patients in Indianapolis and 18 in Ibadan who met the diagnostic criteria for possible or probable Alzheimer's disease. Ten patients in Indianapolis and 8 in Ibadan had vascular dementia. Indianapolis had higher age-adjusted prevalence rates and prevalence rates in all age groups than did Ibadan.

Conclusions.—The Yorubas in Ibadan have a significantly lower prevalence of dementia and Alzheimer's disease than African Americans in Indianapolis, demonstrating the first reported difference in prevalence in populations of the same ethnic group from different environments. After validation of these findings, the interaction of genetic and environmental risk factors may be explored in these 2 populations.

▶ More studies are needed to understand the incidence and prevalence of Alzheimer's disease in African-Americans, particularly in relationship to apolipoprotein E status. Particular interest has been provoked by autopsy studies in Nigeria that have suggested an exceedingly low incidence of Alzheimer's disease. This interesting study compared the prevalence of dementia and, more specifically, the prevalence of Alzheimer's disease in 2 communities: Nigerian Africans and African-Americans in Indianapolis, Indiana. It confirms that Nigerian Africans do get dementia, including Alzheimer's disease, albeit at about a twofold lower risk. As the authors point out, there are many factors, including genetic differences, environmental differences, and their research method, that could explain the results. However, the study is important because it allows us to state that unfortunately no population of humans appears to be free from the risk of Alzheimer's disease, including Nigerians.

P.J. Whitehouse, M.D., Ph.D.

Prevalence of Alzheimer's Disease and Vascular Dementia: Association With Education. The Rotterdam Study
Ott A, Breteler MMB, van Harskamp F, et al (Erasmus Univ, Rotterdam, The Netherlands)
BMJ 310:970–973, 1995   4–13

Background.—The increasing proportion of elderly individuals in the population will have a major impact on health care costs. Given the high frequency of dementing disorders in elderly individuals, it is of great medical and social relevance to know the prevalence rates and determinants of these diseases. The prevalence of dementia was assessed in a population-based, cross-sectional study, with special attention given to the association between dementia and education.

Methods.—The analysis was performed as part of the Rotterdam study, a prospective, population-based study of the neurologic, cardiovascular, locomotor, and ophthalmologic diseases of old age. It included 7,528 research subjects between the ages of 55 and 106 years. A 3-phase approach to the identification of dementia was used: screening with a brief cognitive test, additional testing for subjects with a positive screening result, and confirmatory review of the medical records of patients whose findings suggested the possibility of dementia.

Results.—The overall prevalence of dementia was 6.3%, ranging from 0.4% for subjects aged 55–59 years to 43.2% for those aged 95 years and older. Seventy-two percent of cases of dementia were caused by Alzheimer's disease, which was also the major cause of the marked age-related increase in dementia. Vascular dementia accounted for 16% of cases, Parkinson's disease dementia for 6%, and other dementias for 5%. For these causes, the relative proportion of subjects affected decreased with age. Subjects with lower levels of education had significantly more dementia; the relative risks for individuals in the 2 lowest educational strata were 3.2 compared with those with the highest level of education. The link between dementia and education was not confounded by cardiovascular disease.

Conclusions.—An exponential increase in the prevalence of dementia occurs with age, to the point where approximately one third of individuals 85 years of age and older have dementia. About three fourths of cases of dementia are caused by Alzheimer's disease. Dementia, especially Alzheimer's disease, is more likely to occur in individuals with lower levels of education.

▶ Despite the emphasis on genetic risk factors for Alzheimer's disease, environmental risk factors are also important and are potentially more modifiable. The authors of this study examined dementia, both vascular dementia and Alzheimer's disease, in Rotterdam, The Netherlands. They confirm that education appears to protect individuals from having dementia, particularly Alzheimer's disease, develop. Interestingly, the authors report an inverse dose–response curve relating the amount of education to dementia. It is unclear whether a biological explanation is best invoked (i.e., that more education increases neuronal connectivity or, perhaps, that individuals who obtain more education are born with a more resistant nervous system). It is also possible that factors that correlate with education (e.g., diet or occupational exposure) may also explain this effect. Nevertheless, the results give clinicians reason to continue to encourage their older patients to stay intellectually active and to participate in lifelong learning, not only for its own merit but potentially for its effects in preventing dementia.

P.J. Whitehouse, M.D., Ph.D.

QUALITY OF LIFE

Video Respite: An Innovative Resource for Family, Professional Caregivers, and Persons With Dementia
Lund DA, Hill RD, Caserta MS, et al (Univ of Utah, Salt Lake City)
Gerontologist 35:683–687, 1995   4–14

Introduction.—Research shows that respite time is the most needed, but least available, resource for family and professional caregivers of persons with dementia. Many caregivers are reluctant to use existing respite services, such as day care and in-home respite services, because of inconvenience, guilt, cost, or personal preference. It is difficult to care for persons with dementia because they can be easily agitated, repeat questions endlessly, and need constant attention. Caregivers of such persons need more frequent periods of respite. Video Respite is a videotape created specifically for persons with dementia that is intended to occupy their attention in meaningful activities.

Pilot Study.—It was initially assumed that an effective videotape should include content that focuses on long-term memory specific to the individual, show only 1 person on the screen at a time, encourage interaction from the viewer, and allow time for the viewer to respond. The pilot videotapes used actual family caregivers from local support groups and were specific to individual patients. The tapes included information about the early life experiences of the impaired family member, who was filmed while watching this videotape and an existing television program. These pilot tapes were effective in holding the patient's attention.

Generic Respite Videotapes.—These tapes use professional actors, do not refer to the viewer by name, but still contain the other elements of the pilot tapes. They are slow-paced, simple, conversational, and encourage interaction. They contain positive messages and relate to people and experiences that are likely to be ingrained in long-term memory. The first of these 10 tapes is entitled *Favorite Things* and begins with a friendly visitor who talks and asks questions about parents, babies, growing up, pets, holidays, and gardens. There are pauses so the viewer can respond. The viewer is also asked to sing along to familiar songs. The first 10 tapes have unique themes for men, women, African-American, Jewish, or Spanish-speaking persons or have an event theme, such as patriotic events. The visitors on each tape tell short stories, ask questions, use humor, and encourage the viewer to smile, sing, and perform simple body movements.

Research and Evaluation.—The first videotape, *Favorite Things*, is being evaluated in a 2-year study. Viewers with Alzheimer's disease have been filmed while watching this tape and a Lawrence Welk program. Early results are very positive. Among patients with Alzheimer's disease, 84% remained seated, paid attention, and verbally responded to the videotape; only 56% of patients had these reactions while watching a Lawrence Welk program. Caregivers have used the tapes often and reported that the impaired persons enjoy the tapes every time they watch them.

Discussion.—Potential benefits of these tapes include reducing caregiver burden, reducing a patient's disruptive or problematic behavior, and stimulating other interaction and cognitive functioning in the patient. These videotapes are less effective for persons with early stages of dementia. Each tape includes an instruction booklet. Caregivers should be familiar with the entire videotape and see how the patient responds to it before the patient is left alone with the tape. The videotapes should not be used if they upset the patient or if the caregiver does not like the tape or the effect it has on the viewer.

▶ It is time that we think more cleverly about the use of information technology in the care of patients with dementia. This article takes a step in that direction by describing a program called Video Respite. Individualized videotapes are created for patients to attract their attention, provide pleasurable experiences, and provide time off for the caregiver. A television monitor does attract all types of persons, including those in nursing homes. In this setting, the television in the day room is frequently one of the most noticeable auditory and visual stimuli. We could develop not only videotapes but also CD-ROMs, which could be individually designed for patients to play music, show images, and provide pleasure and perhaps some degree of behavioral control. As dementia progresses, the music could be varied so that as a patient's memories become more distant, the age of the musical collections included on the individualized program increases. In the later stages of the disease, many patients with Alzheimer's disease have difficulty distinguishing a television image from reality. Instead of seeing the television as a form of reality therapy (i.e., watching what we watch to learn about the real world), could not the television program be used as a form of validation, to reflect the issues and time base of the patient's current existence?

P.J. Whitehouse, M.D., Ph.D.

Bathing Persons With Dementia
Sloane PD, Rader J, Barrick A-L, et al (Univ of North Carolina, Chapel Hill; Benedictine Inst for Long-Term Care Research, Mt Angel, Ore; Oregon Health Sciences Univ, Portland; et al)
Gerontologist 35:672–678, 1995   4–15

Introduction.—Bathing individuals with Alzheimer's disease and related disorders can be an extremely stressful experience for both patients and caregivers. Practical guidelines for care providers were developed by staff from 2 studies, sponsored by the National Institutes of Health, on reducing aggressive and agitated behaviors when bathing patients with dementia.

Recommended Approach to Bathing.—Individuals with dementia may interpret baths as assaults and respond to perceived threats with natural, defensive behaviors. Therefore, care must be individualized by knowing the patient's bathing history and preferences, and by focusing on the patient, more so than the task, through appropriate communication techniques. Caregivers must also be flexible and willing to use a different bathing technique or stop the procedure if the patient becomes agitated.

Environment.—A homelike setting is suggested, with a room that feels private and personal. Measures should be taken to keep the patient warm. Music, soft lighting, and noise reduction may relax some patients. Aromas may evoke memories, set the mood, and make the bath more pleasant. Bathing equipment should be comfortable and functional.

Communication.—Distraction, patient persuasion, and providing a reason for the bath (e.g., "your hair is dirty") may help encourage reluctant patients. One individual, rather than several, approaching the patient is much less threatening. Providing information about what is going on and giving positive feedback and rewards for cooperating can make the task easier, as will addressing the patient in familiar terms such as those used by family members.

Summary.—Bathing is not a mechanical task but a complex set of skills. When faced with reluctant patients, caregivers should ask whether the time and conditions are appropriate for bathing. Simple actions, such as providing adequate covering, show respect for the patient's dignity and privacy. Making changes in the way hygiene is approached in institutional settings requires basing care on individually assessed needs rather than rituals of practice.

▶ In this chapter about geriatric neurology, we frequently feature basic research regarding the molecular biology and genetics of Alzheimer's disease, and I share the excitement concerning these studies and their implications for therapeutics. It is also important, however, that we share information about seemingly more mundane interventions that can dramatically affect the quality of life of patients and caregivers. Many of us know that personal hygiene and refusal of bathing are major difficulties in patients with dementia that frequently may precipitate institutionalization. This nicely written summary of a National Consensus Conference presents practical advice that, in the short term, will improve the quality of life of more patients and caregivers than will any molecular biology study.

P.J. Whitehouse, M.D., Ph.D.

ETHICAL AND LEGAL ISSUES

Knowledge and Experience With Alzheimer's Disease: Relationship to Resuscitation Preference
Griffith CH III, Wilson JF, Emmett KR, et al (Univ of Kentucky, Lexington)
Arch Fam Med 4:780–784, 1995   4–16

Background.—Many studies of patient preferences for cardiopulmonary resuscitation (CPR) have found that at least 20% of patients want resuscitation in any scenario. Is there a core group of individuals who, because of religious or personal beliefs, want resuscitation under any circumstances? The hypothesis that, independent of religious beliefs, individuals with greater knowledge of and experience with Alzheimer's disease would be less likely to request CPR in hypothetical scenarios in which they have Alzheimer's disease was investigated.

Methods.—A telephone survey of adult Kentuckians chosen by random digit dialing was done in 1993. The 16 questions about CPR, Alzheimer's disease, and resuscitation preferences were among 213 questions included in the Kentucky Health Survey. A random selection of half the survey respondents were read a short educational paragraph about CPR and the chances of surviving resuscitation (fewer than 10% of older persons survive to leave the hospital). All respondents were then asked about their CPR preferences in 1 of 2 scenarios: (1) in their current state of health, and (2) if they had memory loss and senility (Alzheimer's disease) such that they were no longer able to recognize family and friends.

Results.—Of the 1,581 eligible residents called, 45.2% (661) completed the survey. Overall, 88% said they would want to be resuscitated in their present state of health, and 22% said that they would want to be resuscitated if they had Alzheimer's disease. The following factors were significantly correlated with a *decreased* desire to be resuscitated: increased education, increased income, female sex, nonwhite race, being married, nonrural residence, desiring CPR in current state of health, and greater knowledge of or experience with Alzheimer's disease. Knowledge of Alzheimer's disease superseded level of education as an independent predictor of CPR preferences. The elderly individuals were less likely to prefer CPR in their current state of health (73% vs. 92%) or if they had Alzheimer's disease (15% vs. 22%). In scenarios involving Alzheimer's disease, neither knowledge of resuscitation outcomes (± hearing the data in the CPR educational paragraph) nor one's CPR preference in the current state of health was predictive of CPR preference. Because 88% of the respondents were Christians, the role of different religious beliefs in deciding CPR preferences could not be determined.

Conclusions.—In hypothetical scenarios involving Alzheimer's disease, CPR preference is influenced by an individual's knowledge of or experience with Alzheimer's disease, independent of such factors as knowledge of CPR, income level, or education. When discussing advanced care directives and resuscitation preferences in some future state of health, individuals with little knowledge or experience with Alzheimer's disease may need to be educated about Alzheimer's disease to make informed decisions.

▶ This telephone survey provides interesting information about individual preferences for CPR. Certain demographic variables, such as older age, greater income, female sex, and nonwhite race, predicted a greater likelihood of refusing CPR. Interestingly, knowledge of or experience with Alzheimer's disease was also a high predictor, suggesting that this variable is important to consider in discussions with patients and families. I suspect that the authors are correct in believing that their effort to improve understanding of CPR (they read an educational paragraph to survey participants over the phone) was not a powerful enough intervention to affect decision making. Previous studies have shown that if individuals recognize that likely outcomes from CPR are usually less favorable than most people think, this will affect their desire to have resuscitation.

P.J. Whitehouse, M.D., Ph.D.

Fairhill Guidelines on Ethics of the Care of People With Alzheimer's Disease: A Clinical Summary
Post SG, Whitehouse PJ (Case Western Reserve Univ, Cleveland, Ohio)
J Am Geriatr Soc 43:1423–1429, 1995   4–17

Introduction.—An inductive method was used to formulate ethical principles by listening carefully to those most affected by particular ethical questions involved in the care of patients with dementia. This method of "discourse ethics" contrasted with deductive methods of moral theory making.

Methods.—A focus group of professionals (including nurses, physicians, lawyers, ethicists, and administrators) raised questions and issues and listened to the input of patients with mild dementia of the Alzheimer's type and family members.

Guidelines For Ethical Care of Patients With Dementia.—The patients and their families should always be informed of the diagnosis of probable Alzheimer's disease (AD). Questions should be encouraged and answered fully. Physician recommendations should include information about the resources available to the patient and family. Personal values and the use of life-prolonging technologies should be discussed and a care plan formulated, preferably with both the patient and the family. End-of-life decisions should be discussed with the patient before the progression of dementia, and the choice to refuse treatments should not be equated with assisted suicide. Driving privileges should not be revoked automatically but should be considered in the context of an individualized risk appraisal, possibly with negotiations for the gradual curtailment of driving. In general, privileges should not be limited without identifying alternatives and addressing the sense of loss and of self-control. Autonomy should be supported whenever possible, with capacity assessments varying according to the likely harms and benefits associated with these decisions. Typical behaviors, such as wandering, should not be limited whenever possible. Rather, the environmment should be modified to increase safety. Behavior-controlling medication should be used cautiously for specified symptom control only when clearly beneficial. Quality of life should be assessed on the patient's terms, which requires careful attention to patient responses. When only comfort measures are requested, routine support technologies, such as artificial feeding, should be reassessed.

Conclusions.—As the prevalence of Alzheimer's disease increases, greater attention to the ethical issues involved in the care of patients with dementia will be needed to ensure respect for human dignity and the emotional and relational well-being of patients with dementia.

Public Understanding of Science
Turney J (Univ College, London)
Lancet 347:1087–1090, 1996   4–18

Introduction.—In the past 20 years, there have been greater efforts to increase public understanding of science. However, these efforts have fostered increasing tensions between those who seek public awareness, appreciation, or approval of science and those who consider public understanding of science as the prerequisite for constructive criticism of scientific inquiries. The political issues and research findings related to public understanding of science were reviewed.

Informing the Public.—The traditional approach to advocating public understanding of science has assumed that the public is either ignorant or irrational. However, research has shown that many people have a possibly justifiable belief that science simply has nothing to do with their needs or interests.

Traditionally, science has been treated as revealed truth, and education efforts have focused on disseminating facts. However, this approach implies an assumption of trust, which may be difficult in an era of ambivalence. Although surveys have shown that most people have favorable attitudes toward medical research, current medical research emphasizes predictive medicine, involving assessments of risk and probability. Therefore, an approach that emphasizes understanding the scientific process and interactions between science and society is increasingly being taken.

Increasing the Relevance.—Current social science research has shown that increasing public understanding of science may depend upon increasing understanding of the public. Adult science education should therefore consider what the multiple publics, rather than a single monolithic public, want to know about, rather than force-feeding what scientists believe the public should know. Research shows that individuals are very resourceful in finding the information that interests them, and they use their personal evaluations of the various sources of information to determine how trustworthy the information is. In addition, they may resist absorbing information that is perceived as pertaining to forces beyond their control.

Conclusion.—Because understanding follows motivation, the success of efforts to improve public understanding of science depends upon accurately assessing and addressing the needs or interests of particular publics.

▶ I have resisted commenting on my own articles in this YEAR BOOK, but I wish to present this one (Abstract 4–17) because it represents a new approach to developing ethical guidelines for the care of patients with AD. The process described was a bottom-up approach driven by patients and families to understand the practical, real-life decisions with which they require help from health care professionals. The article reviews patients' and family members' thoughts concerning diagnosis, competence, behavior control, death and dying, quality of life, treatment decisions, and driving privileges. All these issues emerged from conversations with participants who represented a wide variety of professional and nonprofessional groups.

This effort was grounded in a form of ethics referred to as discourse or communicative ethics, in which the emphasis is placed on sincere, effective communication among individuals facing practical, real-life dilemmas. It does not substitute for, but rather complements, the more principle-driven ethics that dominate bioethics in the United States, in which major consideration is given to theoretical principles such as autonomy, beneficence, and justice. The Fairhill guidelines process is being adopted by AD associations in the United States, Canada, and Japan to promote discussion about ethical issues among their members.

The issue of listening to the public goes far beyond AD in terms of its importance for physicians caring for older people and for physicians and scientists in general. As the article from *Lancet* (Abstract 4–18) suggests, scientists often believe that if they could only adequately communicate the content of their material, the public would rush to support them with more tax dollars. What is emphasized in this article is similar to the philosophy of the Fairhill guidelines process: Scientists need to listen to the public and understand them better, rather than just the reverse.

P.J. Whitehouse, M.D., Ph.D.

Assessing the Competency of Patients With Alzheimer's Disease Under Different Legal Standards: A Prototype Instrument

Marson DC, Ingram KK, Cody HA, et al (Univ of Alabama, Birmingham)
Arch Neurol 52:949–954, 1995   4–19

Background.—Although competency is a legal term, determinations of a patient's capability to make judgements regarding medical treatment must be made continually by physicians caring for patients with Alzheimer's disease (AD). These determinations are typically based on subjective clinical assessments and brief mental status testing. The utility of a prototype instrument for the empirical assessment of the competency of patients with AD regarding making medical treatment judgments was evaluated using 5 different legal standards (LSs).

Methods.—Twenty-nine patients with probable AD and 15 normal older control subjects were asked to answer questions related to 2 clinical vignettes. The instrument tested competency under the following 5 LSs: the capacity to make a treatment choice (LS1), to make a reasonable treatment choice (LS2), to appreciate the emotional and cognitive consequences of their choices (LS3), to provide rational reasons for the treatment choice (LS4), and to understand the choices (LS5).

Results.—The control subjects demonstrated competency under all 5 LSs. Compared with the performance of control patients, competency performance was significantly lower on LS3 through LS5 in the AD group. In addition, patients with mild AD performed significantly better than patients with moderate AD. The pattern of compromise in the patients with AD was consistently progressive, related to both the severity of dementia and the stringency of the LS.

Conclusions.—The prototype instrument was reliable and valid in evaluating the competency status of both normal older subjects and patients with AD under well-established legal standards. This method of assessment shows great clinical promise.

Neuropsychologic Predictors of Competency in Alzheimer's Disease Using a Rational Reasons Legal Standard

Marson DC, Cody HA, Ingram KK, et al (Univ of Alabama, Birmingham)
Arch Neurol 52:955–959, 1995   4–20

Background.—Little is known about the natural history or the neuropsychological correlates of competency loss in patients with dementia. To help illuminate the assessment of competency in these patients, the neuropsychological predictors of competency performance under a single specific legal standard were analyzed.

Methods.—Twenty-nine patients with probable AD and 15 normal older controls underwent competency assessment, using 2 clinical vignettes and questions related to legal standards. One of these legal standards, the capacity to provide rational reasons for a medical treatment choice, was analyzed for associations with measurements of the following neuropsychological domains: attention, expressive language, receptive language, short-term verbal memory, delayed verbal memory, abstraction, social comprehension/judgment, executive function, and dementia severity.

Results.—All neuropsychological measures were significantly better in control subjects than in patients with AD. Measures of word fluency were the most important predictors of performance under the rational reason legal standard in both univariate and multivariate analysis. The severity of dementia, as measured by the Mini-Mental State Examination, was not significantly associated with competency status.

Conclusions.—Word fluency is a significant, independent predictor of the capacity to formulate rational reasons for medical decisions. Measures of word fluency have been significantly associated with frontal lobe functioning, suggesting that frontal lobe function governs the ability to formulate rational reasons for making a medical decision.

▶ The assessment of the competency of patients with AD requires more study. Previous national bioethics commissions have developed guidelines for children and prisoners, but not for cognitively impaired individuals, that detail the appropriate means of obtaining informed consent for either research or clinical care.

The group that wrote the 2 articles (Abstracts 4–19 and 4–20) have been pioneers in analyzing the basis of competency in dementia and its assessment. They find, not surprisingly, that word fluency (which is probably a reasonable measure of executive function in AD) is associated with the competency status of older subjects. Thus, AD does appear to cause so-called frontal lobe dysfunction (although it is not as severe as in the frontal lobe dementias), which affects judgment and, therefore, the capacity to consent to medical treatment.

The authors also present information about a prototypical instrument based on clinical vignettes in which a subject's decision making is evaluated using 5 legal standards. This may be somewhat cumbersome for a geriatric clinician to use, but it is important for primary care physicians to be aware that neurologists, psychiatrists, and neuropsychologists are making progress in assisting competency decision making in dementia.

P.J. Whitehouse, M.D., Ph.D.

Vascular Dementia

Vascular Dementia
Amar K, Wilcock G (Bristol Univ, England)
BMJ 312:227–231, 1996   4–21

Introduction.—At the turn of the century, cerebral atherosclerosis was believed to be the most common cause of dementia. Alzheimer's disease was thought to be a rare cause of dementia that only affected younger patients. By the 1950s, it had been discovered that cerebral atherosclerosis could be present in normal persons and those with cognitive impairment. The characteristics of ischemic vascular dementia were reviewed.

Mechanisms.—Vascular dementia is 1 of the 3 most common causes of dementia and may be caused by multiple infarction, a single strategically placed infarction, or white-matter ischemia. Infarctions can be in the cerebral cortex, subcortical regions, or in both cortical and subcortical areas. The site of the infarction has more effect on resulting dementia than the volume of tissue lost. Multiple cortical infarctions often result from thromboembolic disease or cerebral vasculitis. Dementia can also result from multiple lacunar infarctions. Angular gyrus syndrome is a dementia resulting from infarction of the angular gyrus in the inferior parietal lobule. This syndrome was often misdiagnosed as Alzheimer's disease. White-matter ischemia may be the most common mechanism of vascular dementia. White-matter lesions are seen in 70% to 90% of patients with vascular dementia, 10% to 20% of patients with early-onset Alzheimer's disease, and 70% to 80% of those with late-onset Alzheimer's disease.

Risk Factors.—Stroke and age are the most significant risk factors for dementia, and stroke alone increases the risk 9 times. Other risk factors include older age, low education level, history of stroke, diabetes, and left-sided lesions.

Evaluation and Differential Diagnosis.—Evaluation of a patient with possible cognitive impairment should include assessment of vascular risk factors, examination of the cardiovascular system, and neurologic examination. It is important to look for treatable causes of dementia, such as hypothyroidism, neurosyphilis, vitamin B_{12} deficiency, normal-pressure hydrocephalus, frontal lobe tumors, cerebral vasculitis, and even hyperviscosity syndromes and severe bilateral carotid stenosis. Computed tomography or MRI is necessary to exclude some of these possible causes. Vascular dementia must be differentiated from Alzheimer's disease, Lewy body type dementia, progressive supranuclear palsy, corticobasal degeneration, Parkinson's disease dementia, and frontal lobe tumors.

Discussion.—Vascular dementia is preventable, and cognitive functioning may be improved by controlling risk factors such as hypertension and diabetes and by using an antiplatelet drug. Ongoing research is examining the role of white-matter disease in dementia. Further research regarding the relation of structural pathologic changes to signs and symptoms in subtypes of vascular dementia is needed. The use of thrombolytic drugs to treat acute stroke may also have implications for vascular dementia.

▶ The discussion about the definition of vascular dementia and its relationship to Alzheimer's disease continues. Several diagnostic criteria have been proposed (e.g., by the Alzheimer's Disease Diagnostic and Treatment Center in California, the National Institute of Neurological and Communicative Disorders and Stroke, and the European Panel of Experts), but the application of these criteria in practice is difficult. Some novel methods are being brought to bear in drug studies of this condition.

Many medications are useful in treating vascular dementia, but there have been few studies of this condition. Fortunately, that neglect seems to be changing, and in the process we are considering how to ensure that we adequately categorize patients to examine potential effects of different drugs. One suggestion is that we grade the likelihood that vascular dementia is contributing to the cognitive impairment. The importance of this approach is illustrated by Sevush et al. (see Abstract 4–22), who studied almost 100 patients who came to autopsy, using the standard rules for diagnosis of cerebral vascular disease (history, focal deficits on examination, and neuroimaging). These criteria showed exceedingly low sensitivity and specificity.

We have become overly obsessed with differentiating Alzheimer's disease from vascular dementia. We must broaden our studies to include a wider range of individuals and see whether some of the drugs being studied for Alzheimer's disease can help patients whose dementia has vascular components.

P.J. Whitehouse, M.D., Ph.D.

Clinicopathologic Study of Probable Alzheimer Disease: Assessment of Criteria for Excluding Cerebrovascular Disease

Sevush S, Duara R, Rivero J, et al (Univ of Miami, Fla; Mount Sinai Med Ctr, New York)

Alzheimer Dis Assoc Disord 9:208–212, 1995   4–22

Background and Objective.—The National Institute of Neurological and Communicative Disorders and Stroke/Alzheimer's Disease and Related Disorders Association requires that other cognition-impairing conditions be excluded before probable Alzheimer's disease can be diagnosed. However, the Institute provides no exclusion rules. Specific exclusion criteria would improve the reliability of diagnostic decisions. Exclusion rules for probable Alzheimer's disease–cerebrovascular disease must identify pure cerebrovascular disease, as well as mixed Alzheimer's disease and cerebrovascular disease. Exclusion rules for cerebrovascular disease, the most common of the non–Alzheimer's disease cognition-impairing conditions, were defined.

Methods.—A provisional set of exclusion rules for cerebrovascular disease was defined on the basis of history of strokelike episodes, history of stepwise cognitive decline, focal deficits on neurologic examination, and significant cerebrovascular disease on neuroimaging. These rules were applied retrospectively to the cases of 92 patients with cognitive decline who met criteria for probable Alzheimer's disease and whose brains were examined after death. The effectiveness of the exclusion rules was determined by comparing the clinical records with the autopsy diagnoses.

Results.—The exclusion rules predicted cerebrovascular disease on autopsy significantly better than chance, but the overall accuracy was only 50%; the sensitivity, also low, was 52.6%. Independent examination of the exclusion rules as predictors of cerebrovascular disease showed that the neuroimaging and the criteria for stepwise decline predicted cerebrovascular disease better than chance. The other criteria did not predict findings from autopsy better than chance.

Discussion.—These exclusions rules must be modified to improve accuracy and sensitivity; however, the accuracy and sensitivity may have been affected by study design and limitations in the exclusion rules themselves. Techniques more discriminating than histologic inspection alone are needed to determine levels of autopsy evidence of cerebrovascular disease that should be considered clinically significant. Neuropathologic evaluation is inadequate for predicting changes in cognition and behavior.

▶ The discussion about the definition of vascular dementia and its relationship to Alzheimer's disease continues. Several diagnostic criteria have been proposed (by, e.g., the Alzheimer's Disease Diagnostic and Treatment Center in California, the National Institute of Neurological and Communicative Disorders and Stroke, and the European Panel of Experts), but the application of these criteria in practice is difficult. Some novel methods are being brought to bear in drug studies of this condition.

Many medications are useful in treating vascular dementia, but there have been few studies of this condition. Fortunately, that neglect seems to be changing, and in the process we are considering how to ensure that we categorize patients adequately to examine potential effects of different drugs. One suggestion is that we grade the likelihood that vascular dementia is contributing to the cognitive impairment. The importance of this approach is illustrated by Sevush et al., who studied almost 100 patients who came to autopsy by using the usual rules concerning diagnosis of cerebral vascular disease (history, focal deficits on examination, and neuroimaging). These criteria showed exceedingly low sensitivity and specificity.

We have become overly obsessed with differentiating Alzheimer's disease from vascular dementia. We must broaden our studies to include a wider range of individuals and see whether some of the drugs being studied in Alzheimer's disease can help patients whose dementia has vascular components.

P.J. Whitehouse, M.D., Ph.D.

Cortical Abnormalities Associated With Subcortical Lesions in Vascular Dementia: Clinical and Positron Emission Tomographic Findings
Sultzer DL, Mahler ME, Cummings JL, et al (Univ of California, Los Angeles; Veterans Affairs Med Ctr, West Los Angeles)
Arch Neurol 52:773–780, 1995   4–23

Background.—The pathophysiologic causes of the cognitive deficits, psychiatric symptoms, and behavioral disturbances that occur in patients with vascular dementia (VaD) are not known. Although most patients with VaD have subcortical lesions, the clinical significance of these lesions is not clear. The relationship between subcortical lesions, detected on MRI, and regional cortical metabolic deficits, detected on positron emission tomography (PET), was studied in patients with VaD who had subcortical, but not cortical, lesions. The relationship between subcortical lesions and neuropsychiatric symptoms was also examined.

Methods.—Eleven patients with VaD, who had no cortical lesions on MRI, were evaluated with PET and a psychiatric assessment. Investigators blinded to patient identity examined the MR and PET images. Psychiatric assessment used the Neurobehavioral Rating Scale (NRS), which measures the severity of cognitive deficits, psychiatric symptoms, and behavioral disturbances.

Results.—There was substantial variability in the location and extent of subcortical lesions and in the severity of regional cortical metabolic deficits. However, there were associations between the overall severity of subcortical lesions and cortical hypometabolism and between the global hypometabolism index in the cortex and the severity of total ipsilateral subcortical white matter lesions. In particular, the severity of white matter lesions was associated with the hypometabolism index in the temporal cortex and in the parietal cortex. Lacunar lesions in the basal ganglia or thalamus were associated with a reduced metabolic rate in the frontal cortex. The severity of white matter lesions was significantly correlated with the Neurobehavioral Rating Scale total score, the Verbal Output Disturbance score, and the Anxiety/Depression score and tended to corelate with the Cognition Factor score.

Conclusions.—There is a relationship, although limited and variable, between subcortical pathologic changes and cortical metabolic function, even in the absence of cortical infarcts. Neuropsychiatric symptoms are also related to white matter ischemic injury.

▶ Vascular dementia (VaD) is often ignored in our excessive focus on Alzheimer's disease. However, VaD has played an interesting role in discussions about the mechanisms that produce dementia, particularly the relative role of the subcortex and cortex. This paper confirms what would appear to be sensible anatomically: lesions in the subcortical areas can cause impairments in cortical cerebral metabolism. These mechanisms presumably involve brain-stem systems (e.g., the basal forebrain) as well as more traditional subcortical structures (e.g., the thalamus and basal ganglia). These findings illustrate the importance of thinking about the relationships between cortex and subcortex in producing normal cognition rather than categorizing dementia into subcortical and cortical forms.

P.J. Whitehouse, M.D., Ph.D.

Comparison of Different Diagnostic Criteria for Vascular Dementia (ADDTC, DSM-IV, ICD-10, NINDS-AIREN)

Wetterling T, Kanitz R-D, Borgis K-J (Univ School of Medicine, Lübeck, Germany)

Stroke 27:30–36, 1996

4–24

Background.—Vascular dementia (VD) is an unclear term. Several groups of institutions have recently proposed detailed criteria for diagnosis of VD. The clinical feasibilities of these different sets of criteria were examined in an unselected sample of 167 elderly patients (mean age, 72 years) undergoing evaluation for probable dementia.

Methods.—Four sets of diagnostic criteria were compared: *Diagnostic and Statistical Manual of Medical Disorders*, Fourth Edition, 1994 (DSM-IV); *International Classification of Diseases*, Tenth Revision, 1992, 1993 (ICD-10); National Institute of Neurologic Disorders and Stroke-Association Internationale pour la Recherche et l'Enseignement en Neurosciences, 1993 (NINDS-AIREN); and Alzheimer's Disease Diagnostic and Treatment Centers, 1992 (ADDTC).

Results.—Concordance between the 4 sets of criteria for VD was very poor. Vascular dementia was diagnosed in 45 patients via DSM-IV criteria, 21 patients via ICD-10 criteria, and 12 patients via NINDS-AIREN criteria. Ischemic VD as defined by ADDTC criteria was diagnosed in 23 patients. Only 5 patients met the criteria for VD of all 4 sets of diagnostic guidelines.

Discussion.—Determination of diagnostic criteria for VD is complicated by the need to define both the terms "vascular" and "dementia." For example, the ADDTC criteria are limited to ischemic brain injury, whereas the DSM-IV criteria contain no specification of underlying vascular process. Diagnosis of dementia is similarly defined in the DSM-IV, ICD-10, and NINDS-AIREN criteria but is not clearly defined in the ADDTC criteria. Widely divergent results are obtained from these sets of criteria because cognitive deficits considered typical of VD differ; requirements for previous stroke or ischemic attack differ; all methods consider focal neurologic signs to be consistent with VD, although patients with white matter lesions frequently lack such signs; and only the ADDTC and NINDS-AIREN criteria include information from CT and MR studies. The multifactorial etiopathologic origins of dementia also complicate diagnosis. Perhaps less problematic and more promising would be the establishment of neuropathologically verified criteria for each subtype of VD.

▶ Diagnostic criteria for Alzheimer's disease are well developed and agreed on, but the diagnostic criteria for VD are in an early stage of development. This important article compares 4 such criteria developed by different international groups. Out of 167 elderly patients with cognitive dementia, 45 received a diagnosis of VD by DSM-IV but only 12 by NINDS-AIREN. Concordance was exceptionally poor, with only 5 cases meeting the criteria of both sets of diagnostic guidelines. Clearly, a number of factors can contribute to VD, and different criteria may be sensitive to different types of VD. For example, DSM-IV does not allow subtypes to be designated according to brain imaging studies. Moreover, there are still basic differences in how VD itself is defined. Much more work is needed to clarify the diagnosis of this important disease.

P.J. Whitehouse, M.D., Ph.D.

Cerebrovascular Disease

US National Survey of Physician Practices for the Secondary and Tertiary Prevention of Ischemic Stroke: Design, Service Availability, and Common Practices
Goldstein LB, Bonito AJ, Matchar DB, et al (Duke Univ, Durham, NC; Veterans Affairs Med Ctr, Durham, NC; Research Triangle Inst, Research Triangle Park, NC; et al)
Stroke 26:1607–1615, 1995   4–25

Purpose.—Although many cases of stroke are preventable, few studies have examined the extent to which physicians use diagnostic and treatment methods for stroke prevention in clinical practice. Such information would be valuable for allocating resources and targeting educational efforts. A nationwide sample of physicians was surveyed to determine their practice relating to stroke prevention, as well as their beliefs about various secondary and tertiary approaches to stroke prevention.

Methods.—A stratified random sample of 2,000 physicians from the membership of the American Medical Association were sent a questionnaire regarding their stroke prevention practices. This instrument asked about the availability and use of basic and advanced stroke prevention services for patients at risk for stroke. Data on physician and practice characteristics were requested as well.

Results.—The response rate was 67%. All of the following diagnostic methods were readily available to 90% or more of physicians responding: carotid ultrasound, transthoracic echocardiography, Holter monitoring, and brain CT and MRI scanning. Approximately 70% said that MR angiography and transesophageal echocardiography were readily available, but approximately 10% said that cerebral arteriography and carotid endarterectomy were not. The availability of these services varied with specialty, practice setting, and/or region of the country. Compared with physicians in the South, those in the central, northeastern, and western United States were 2.5–3.5 times more likely to have ready access to carotid endarterectomy.

The prescribed dose of aspirin for stroke prevention was 325 mg for 61% of respondents, less than 325 mg for 33%, and 650 mg or more for 4%. Of physicians who prescribed warfarin, 71% said they monitored anticoagulation using international normalized ratios. Seventy-eight percent monitored their patients receiving anticoagulation at least once monthly. More than 80% of the respondents knew the perioperative carotid endarterectomy complication rates at the hospital where they performed or referred patients for this operation.

Conclusions.—Although most physicians report that basic and advanced stroke prevention services are readily available, general practitioners and rural physicians may lack access to certain services. Some physicians still do not use international normalized ratios to monitor their patients receiving warfarin therapy. Carotid endarterectomy may be less available in the southern United States, which has a high incidence of cerebrovascular disease, than in other regions of the country. Physicians seem to lack important knowledge about the complication rates associated with carotid endarterectomy in their area. This study uncovers problems in the secondary and tertiary prevention of stroke, which could be addressed through physician education and changes in the way services are provided.

Implementation of Guidelines on Stroke Prevention
Steffensen FH, Olesen F, Sørensen HT (Univ of Aarhus, Denmark)
Fam Pract 12:269–273, 1995   4–26

Objective.—Chronic atrial fibrillation (AF) becomes much more prevalent in old age, reaching 9% for individuals in their eighties. The risk of stroke is increased even in patients without valvular heart disease. Several recent randomized trials have shown that warfarin anticoagulation effectively prevents stroke in patients with nonvalvular AF, and that antiplatelet therapy with aspirin is less effective. These data were used to formulate new Danish national guidelines for oral anticoagulation therapy for patients with AF. A survey study was performed to determine the impact of these guidelines, which were sent to all internal medicine specialists and otherwise publicized to Danish physicians.

Methods.—An anonymous questionnaire was sent to a sample of Danish physicians, including 315 general practitioners, 79 heads of medicine and cardiology departments, and 20 heads of neurology departments. The physicians were presented with 6 standardized case histories of patients with AF and asked for their treatment recommendations.

Results.—The response rate was 51% for the general practitioners, 79% for the medical department heads, and 90% for the neurology department heads. The percentage of respondents recommending anticoagulant therapy for the cases in which it was indicated ranged from 14% to 57% for the general practitioners and from 42% to 89% for the specialists. All respondents were more likely to recommend anticoagulant therapy for cases involving a previous transient ischemic attack or ischemic stroke, i.e., for secondary prevention. The reasons cited for not recommending anticoagulant therapy included lack of knowledge about the AF-related risk of stroke, concerns about the treatment risks, and lack of knowledge about the benefits of treatment.

Conclusions.—Even with strong research support and intensive implementation of practice guidelines, physicians' knowledge of new research findings is variable but generally limited. Strategies to maximize the benefits of new research findings should include energetic efforts to implement and build close cooperation between research and postgraduate education. The Danish guidelines for anticoagulation therapy to prevent AF-related stroke are reprinted in an appendix.

▶ Despite our enthusiasm for developing new thrombolytic and neuroprotective therapies, prevention of stroke should continue to be the major priority. Treatment of stroke once a stroke has occurred is an expensive process that is not as effective as implementing the guidelines that have been proposed around the world. Both of these rather different studies, one from the United States (Abstract 4–25) and one from Denmark (Abstract 4–26), found that physicians' knowledge of preventive measures was inadequate. These discouraging findings imply that we need to pay much more attention to helping physicians in practice use the information that we already have.

P.J. Whitehouse, M.D., Ph.D.

Detection of Carotid Stenosis: From NASCET Results to Clinical Practice
Chang Y-J, Golby AJ, Albers GW (Stanford Stroke Ctr, Calif)
Stroke 26:1325–1328, 1995   4–27

Background.—Carotid endarterectomy is beneficial for patients with symptomatic carotid artery stenosis of 70% or more, as calculated according to strict North American Symptomatic Endarterectomy Trial (NASCET) criteria. If individual institutions are to apply the results of the NASCET study, they should investigate the correlation between their ultrasonographic and angiographic measurements of carotid stenosis. Ultrasound and angiographic results were compared at the Stanford Stroke Center, and the degree of stenosis as determined by both methods was compared with measurements obtained using NASCET criteria.

Methods.—The records of all patients who underwent both carotid duplex ultrasound and cerebral angiography during a 6-month period at Stanford University Hospital and at the affiliated Palo Alto Veterans Affairs Medical Center were reviewed. An evaluator who was blinded to the ultrasound and angiography reports determined the degree of stenosis from angiographic films using NASCET criteria.

Results.—Studies of 171 arteries from 92 patients were available for review. In 91% (155) of the cases, the ultrasonographic and angiographic reports were in agreement as to whether the stenosis was less than 70% or 70% or more. In 11 of the 16 cases in which the reports disagreed, the ultrasound measurements were in closer agreement with the results obtained using NASCET criteria. Compared with NASCET measurements, the angiography reports overestimated the stenosis in 9 cases and underestimated it in 2 cases. The ultrasound reports overestimated the stenosis in 3 cases and underestimated it in 2 cases.

Conclusions.—At the Stanford Stroke Center, duplex ultrasonography is highly sensitive for detecting significant carotid artery stenosis. However, angiography reports often overestimate the stenosis when compared with measurements obtained using strict NASCET criteria. To apply the NASCET results accurately, individual institutions that evaluate patients for carotid endarterectomy should investigate the correlation between their ultrasound and angiographic studies.

▶ It has been established that patients with symptomatic high-grade stenosis of the carotid arteries can benefit from carotid endarterectomy. However, the evaluations performed in recent randomized clinical trials need to be compared with the evaluations done in standard clinical practice. This study represents work from only 1 institution, and the authors correctly invite other health care systems to review their noninvasive evaluations of carotids and see whether they are adequate in predicting who will benefit from surgery. The message for the clinician is to get to know not only your surgical referrals and their operative risks, but also your neurology and neuroradiology teams to understand their philosophies and supporting data about how they detect carotid stenosis.

P.J. Whitehouse, M.D., Ph.D.

Reduced Length of Stay Following Carotid Endarterectomy Under General Anesthesia

Friedman SG, Tortolani AJ (North Shore Univ Hosp, Manhasset, NY)
Am J Surg 170:235–236, 1995   4–28

Objective.—Traditionally, patients are admitted at least 1 day before carotid endarterectomy (CEA) for angiography, and they remain hospitalized for 2–7 days after the procedure. A prospective study of 72 patients was done to determine whether discharge on the first postoperative day is feasible.

Patients.—Sixty-two men and 10 women (average age, 68 years) underwent CEA. Eleven patients had sustained stroke. One fifth of the operations were done for high-grade stenosis in asymptomatic patients. Approximately half the patients had coronary artery disease, and more than 40% were hypertensive.

Management.—Whenever possible, cerebral angiography was replaced by MR angiography and duplex scanning, which were performed on an outpatient basis. Conventional cerebral angiography was done in 47% of patients, mainly early in the study period. All operations were done with the patient receiving general anesthesia.

Outcome.—There were no complications from imaging studies, and no patient died or had a stroke after CEA. Two patients described transient ischemic attacks the morning after surgery. Ten patients received nitroprusside IV in the recovery room, but only 3 patients required blood pressure control until the next day. In all, 66 (88%) of patients were discharged on the first day after CEA, 8 (11%) on the second day, and 1 (1%) patient on the third day. The overall average length of stay was 1.1 days. No patient was readmitted on an emergency basis. Five of the 9 later discharges were warranted. No further transient ischemic attacks occurred during an average follow-up of 1 year, but 1 patient had a stroke 9 months postoperatively and was found to have thrombosis at the site of endarterectomy.

Conclusion.—It is both safe and cost-effective to discharge patients the first day after CEA is performed under general anesthesia.

▶ This brief report confirms that in a high percentage of cases, patients undergoing CEAs can be discharged the day after surgery. This report is, however, different than previous reports of short stays in that the patients had general anesthesia rather than cervical block anesthesia. As pressures to reduce length of stay continue, it will be important to conduct these kinds of studies at our own institutions to develop the best care pathways for patients undergoing carotid endarterectomy.

P.J. Whitehouse, M.D., Ph.D.

Results of a Computerized Screening of Stroke Patients for Unjustified Hospital Stay
Goldman RS, Hartz AJ, Lanska DJ, et al (Clement J Zablocki VA Med Ctr, Milwaukee, Wis; Med College of Wisconsin, Milwaukee; Univ of Kentucky, Lexington, et al)
Stroke 27:639–644, 1996   4–29

Background and Objective.—Monitoring hospital length of stay can create an environment that emphasizes cost control at the expense of quality. It is important for monitoring procedures to distinguish between a long stay and an unjustified stay. One common approach to monitoring uses risk-adjusted outcomes; another uses clinical judgment. Approaches that use clinical judgment can be expensive if extensive data collection or the time of a clinician is required. A computerized procedure to monitor length of hospital stay in patients who have had stroke without compromising quality of care was devised.

Methods.—An algorithm was developed to calculate medically justified or unjustified length of stay for 177 patients who had had ischemic stroke. In a subset of 46 patients, the algorithm was tested by comparing the number of unjustified hospital days, as determined by the algorithm and by 2 neurologists.

Results.—Of the 177 patients, 68% had some hospital days that were rated unjustified by the algorithm. In 41% of the 177 patients, all hospital days were rated unjustified by the algorithm. By using the decision of the neurologists as the standard, the sensitivity of the algorithm was 89% and the specificity was 91%. The correlation between the neurologists and the algorithm was 76%.

Discussion.—The amount of agreement between the neurologists and the algorithm was the same as that between the 2 neurologists. The algorithm was designed to evaluate unjustified length of stay because of errors in discharging the patient or other services; it was not designed to address unnecessary hospitalization or other issues. A benefit to the algorithm is that it addresses course of disease and treatment, not just length of stay. Algorithms may be valuable in monitoring length of stay in patients who have had stroke.

▶ As clinicians, we are aware of the need to reduce unjustified hospital stays and of the numerous efforts being made to predict and assess the reasonableness of the length of hospital stays. This particular project is interesting because an algorithm was developed and compared with neurologists' judgments concerning the appropriateness of the hospitalization standard. The study is weakened because the neurologists used no explicit criteria and because the neurologists helped create the algorithm. Length of stay was shorter in the neurology service, but this service may have represented a different population of patients; patients who have had stroke and are admitted to medical services frequently have more concomitant illnesses. The correlation between the 2 neurologists was reasonably high—0.8. The inclusion of only 2 neurologists limits our ability to validate the algorithm, but this study shows an interesting approach that may become more widely adopted. It would be important for clinicians to have input into the development of algorithms because we are the ones affected by decisions made on the basis of their application.

P.J. Whitehouse, M.D., Ph.D.

Is the Stroke Belt Disappearing: An Analysis of Racial, Temporal, and Age Effects
Howard G, Evans GW, Pearce K, et al (Wake Forest Univ, Winston-Salem, NC)
Stroke 26:1153–1158, 1995   4–30

Background.—Since approximately 1939, white residents of the "Stroke Belt" (coastal plain of North Carolina, South Carolina, and Georgia) have been reported to have a stroke risk between 1.3–2.0 times the national average. The following questions were investigated: (1) whether blacks have a similar increased stroke risk in this region, (2) whether this risk has decreased over time, and (3) whether this excess risk is consistent across age groups.

Methods.—The basis for this report was data from the Compressed Mortality File from the National Center for Health Statistics. This file includes the number of deaths by cause of death and population of each county in the United States, for each year from 1968 to 1991. The data were used to estimate the annual relative stroke mortality risk for residents from 153 coastal plain counties (the Stroke Belt) and to compare these rates with those of the rest of the United States.

Results.—For both black residents and white residents of the Stroke Belt, and for both men and women, the relative geographic excess risk of stroke death was similar. The mortality rates were highest in black men, followed by black women, white men, and white women. Compared with non–Stroke Belt regions, the excessive mortality in the Stroke Belt was higher in black men (1.43–1.50 across 4-year periods) than in white men (1.33–1.43), black women (1.32–1.42), or white women (1.27–1.33). For white women, the excess stroke mortality rate was relatively constant over time and age groups. For white men, the mortality ratios decreased slightly for those younger than 85 years of age. Over time, the relative risks for mortality from strokes have decreased for younger blacks in the Stroke Belt and have increased for older blacks. Although the stroke mortality rates have decreased, the relative increased risk for stroke death in the Stroke Belt compared with the rest of the United States has remained constant from 1968 to 1991.

Conclusions.—The Stroke Belt continues to exist for both blacks and whites and for both men and women. The specific cause (or causes) of the Stroke Belt is not known. However, the health and economic effects are remarkable, with a greater-than-40% excess risk of stroke mortality and more than 1,200 excess stroke deaths yearly.

▶ Although the incidence of stroke is declining nationally, additional epidemiologic studies can contribute to our understanding of its public health impact and can suggest risk factors. This article describes the so-called Stroke Belt, the clustering of high rates of stroke in the southeastern United States, which still exists for all ages, both sexes, and blacks and whites alike. Interestingly, the increased risk has been relatively stable over time. The authors speculate that the increased risk in this geographic area is associated with higher incidences of hypertension, diabetes, and smoking.

P.J. Whitehouse, M.D., Ph.D.

Temporal Patterns of Stroke Onset: The Framingham Study
Kelly-Hayes M, Wolf PA, Kase CS, et al (Boston Univ; Natl Heart, Lung, and Blood Inst, Framingham, Mass)
Stroke 26:1343–1347, 1995   4–31

Background.—Previous studies have indicated that stroke onset varies by season, day of the week, and time of day. These temporal patterns were, however, observed primarily in clinical series, which are susceptible to selection bias. Temporal patterns were, therefore, evaluated in a community-based cohort in an effort to help clarify their role in the onset of stroke.

Patients and Methods.—A total of 5,060 individuals enrolled in the Framingham Study, all of whom were free of stroke and cardiovascular disease at entry, have been followed for 40 years. The individuals were 30–62 years of age at enrollment. Over the 40-year period, 637 completed initial strokes have been documented. A systematic evaluation of the month, day of the week, time of day, and place of stroke occurrence was done. The findings were then related prospectively to stroke incidence, subtype, and sex.

Results.—Winter was identified as the peak season for cerebral embolic strokes, and significantly more stroke events occurred on Monday. This latter finding was particularly true for working men. A third of the intracerebral hemorrhages took place on Mondays in both men and women. All strokes, regardless of subtype, most commonly occurred between 8 AM and noon, and this pattern was found to persist even after excluding individuals whose onset occurred while asleep or on awakening. Strokes, in general, occurred most often at home. Hemorrhagic strokes were found to take place outside the home, and cerebral embolism was more frequently found to take place in the hospital when compared with other subtypes.

Conclusion.—Preventive strategies targeted at periods of increased risk of stroke may prove useful.

▶ This study examines the Framingham Study of more than 5,000 patients, in which more than 600 completed initial strokes occurred over 40 years. The investigators asked the question "When do strokes occur?" (i.e., in which season, in which month, on which day of the week, and at which time of day). Although this seems rather mundane, if we are to continue our efforts to prevent stroke, and treat acute events, we should know when—as well as toward whom—we should focus our efforts. Some of the conclusions are perhaps not surprising (e.g., cerebral embolism occurring in the hospital). However, I found it particularly interesting that one third of strokes occur on Mondays, particularly in working men. It is important to be sure that patients do not take a weekend rest from their stroke prophylaxis programs. Perhaps we should be sure EMS personnel with special training to treat brain attack are on duty on Mondays!

P.J. Whitehouse, M.D., Ph.D.

Parkinson's Disease

Prevalence of Parkinsonian Signs and Associated Mortality in a Community Population of Older People
Bennett DA, Beckett LA, Murray AM, et al (Rush Univ, Chicago; Harvard Community Health Plan, Boston)
N Engl J Med 334:71–76, 1996   4–32

Introduction.—Few population-based studies of parkinsonism have been conducted, and most estimates of the prevalence of parkinsonian signs are based on studies of individuals seeking medical care. The prevalence of parkinsonian signs among older individuals living in the community and the relation of these signs with mortality was investigated.

Design.—Four hundred sixty-seven residents of East Boston, aged 65 years or older, underwent structured neurologic examinations. The prevalence of 12 parkinsonian signs in 4 categories (bradykinesia, gait disturbance, rigidity, and tremor) was evaluated. The presence of signs in 2 or more of these categories was indicative of parkinsonism. Parkinson's disease was not distinguished from other conditions causing parkinsonism.

Findings.—Parkinsonism was diagnosed in 159 participants. Parkinsonism was absent in 301 participants; diagnosis was not possible in 7. Participants who were 65–74 years of age showed an overall prevalence estimate of parkinsonism of 14.9%. Overall prevalence estimate increased with advancing age to 29.5% for those 75–84 years old and to 52.4% for those aged 85 or older. Of the 12 parkinsonian signs evaluated, estimated prevalence was lowest for resting tremor. After a mean follow-up period of 9.2 years, 78% of participants with parkinsonism and 49% of participants without it had died. After adjusting for age and sex, overall risk of death among those with parkinsonism was twice that among those without it. Increased risk of death was also associated with the presence of gait disturbance in individuals with parkinsonism.

Discussion.—Severity of parkinsonism was not studied beyond determining the number of signs present. Much of the parkinsonism detected probably was mild. Prevalence estimates were higher than those of previous population-based studies, perhaps resulting from differences in definitions of parkinsonism. If individuals living in institutions were included in the analysis, estimates of the prevalence of parkinsonism would likely increase.

▶ Considerable attention has been paid recently to the epidemiology of Alzheimer's disease and other dementias. This stratified sample of residents in East Boston provides similar data about the frequency of Parkinson's disease in later life. The same East Boston population had been examined previously for the prevalence of Alzheimer's disease, and a similar increase in risk with age had been found, approaching 50% for those older than 85 years.[1] The current article demonstrates that Parkinson's disease is associated with an increased risk for death, particularly when a gait disturbance is present.

P.J. Whitehouse, M.D., Ph.D.

Reference

1. Evans DA, Smith LA, Scherr PA, et al: Risk of death from Alzheimer's disease in a community population of older persons: Higher than previously thought. *JAMA* 262:2551–2556, 1989.

The Frequency and Associated Risk Factors for Dementia in Patients With Parkinson's Disease

Marder K, Tang M-X, Cote L, et al (Gertrude H Sergievsky Ctr, New York; Columbia Univ, New York)

Arch Neurol 52:695–701, 1995   4–33

Background.—For patients with Parkinson's disease (PD), the risk factors for dementia include older age at onset of motor manifestations, a family history of dementia, severity of extrapyramidal signs, depression, psychologic stress, low socioeconomic or educational attainment, and hypertension. Patients with PD were prospectively compared with control subjects living in the same community to evaluate the risk of dementia developing.

Findings.—In a community in New York City, 140 patients with idiopathic PD (mean age, 71.1 years) and 572 other individuals (mean age, 73.9 years), all of whom did not have signs of dementia, underwent neurologic and neuropsychologic evaluations and follow-up examinations for 3.5 years. Within 2 years, dementia occurred in 27 patients with PD (19.2%) and 87 control subjects (15.2%). After adjusting for age, education, and sex, the relative risk of dementia developing in patients with PD was 1.7, almost twice the risk shown by the control group. Incident dementia was predicted by an extrapyramidal score greater than 25 or a Hamilton Depression Rating Scale score greater than 10. Patients with PD in whom dementia developed were significantly older at the time motor signs of PD began than were those patients with PD who did not become demented. Patients with PD in whom dementia either did or did not occur showed no significant differences in disease duration, sex, or education.

Conclusions.—This study is unique in its use of a full neuropsychologic battery rather than a screening mental status examination for the evaluation of criteria for dementia. Development of dementia in patients with PD may be predicted by the severity of extrapyramidal signs and, possibly, by depressive symptoms. Dementia is more likely to develop in patients with PD than in patients without PD, patients with PD and severe extrapyramidal signs seem to be particularly vulnerable.

▶ For some time, clinicians have believed that dementia occurs more frequently in individuals with PD than in healthy, age-matched controls. However, the magnitude of the increased risk has been difficult to estimate. This prospective cohort study tells us that the relative risk is almost double after adjusting for age, education, and sex. Moreover, it suggests that more severe extrapyramidal symptoms and depression may be present in patients who are more likely to have dementia develop. Damage to nonnigrostriatal dopaminergic pathways (e.g., the mesocortical system), along with damage to the serotonergic system, may underlie motor and affective signs and may be a pathologic substrate for some of the cognitive impairments.

P.J. Whitehouse, M.D., Ph.D.

Tremor and Longevity in Relatives of Patients With Parkinson's Disease, Essential Tremor, and Control Subjects

Jankovic J, Beach J, Schwartz K, et al (Baylor College of Medicine, Houston)
Neurology 45:645–648, 1995   4–34

Objectives.—The occurrence of postural tremor, a typical presentation in patients with essential tremor (ET), is frequent in parents and siblings of patients with Parkinson's disease (PD). This observation suggests that PD and ET are pathogenetically related. The history of tremor in family members of patients with PD, ET, and a combination of ET and PD was compared with that of patients with progressive supranuclear palsy (PSP) and normal controls to explore the possible relationship between ET and PD.

Patients.—The family histories of tremor from 391 patients with PD, 140 patients with ET, 125 patients with a combination of ET and PD, 99 patients with PSP, and 104 normal matched controls were compared. The patients were questioned regarding the location and nature of tremor in their relatives and other neurological symptoms.

Results.—Associations of familial tremor with both PD and increased longevity were found. A family history of tremor was noted in 20.7% of patients with PD, 70% of patients with ET, 64% of patients with a combination of PD and ET, 11.1% of patients with PSP, and 10.6% of normal controls. The presence of tremor was recorded in 5.1% of 1,874 parents and siblings of patients with PD, 23.4% of 650 relatives of patients with ET, 20.7% of 439 relatives of patients with ET-PD, 2.6% of 462 relatives of patients with PSP, and 2.2% of 448 relatives of normal controls. The fathers with tremor lived a median of 10 years longer than those without tremor, and the mothers with tremor lived a median of 5 years longer than those without tremor.

Conclusions.—The results suggest an association of both longevity and PD with familial tremor. The most common familial tremor was ET, suggesting that ET and PD are pathogenetically related.

▶ One of the common errors in clinical practice is to diagnose PD on the basis of a tremor alone. Frequently, ET, particularly that with a family history, is mistaken for the resting tremor in PD, and patients are inappropriately given parkinsonian medications. However, this study does demonstrate that ET and PD appear to be related. Therefore, it is important to remember that the resting tremor is not the only tremor associated with PD. Interestingly, this study found that familial tremor was associated with increased longevity, although given how the samples of patients and controls were ascertained, other factors may play a role in creating this difference.

P.J. Whitehouse, M.D., Ph.D.

Comparison of Therapeutic Effects and Mortality Data of Levodopa and Levodopa Combined With Selegiline in Patients With Early, Mild Parkinson's Disease

Lees AJ (Natl Hosp for Neurology and Neurosurgery, London)
BMJ 311:1602–1607, 1995   4–35

Background.—In 1985, the Parkinson's Disease Research Group of the United Kingdom compared the effects of levodopa (with a dopa decarboxylase inhibitor), levodopa combined with selegiline hydrochloride, and bromocriptine on the natural course of Parkinson's disease. Baseline disabilities improved with all 3 regimens after 1 year of continuous treatment, but functional disability and physical signs had deteriorated after 3 years. Mortality did not differ significantly between groups after 3 years. Results of an interim analysis in 1994 were reported.

Design.—Participants in the open, long-term, prospective randomized trial included 520 patients with early Parkinson's disease who were not receiving dopaminergic treatment. Patients in arm 1 of the study received 62.5 mg of levodopa and benserazide 3 times a day after meals. The dose was increased to 125 mg 3 times daily for 3 months; further dose increases were left to the discretion of individual physicians. Patients in arm 2 of the study received selegiline, 5 mg once in the morning for 1 week, then 5 mg twice daily for 3 more weeks. The patients continued to receive selegiline at the same dose while additional treatment with levodopa and benserazide was begun, as with patients in arm 1.

Results.—Interim follow-up analysis after 5.6 years revealed that the mortality ratio among patients in arm 2 compared with that of patients in arm 1 was 1.57; difference in survival was significant. The hazard ratio was 1.49 after adjustment for age and sex but increased to 1.57 after adjustment for other baseline factors. Patients in arm 1 showed slightly, but nonsignificantly, worse disability scores than did patients in arm 2. Patients in arm 2 experienced more frequent functionally disabling peak dose dyskinesias and on/off fluctuations than did patients in arm 1. The dose of levodopa required to produce optimum motor control steadily increased in arm-1, but not in arm-2, participants.

Conclusions.—Patients with mild, previously untreated Parkinson's disease seemed to derive no clinically detectable benefit from treatment with selegiline in addition to levodopa. Mortality was significantly increased in patients receiving both drugs compared with those receiving only levodopa. Participants in arm 2 of this ongoing study were advised to discontinue use of selegiline. Follow-up of these patients and the other participants continues.

▶ A few years ago, after the DATATOP study was published, neurologists treated Parkinson's disease with selegiline in great numbers with the hope that this treatment would slow the progression of disease. Recently, however, the DATATOP study has been reinterpreted, and prescriptions for selegiline apparently have decreased. This study provides additional evidence that the combination of levodopa and selegiline may not be a good idea. Not only did the combination seem not to improve the clinical symptoms, but mortality was increased in the population taking both drugs. However, this mortality data is open to different interpretations and needs to be confirmed.

P.J. Whitehouse, M.D., Ph.D.

Effect of GPi Pallidotomy on Motor Function in Parkinson's Disease
Lozano AM, Lang AE, Galvez-Jimenez N, et al (Morton and Gloria Shulman-Movement Disorders Centre, Toronto; Univ of Toronto)
Lancet 346:1383–1387, 1995   4–36

Objective.—There is new interest in the performance of ventrolateral medial pallidotomy for patients with severe, advanced Parkinson's disease (PD), but careful evaluation is needed before this operation is widely adopted. In PD, the major motor disturbances seem to arise from overactivity of the large segment of the globus pallidus (GPi), largely because of excessive drive from the subthalamic nucleus. The characteristic slowness, rigidity, and poverty of movement seen with PD is thought to result from "braking" of the motor thalamus and cortical motor system by the excessive inhibitory activity of the GPi. By directly reducing GPi activity, GPi pallidotomy may be able to improve motor function. Only 1 limited study has sought to evaluate the effects of pallidotomy in blinded fashion, however. The effects of GPi pallidotomy in 14 patients were evaluated.

Methods.—The operation was performed in 8 men and 6 women with PD, all of whom had severe motor fluctuations and resulting disability despite receiving optimal medical therapy. Unilateral GPi lesions were created after the location of the GPi was confirmed by microelectrode recording. Standardized videotape recordings were made before and after pallidotomy to be scored in blinded fashion by an evaluator using the Core Assessment Program for Intracerebral Transplantation protocol, which includes the Unified Parkinson's Disease Rating Scale (UPDRS).

Results.—At the 6-month postoperative assessment, the patients showed a 30% improvement in total motor score in the "off" state, as well as a 33% improvement in total akinesia score. There was also a 15% improvement in gait score in the "off" state and a 23% improvement in a composite postural instability and gait score. The UPDRS total activities of daily living score improved by 31%. Drug-induced involuntary movements, i.e., dyskinesias, were almost completely eliminated at follow-up. This reduction reached 92% on the contralateral side compared with just 32% on the ipsilateral side. There were no visual or corticospinal complications.

Conclusions.—For patients with severe, advanced PD, GPi pallidotomy appears to improve many of the "off" period symptoms. Aside from a remarkable reduction of drug-induced dyskinesias on the contralateral side, there is little change during the "on" state. Although the long-term effects remain to be determined, GPi pallidotomy appears to be a safe and effective treatment for cognitively intact PD patients who remain responsive to levodopa but who have disabling "off" periods or problematic levodopa-induced dyskinesias.

▶ Considerable efforts are being made to develop better pharmacologic treatment for PD. An old therapeutic intervention that has been revised is the ventral lateral medial pallidotomy. As this brief article shows, it is appropriate for clinicians to keep an open mind about surgery. In severe cases, it can indeed provide significant benefit for patients with PD. However, careful patient selection and monitoring is necessary to determine whether this costly intervention is warranted.

P.J. Whitehouse, M.D., Ph.D.

General Geriatric Neurology

The Contribution of Predisposing and Situational Risk Factors to Serious Fall Injuries
Tinetti ME, Doucette JT, Claus EB (Yale Univ, New Haven, Conn)
J Am Geriatr Soc 43:1207–1213, 1995   4–37

Background.—Eight percent to 10% of individuals older than 75 years of age reportedly experience a serious injury as a result of falling each year, resulting in increased health care utilization and functional impairment. Predisposing and situational risk factors related to experiencing serious fall injuries were, therefore, evaluated to determine whether, and to what degree, these factors independently contribute to the occurrence of serious fall injuries.

Participants and Methods.—Five hundred sixty-eight members of a representative sample of community-living individuals were studied. All participants were 72 years of age or older, and all had experienced a fall during a median follow-up of 36 months. The demographic, cognitive, medical, and physical performance measures associated with an increased risk of serious injury among fallers, which were identified in a previous analysis of the cohort, served as the candidate predisposing factors. The potential situational risk factors included acute host, behavioral, and environmental factors present at the time of the first reported fall. The occurrence of a serious fall injury during the first fall documented during follow-up was the main outcome measure. Serious injuries were defined as fractures, joint dislocations, or head injuries resulting in loss of consciousness and hospitalization.

Results.—Sixty-nine individuals sustained a serious injury during their first reported fall. No association between acute host factor and increased injury risk was noted. Falling on stairs, falling when engaged in an activity that displaced the center of gravity, and falling from at least body height were environmental and activity factors found to be independently associated with serious injury in multivariate analysis. Corresponding relative risks were 2.0, 1.8, and 2.1, respectively. Independent predisposing factors included female sex, low body mass index, and cognitive impairment, with relative risks of 2.1, 1.8, and 2.8, respectively. Overall, 12% of falls resulted in a serious injury. As the number of predisposing and situational risk factors increased from 0 to 3, this percentage was found to range from 0% to 36% and from 5% to 40%, respectively. In addition, for any given number of predisposing risk factors, the proportion of fallers with serious injury increased with the number of situational risk factors.

Conclusions.—Several environmental and behavioral factors contribute to the risk of serious injuries resulting from falls, independent of the effect of chronic predisposing factors. Such injuries may be best reduced by developing preventive strategies that take into account both predisposing and situational risk factors.

Risk Factors for Serious Injury During Falls by Older Persons in the Community

Tinetti ME, Doucette J, Claus E, et al (Yale Univ, New Haven, Conn)
J Am Geriatr Soc 43:1214–1221, 1995   4–38

Background.—Fall injury among older persons is a common cause of morbidity and mortality. In a prospective study, the frequency of and the chronic risk factors associated with a serious fall in elderly persons were identified.

Methods.—A cohort of 1,103 noninstitutionalized residents of New Haven, Connecticut, who were at least 72 years of age, participated in the study. Demographic, health behavior, fall history, psychosocial, medical, and functional data were obtained at the outset of the study. Each subject recorded his/her fall record and was assessed again by interview after 1 year. The median follow-up was 31 months.

Results.—Forty-nine percent of the subjects reported at least 1 fall in the median 31-month follow-up. An incidence density of 464.5 falls per 1,000 person-years was calculated from the total 1,300 falls reported by 1,103 subjects. Fourteen percent (183) of the 1,300 falls were serious, representing an incidence density of 65.4 serious fall injury events per 1,000 person-years. The factors identified as conveying a risk of serious injury during a fall included the presence of at least 2 chronic conditions, low body mass index, cognitive impairment, balance and gait impairment, and female sex.

Conclusions.—Almost half of the elderly individuals studied were at risk of falling, but only 14% experienced serious injury. The risk factors associated with these falls should help identify those persons who would benefit from prevention efforts.

▶ Unintentional injury, most often resulting from falls, is the sixth leading cause of death in persons older than 65 years of age, and as many as 10% of persons in the older age group will have a serious fall. These 2 articles (Abstracts 4–37 and 4–38) will help clinicians counsel patients regarding the behavioral and environmental factors associated with falls. The risk factors that emerge in both studies are cognitive impairment, the presence of 2 or more chronic conditions, balance and gait impairment, low body mass index, female sex, and situational factors such as stairs. Although it is not discussed, one would also imagine that a history of a previous fall would warn the clinician that a subsequent fall is more likely.

P.J. Whitehouse, M.D., Ph.D.

Peripheral Neuropathy: A True Risk Factor for Falls
Richardson JK, Hurvitz EA (Univ of Michigan, Ann Arbor)
J Gerontol 50A:211M–215M, 1995   4–39

Introduction.—Recently, several studies have linked peripheral nerve dysfunction in elderly individuals with postural instability and falls. Given the potentially high association between peripheral neuropathy (PN) and other diseases and impairments, it has been hypothesized that PN is not a risk factor for falls but is, rather, a marker for a comorbidity, such as CNS dysfunction, that is the true cause of falls in elderly individuals.

Methods.—Twenty patients with electromyographically documented axonal PN affecting the lower extremities were matched by age and sex with 20 individuals with normal lower extremity nerve conduction responses. The mean patient age was 67 years for both groups. All participants underwent a focused history and physical examination designed to identify factors other than PN that might cause falls. All participants were asked about history of falls or postural instability during the previous year.

Findings.—Eleven (55%) patients with PN reported falling within the previous year compared with only 2 individuals (10%) in the control group (odds ratio, 17; 95% confidence interval [CI], 2.5, > 100). In addition, 7 patients who had PN reported repetitive stumbles or a sense of unsteadiness within the previous year, but none of the control group individuals did (odds ratio, 13; 95% CI, 1.5, > 100). The total number of risk factors associated with falls did not differ significantly between the PN and control groups. The PN group took significantly more medications associated with falls, but the pattern of use among those who did and did not fall within the PN group suggested that the medications did not play a primary role in the falls. Compared with control group individuals, patients with PN had significantly decreased unipedal stance time: more frequent abnormal Romberg testing, areflexia at the ankle: decreased proprioception at the great toe: and decreased vibratory sensation at the toe, ankle, and finger. Among those in the PN group, those who reported falling in the previous year demonstrated significantly worse vibratory sensation at the ankle and finger and markedly decreased unipedal stance time than did those who did not fall.

Conclusions.—Peripheral neuropathy in elderly individuals is associated with an increased risk for falling, independent of other risk factors that might be expected to accompany PN, including coincident CNS dysfunction, foot abnormality, or use of drugs associated with falls. A markedly impaired vibratory sense and a substantially diminished ability to maintain unipedal stance may identify patients with PN at particularly high risk for falls.

▶ There are multiple determinants of balance difficulties in elderly individuals, but PN has been suggested as one cause. In this study of a relatively small sample, falls in individuals with well-documented PN were analyzed. The PN was an independent risk factor, even though patients had other risk factors, including medication use. This suggests that it is important for clinicians to assess vibratory sense and unipedal stance in patients who are having a problem with falling.

P.J. Whitehouse, M.D., Ph.D.

Preventive Health Care
Patterson C, Chambers LW (McMaster Univ, Hamilton, Ontario, Canada; Hamilton-Wentworth Dept of Public Health Services, Hamilton, Ontario, Canada)
Lancet 345:1611–1616, 1995   4–40

Introduction.—It has been suggested that 70% of disease is preventable. Prevention may be primary, secondary, or tertiary, and it may follow a "high-risk" or "population" strategy. In clinical practice, preventive health care should be considered when the resources to offer advice and care are available, and when there is evidence that selective screening is more cost-effective than population screening and that the intervention will do more good than harm. Reported, research-based guidelines for primary and secondary clinical preventive health care were reviewed.

Primary Prevention.—Several types of lifestyle modifications may help prevent disease. Lipid modification may reduce the incidence of coronary artery disease, but no specific diets have been shown to benefit asymptomatic elderly individuals with or without hyperlipidemia. However, a low-fat, high-fiber diet is currently recommended, along with increased calcium for postmenopausal women. Sodium reduction is advocated as well. Simple education interventions may enhance compliance with dietary advice. Regular aerobic exercise is a key component of primary prevention; even gentle aerobic activity such as walking appears to have important benefits for cardiovascular fitness. Every attempt should be made to encourage elderly individuals to quit smoking, despite the lack of data from randomized, controlled trials to support the benefits. Physicians should also be aware of whether their elderly patients drive. Annual strain-specific influenza inoculation should be offered to all elderly patients.

Secondary Prevention.—Studies have found that treating patients with blood pressures of more than 160 mm Hg systolic and 90 mm Hg diastolic reduces the risks of stroke, cardiac events, and death. Excessive alcohol intake has been linked to many different disorders, and case finding and brief counseling may be helpful in these patients. Hearing impairment is common in elderly individuals. Patients can be advised to avoid risk factors for hearing loss, and hearing aids can bring significant improvements in quality of life and cognitive performance. Visual problems are also common; patients with reduced visual acuity can be identified by Snellen type testing. Glaucoma screening is no longer recommended. For women 50–69 years of age, regular mammography and clinical examination can aid in the early detection of breast cancer. Regular cervical cytology screening can help prevent invasive carcinoma of the cervix. All postmenopausal women should receive counseling about the risks and benefits of hormone replacement therapy. Older adult patients should receive regular review of the risk factors for falls and their management.

Other Issues.—Screening for diabetes mellitus or hyperlipidemia or by routine urine culture is not indicated in asymptomatic older adults. Data are nonexistent or inconclusive regarding the benefits of screening for certain conditions, including colorectal cancer, prostate cancer, cognitive impairment, and abdominal aortic aneurysm. Other potentially important issues related to preventive health care for elderly individuals include abuse, disability screening, caregiver stress, home interventions, and costs.

Discussion.—Research-based recommendations for preventive health care with elderly patients are reviewed. On the whole, relatively few preventive activities have been proven effective. It can be very difficult to target the elderly individuals who are at greatest risk for preventable conditions, and inconsistent guidelines reduce the effectiveness of preventive efforts. Every clinical encounter with an elderly patient presents an opportunity for prevention.

▶ This brief but appealing article is an excellent review for the clinician of the benefits of preventive medicine in geriatrics. It discusses primary and secondary prevention as well as some of the consensus processes that have led to previous recommendations concerning preventive health maneuvers. The reader is left with the impression, however, that preventive health measures are not only as appealing as motherhood as a central value, but are also as difficult to implement in real clinical practice.

P.J. Whitehouse, M.D., Ph.D.

5 Gerontologic Research

Introduction

As biology (of aging) watchers in the late 1990s, we continue to be impressed that the advances in understanding of cell-to-cell communication in disease states provides a myriad of new opportunities for therapeutic intervention. The classic hormone systems, growth factors, and signaling molecules of the extracellular matrix interact widely. Novel features of intercellular communication appear regularly, including the role of cell receptors in mediating the damage of glycoxidation. The built-in specificity of the communication systems makes us optimistic that the new therapies based on them will be adequately specific. The intracellular events associated with cell senescence, apoptosis (programmed cell death), shear stress, and other aging phenomena are being elucidated and open new opportunities for interventions, although specificity may not be as easy to achieve.

We expect that the extraordinary benefits of calorie restriction and exercise on longevity will also be explainable as the sum of a finite number of definable cellular events in specific cells. We should emphasize the increasingly powerful role of genetics in helping to define longevity and aging genes, the multiple steps in apoptosis, the genetic basis of disorders of premature aging, and the genes that confer susceptibility to the common disorders of old age (e.g., atherosclerosis, Alzheimer's disease, diabetes, and osteoporosis).

Positional cloning, a very powerful tool used to define the Werner-syndrome gene, is finding wide application in several areas, including the genetics of diabetes mellitus, osteoporosis, and malignancy. The articles in this chapter are excellent examples of how the application of techniques in molecular biology facilitate defining specific intracellular regulatory processes that, until now, were not approachable by conventional protein biochemistry. For one, polymerase chain reaction methodology now permits the amplification and characterization of gene products that are present in such minute quantities as to have previously escaped detection. These are heady times for the research of aging.

Jesse Roth, M.D.

Jay R. Shapiro, M.D.

Cancer

Allelic Loss on Chromosome 8p12-21 in Microdissected Prostatic Intraepithelial Neoplasia

Emmert-Buck MR, Vocke CD, Pozzatti RO, et al (Natl Cancer Inst, Bethesda, Md; Mayo Clinic and Found, Rochester, Minn)
Cancer Res 55:2959–2962, 1995   5–1

Background.—Before evolving into overtly invasive cancer, human prostate carcinoma may progress through an in situ tumor phase called prostatic intraepithelial neoplasia (PIN). Previous studies have reported that PIN arises in the peripheral zone of the prostate and that histologic similarities exist between the cells of PIN and invasive prostate cancer cells. The exact relationship between PIN and invasive prostate cancer, however, is uncertain. To examine loss of heterozygosity (LOH), DNA of cancer cells and those in adjacent foci of PIN were amplified by polymerase chain reaction at 3 loci on chromosome 8p12–21.

Methods.—Thirty cases of prostate cancer with concomitant high-grade PIN were selected from tumor samples obtained from more than 100 patients who underwent transurethral prostatectomy or radical prostatectomy. Fourteen of the 30 cases contained multiple foci of PIN. Normal epithelium, PIN, and tumor cells were analyzed in each patient. The criterion for LOH was complete or near-complete loss of 1 allele, as determined under direct microscopic visualization. Tissue microdissection procured essentially pure populations of cells of interest.

Results.—In 26 of 29 informative cases, LOH on chromosome 8p12–21 occurred in at least 1 focus of PIN. Eleven of the 14 cases with multiple foci of PIN showed different patterns of allelic loss among the foci. Overall, 34 of 54 foci of PIN demonstrated 8p12–21 LOH. Allelic loss on chromosome 8p12–21 was detected in 29 of 32 tumor samples; in 26 of those 29, a similar loss was detected in at least 1 focus of PIN.

Conclusions.—Chromosomal differences among PIN foci suggest that PIN arises multifocally within the prostate. The high rate of chromosome 8p12–21 LOH in PIN and matched cancers implicates PIN as a precursor of carcinoma and suggests that the chromosome contains a tumor suppressor gene involved in the development of prostate cancer.

▶ The development and progression of common cancers, such as those of prostate and colon, are thought to be the result of a series of genetic abnormalities in the tumor cells. In particular, oncogenes abnormally stimulate cell growth with a gain of function while suppressor gene functions are lost, removing some of the normal restraints on cell growth. In this study, the authors examined PIN, a precancerous lesion, to determine whether some of the genetic alterations that occur in the invasive forms of this cancer are already present in early lesions as a way of deciding how important they are in the genesis of the cancer. In particular, the authors searched for the loss of a piece of a particular chromosome that is known to occur with the invasive cancer; the lost piece is believed to be the site of a suppressor gene whose loss of function contributes to tumorigenesis. The loss of a piece of 1 chromosome can be recognized as an LOH in that region.

The authors chose to examine a particular region on the short arm of chromosome 8, i.e., the region designated as 8p12–21, because this region had been associated with defects in prostatic cancer cells. Their finding that a high fraction of samples of precancerous lesions have this type of allelic loss suggests that loss of function from that region of the chromosome may be an early event that is causally related to the cancerous process, allowing progression. In addition, if further work substantiates an early, close link between this locus and cancer, then this deletion may become a useful marker in trying to evaluate the seriousness of early histologic abnormalities as an approach to early treatment. More optimistically, if the function that is lost can be defined, early replacements could possibly be used to prevent the cancer.

J. Roth, M.D.

Stimulation of Human Prostate Cancer Cell Lines by Factors Present in Human Osteoblast-like Cells But Not in Bone Marrow
Lang SH, Miller WR, Habib FK (Western Gen Hosp, Edinburgh, Scotland)
Prostate 27:287–293, 1995   5–2

Background.—Primary prostate cancer tumors are slow-growing, whereas secondary tumors grow much more quickly. It has been suggested that the increased growth of secondary tumors may be related to the presence of specific growth factors secreted by the secondary organ. A previous study showed that osteoblasts can be stimulated by soluble prostate-derived factors. Most patients with prostate cancer have skeletal metastases with osteoblastic lesions. Therefore, the effects of culture medium of osteoblast-like cells and of bone marrow on prostate cancer cell lines were assessed.

Methods.—Culture medium was "conditioned" (i.e., enriched with cell-derived factors) by several days' exposure to osteoblast-like cells (derived from human proximal femur) in serial dilutions, bone marrow cells (also derived from human proximal femur), or human skin fibroblasts. Prostate carcinoma cell lines and cells of nonprostatic origin were incubated with each of these conditioned media and with unconditioned (i.e., fresh) medium, and the mitogenic activity was assayed.

Results.—The growth of hormone-insensitive prostate carcinoma cell lines (PC-3 and DU-145) was stimulated by the osteoblast-like conditioned medium in a dose-dependent and time-dependent fashion. Dilutions of at least 12.50% of this medium also stimulated growth of the androgen-sensitive prostate carcinoma cell line (LNCaP). No concentrations of this medium affected the growth of the nonprostatic cells. There was no stimulatory effect on the prostate carcinoma cell lines with either the skin fibroblast conditioned medium or the bone marrow conditioned medium.

Conclusions.—Prostate carcinoma cell lines are stimulated by soluble factors from osteoblast-like cells and are unaffected by bone marrow mitogens. This osteoblast-specific stimulation may explain the osteoblastic nature of prostate cancer skeletal metastasis.

▶ In the olden days, it was believed that cancer cells underwent "uncontrolled growth." Now we know that cancer cells are being stimulated and inhibited in mitosis by cellular signalling mechanisms. These mechanisms include soluble hormone-like signals, specific components of the intercellular matrix, and endogenous intracellular signals. The present study raises the possibility that prostate cancer cells that are metastatic to bone flourish because the osteoblast-like cells release factors that enhance the growth of the prostate cells. This provides an excellent mechanism for therapy; if any of these factors is essential for growth, then a drug that antagonizes it should be effective in restoring a restrained growth pattern. This then will be the challenge for molecular biologists in the next few years.

J. Roth, M.D.

Distant Metastases From Prostatic Carcinoma Express Androgen Receptor Protein
Hobisch A, Culig Z, Radmayr C, et al (Univ of Innsbruck, Austria)
Cancer Res 55:3068–3072, 1995   5–3

Background.—Metastatic spread is present in more than half of prostatic carcinomas at the time of diagnosis. Endocrine therapy—the usual method of managing metastatic carcinoma of the prostate—is designed to reduce the level of circulating androgen and/or inhibit the function of androgens at the receptor level. Although nearly all primary prostatic carcinomas express the androgen receptor (AR) protein (irrespective of their sensitivity to hormone treatment), expression of the AR in distant metastases has not been extensively studied. Specimens obtained from the metastases of 18 patients who had prostate cancer were examined for AR expression.

Methods.—Twenty-two metastatic lesion specimens were obtained at the time of surgical intervention, which was primarily performed to provide some relief in the affected region. Four patients underwent surgery twice, and metastatic specimens were obtained on both occasions. The location of the lesions was bone in 18 cases, the epidural space in 3 cases, and the periosteum in 1 case. All but 1 patient had received preoperative endocrine therapy. Paraffin-embedded tissue sections from the metastatic specimens were stained for AR, using a streptavidin-biotin-peroxidase protocol with the polyclonal antibody PG-21.

Results.—Good-quality staining was achieved in all specimens with the polyclonal antibody PG-21. Expression of AR was detected exclusively in the nuclei of adenocarcinoma cells in all specimens. Although a single AR-positive, poorly differentiated metastatic lesion did not stain for prostate-specific antigen, this protein, which is regulated by means of the AR, was identified in all other metastases by immunohistochemistry. Based on a 4-point scale designed to describe the quantity of AR-positive cells, more than 50% of tumor cells were AR positive in 8 metastases, 10% to 50% were AR positive in 10 metastases, and fewer than 10% of tumor cells expressed the AR in 4 metastases.

Conclusion.—Distant metastases of prostatic carcinoma express the immunoreactive AR protein, as do the primary tumors. This finding may have been unexpected because the metastatic specimens were derived from progressive prostatic carcinomas, which are thought to acquire an androgen-independent growth pattern after endocrine therapy. The presence of AR in these specimens supports the hypothesis that the AR, possibly in an altered form, plays a role in progression of prostatic tumors.

▶ When first diagnosed, prostate cancers are often responsive to endocrine therapy (i.e., lowering the level of circulating androgen and inhibiting the function of the AR). With time, the effectiveness of this therapy disappears. The majority of progressive cancers still react positively for the presence of the AR. On the basis of studies of tissue cell lines, it had been believed that metastatic prostatic carcinoma lacks the AR. In this study, the authors show that tumor metastases in the vast majority of cases continue to show the presence of AR. Is this loss of sensitivity to endocrine therapy the result of new mutations unrelated to the AR or are there mutations in the AR that leave it in an activated form, even in the absence of androgen or in the presence of an androgen antagonist?

A better understanding of what a normal hormone does to a normal receptor to activate it and how mutations can activate the receptor without the hormone should lead to new therapeutic approaches. For example, new ligands can be developed to turn off the activated receptor—so-called inverse agonists. An alternative strategy might be to introduce into the cancer cells artificial receptors that themselves are not active and that, when they interact with natural receptors, cause them to be inactive; these are known as "dominant negatives." There is growing evidence that many cancers are associated with multiple mutations and that as cancers progress, they accumulate further mutations that permit them to invade and others that permit them to metastasize.

When research yields a precise delineation of the defects, specific therapeutic approaches can be devised. A potential advantage of these future therapies is that they have precisely defined biochemical targets, compared with the conventional therapies, such as radiation or chemotherapy, to which cancer cells and normal cells are both susceptible, resulting in a therapeutic index that is relatively low.

J. Roth, M.D.

Endogenous Interleukin 6 Is a Resistance Factor for *cis*-Diamminedichloroplatinum and Etoposide-Mediated Cytotoxicity of Human Prostate Carcinoma Cell Lines

Borsellino N, Belldegrun A, Bonavida B (Univ of California, Los Angeles)
Cancer Res 55:4633–4639, 1995   5–4

Background.—Most patients who have prostate cancer have an advanced stage of the disease at diagnosis. Although hormone therapy is initially beneficial in such cases, the cancer commonly recurs with hormonally independent disease that is resistant to current treatments. Using 2 hormone-independent prostate cell lines, researchers sought to determine the role of interleukin 6 (IL-6) in regulating prostate tumor growth and tumor cell sensitivity to drugs. Recent studies have shown this cytokine to be a growth factor for myeloma and other tumors.

Methods.—The human hormone-independent prostatic carcinoma cell lines used in the study were PC-3 and DU145. These cell lines express IL-6 messenger RNA (mRNA) and secrete IL-6 and are relatively resistant to *cis*-diamminedichloroplatinum (CDDP), etoposide (VP-16), and doxorubicin (Adriamycin [ADR]).

Results.—Both PC-3 and DU145 were growth inhibited when tumor cell lines were cultured for 48 hours in the presence of various dilutions of anti-IL-6 antibody. Growth inhibition was maximal at the highest concentration used and was greater in the DU145 cell line than in the PC-3 line. The effect of anti–IL-6 antibody treatment did not continue after day 2, but the addition of antibody at this time yielded a significant concentration-dependent inhibition of cell growth that continued for 4 days. Coaddition of anti–IL-6 antiserum and CDDP or VP-16 significantly increased cytotoxicity, with a marked synergy when the 2 drugs were given together. In contrast, the combination of anti–IL-6 and ADR or suramin produced only additive effects. Treatment of tumor cells with CDDP downregulated IL-6 mRNA expression and secretion of IL-6 in both lines, an effect not achieved with V-16.

Conclusion.—The cytokine IL-6 was found to be an autocrine/paracrine growth factor for DU145 and PC-3 prostate cancer cell lines. Growth of both cell lines was significantly inhibited, and anti–IL-6 sensitized the tumor cells to cytotoxicity by CDDP and VP-16. Combination treatments produced a significant synergy. Drug resistance in patients with advanced prostate cancer may be overcome by agents that inhibit or downregulate the protective factors in tumors.

▶ In an attempt to understand the mechanisms by which human prostatic cancers gain resistance to drug treatment, these investigators examined the effect of IL-6 on cell lines derived from prostatic cancers. The authors chose to look at IL-6 because it is a growth factor and because it blocks apoptosis (programmed cell death) in several systems. The authors showed that the 2 prostatic cell lines produced IL-6 and that anti–IL-6 antibodies inhibited growth of the tumors and promoted cytotoxicity induced by other agents.

Recognition of the molecular mechanisms of promoting cell growth or preventing cell death—especially when they involve specific growth factors with specific receptors—should enable investigators to devise specific therapies to aid in the treatment of these cancers. Treatment of prostate cancer that is resistant to endocrine therapy is daunting; the results of this study provide a promising new approach, despite concerns about extrapolating the results from cancer cell lines to cancers in vivo.

J. Roth, M.D.

Association of *p53* Mutations With Metastatic Prostate Cancer
Eastham JA, Stapleton AMF, Gousse AE, et al (Baylor College of Medicine, Houston; Methodist Hosp, Houston; Veterans Affairs Med Ctr, Houston)
Clin Cancer Res 1:1111–1118, 1995   5–5

Introduction.—Mutations in the tumor suppressor gene *p53* have been found in the tumor tissue of a number of human cancers. Recently, *p53* mutations have been associated with advanced prostate cancer that is predominantly localized to bone and resistant to hormone treatment. To further explore the involvement of *p53* mutations in prostate cancer, the status of the *p53* gene was assessed in patients with prostate cancer who had complete clinical and pathologic information.

Methods.—The medical records of 86 patients who had adenocarcinoma of the prostate were reviewed. Archival formalin-fixed, paraffin-embedded tissue was obtained from each patient and was examined immunohistochemically for the nuclear accumulation of the p53 protein. These sections were analyzed by polymerase chain reaction (PCR) amplification of the DNA and then by single-strand conformation polymorphism (SSCP) analysis of exons 5, 7, and 8 and direct sequencing.

Results.—Of the 86 patients, 18 had disease that was confined to the prostate, 21 had locally advanced disease (with either extracapsular extension or seminal vesicle invasion), and 47 had metastatic prostate cancer. Only 4 of the patients who had metastatic disease had received hormone treatment. Staining for p53 protein was present in none of the tumors from patients who had disease confined to the prostate, in 2 (9.5%) of the tumors from patients with locally advanced prostate cancer, and in 4 (8.5%) of the primary tumors and 11 (23%) of the metastatic tumors. The staining in metastatic tumors included 8 pelvic lymph node metastases, 1 bone metastasis, and 1 lung metastasis. The PCR-SSCP evaluation suggested a mutation in exon 7 in 1 of the 2 patients with locally advanced prostate cancer and a mutation in exon 5 in 3 of the metastatic tumors.

Conclusions.—Mutations in the *p53* gene were more common in metastatic than in primary tumors in these patients who had prostate cancer, and they were particularly common in lymph node metastases. These mutations were unrelated to hormone therapy.

Intratumor Cellular Heterogeneity and Alterations in *ras* Oncogene and p53 Tumor Suppressor Gene in Human Prostate Carcinoma

Konishi N, Hiasa Y, Matsuda H, et al (Nara Med Univ, Japan; Mie Univ, Japan; Chiba Univ, China; et al)
Am J Pathol 147:1112–1122, 1995   5–6

Introduction.—Prostate carcinoma is distinctly heterogeneous, and it is difficult to predict biological behavior from the morphologic classification. Relatively little is understood about its pathogenesis; however, mutations in the *ras* and *p53* genes have been implicated, although the findings have been conflicting. Recent studies have found both *ras* and *p53* aberrations in colon, lung, and endometrial tumors, suggesting an association between these mutations and histogenesis of tumor-cell populations. Therefore, the possibility of an interrelationship between altered *ras* and *p53* genes and histogenesis of tumor-cell heterogeneity was investigated by examining gene alterations in areas of different growth patterns within larger tumor masses.

Methods.—Nine excised tumors were obtained from patients who, except for 1, had undergone no chemotherapy or hormonal treatments before surgery. Between 5 and 10 areas of each tumor were examined. Tissues were immunohistochemically stained to detect p53 and *ras*. Samples of DNA were extracted from the stained areas and amplified with the polymerase chain reaction; they were then analyzed with single-strand conformational polymorphisms with direct sequencing and restriction fragment length polymorphism analysis.

Results.—The areas examined within each tumor demonstrated considerable heterogeneity in growth patterns. The staining revealed the localization of *ras* p21 in the cytoplasm and of p53 in the nucleus. All tumor sections with a *ras* mutation also stained for activated *ras* p21 protein, whereas p53 gene mutational status did not always correlate with the expression of p53 protein. Three patients had point mutations in the *ras* gene, with mutations at the *K-ras* codon 13 and the *H-ras* codon 61 found in specific foci, which occurred in areas of invasive growth in 2 of the 3 tumors. Mutations of the *p53* gene were detected in 3 tumors. There was loss of heterozygosity in codon 72 of exon 4 of the *p53* gene in 2 tumors within foci with the invasive growth pattern.

Discussion.—Mutations in the *ras* and *p53* genes appear to be independent genetic events in prostate tumors. The heterogeneity of these multifocus tumors may reflect a multistep carcinogenetic process, in which separate clonal populations may undergo independent genetic changes, which may in turn induce aggressive growth. It therefore appears necessary to perform a systematic analysis of all areas of a tumor to detect mutations.

▶ I have combined my comments on the preceding 2 articles (Abstracts 5–5 and 5–6) because they focus on the same problem, although from different perspectives. These articles were chosen because they address the question of the role of mutations of the *p53* gene in the genesis of prostatic cancer and in the development of its metastatic potential. Previous studies have implicated *p53* mutations in the development or progression of more than 50% of colon, lung, and breast cancers. Earlier studies indicate that *p53* mutations are uncommon in early prostate cancers but are found in approximately 20% to 25% of advanced prostatic cancers.[1]

These papers analyzed paraffin-embedded tumor tissue for the presence of *p53* mutations by immunohistochemistry and by PCR amplification of extracted DNA, followed by SSCP analysis and direct DNA sequencing to define the mutation. The Konishi study analyzed exons 4–9, and found mutations in exons 6, 7, and 8. The Eastham study, which analyzed both the primary tumor and metastatic lesions in the same patient, detected mutations in exon 5 by SSCP, and in exons 5 and 7 by DNA sequence analysis of PCR products.

There are 3 major points to be gained from these papers. First, both studies agree with previous reports indicating that *p53* mutations are found with a higher frequency in metastatic lesions than in the primary tumors. Second, Eastham concludes that screening tumor tissue with immunohistochemistry and SSCP will miss a significant number of mutations. Similarly, Konishi concluded that the heterogeneity of the prostatic cancer tissue is one explanation for the variable results reported for mutational analysis and cautions one against relying on a single needle biopsy for diagnostic or prognostic purposes. An additional point is that, compared with other malignancies, the frequency of *p53* mutation is relatively low, and the frequency of *ras* mutations, as described by Konishi, is very low and unrelated to that for *p53*. Therefore, with the exception that *p53* appears to be related to a subset of prostatic cancers, the cause for the majority of these cancers remains to be defined.

J.R. Shapiro, M.D.

Reference

1. Bookstein R, MacGrogan D, Hilsenbeck SG, et al: p53 is mutated in a subset of advanced-stage prostate cancers. *Cancer Res* 53:3369–3373, 1993.

Expression of Plasminogen Activator Inhibitor Type 1 by Human Prostate Carcinoma Cells Inhibits Primary Tumor Growth, Tumor-Associated Angiogenesis, and Metastasis to Lung and Liver in an Athymic Mouse Model
Soff GA, Sanderowitz J, Gately S, et al (Northwestern Univ, Chicago)
J Clin Invest 96:2593–2600, 1995   5–7

Purpose.—Cancer cells that express urokinase-type plasminogen activator (uPA) have an aggressive phenotype, with increased invasiveness, tumor-related angiogenesis, and metastases. Some aggressive cancers show no evidence of plasminogen activator inhibitor type 1 (PAI-1) in their cells,

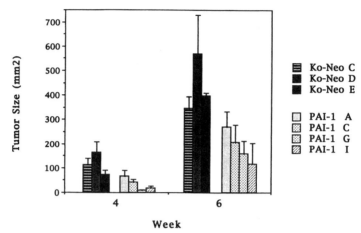

FIGURE 3.—Primary tumor size. A marked inhibition of primary tumor growth was observed by PAI-1–transfected clones, when compared with control Ko-Neo clones. This difference was initially observed throughout the time course of the experiments. (Reproduced from *The Journal of Clinical Investigation*, 1995, vol 96, pp 2593–2600, by copyright permission of The American Society for Clinical Investigation.)

although this inhibitor may be found in the stroma of the tumor-associated microvasculature. The function of the uPA/PAI-1/plasmin system in primary growth and metastasis was examined using an athymic mouse model of prostate cancer.

Findings.—The aggressive human prostate carcinoma line PC-3 was transfected to cause a marked increase in PAI-1 expression, as confirmed by Northern blotting. The PAI-1 transfected clones expressed approximately 9 times more PAI-1 protein than control-transfected clones in the conditioned media, and approximately 4 times more in the cell lysates. A clone designated Ko-Neo B (the only clone that expressed sufficient PAI-1 to produce a uPA-PAI-1 complex on zymography) was selected for in vivo characterization in athymic mice. In vitro analysis found no effect of PAI-1 expression on invasiveness, compared with control cells.

Injection of clones into athymic mice produced palpable tumors in all animals. However, tumors growing from PAI-1 clones were smaller and slower-growing than those from control Ko-Neo clones (Fig 3). None of the control or PAI-1–expressing tumors showed any gross evidence of metastases. However, the PAI-1 tumors showed fewer necrotic areas, less mitosis, and less vascularity. There was also a small decrease in vascular density on immunostaining for collagen type IV and laminin, perhaps reflecting inhibition of tumor-associated angiogenesis by PAI-1. In repeated mouse experiments designed to produce metastases, there were significantly fewer lung metastases from the PAI-1 clones than from the control clones. Expression of PAI-1 was also associated with a significant reduction in liver metastases.

Conclusions.—Inhibition of uPA activity in prostate cancer cells is associated with reduced and slower tumor growth, inhibition of tumor-associated angiogenesis, and reduced metastases to the lung and liver. Impairment of pericellular proteolysis, as mediated by PAI-1, results in reduced tumor invasiveness and metastasis. Future studies should examine the value of trying to inhibit uPA activity by means of drug or gene therapy for prostate cancer. Available inhibitors of the uPA/plasmin system include aprotinin, epsilon aminocaproic acid, and tranexamic acid.

▶ This is an excellent article. The malignant potential of an aggressive human prostate cancer cell line (PC-3) grown in athymic mice was altered by stable transfection of the cancer cells with a vector conferring expression of human PAI-1 mRNA and PAI-1 protein. Plasminogen activator inhibitor-1 is a physiologic inhibitor of UPA, which is known to be expressed by aggressive and invasive cancers, particularly those of the lung, breast, colon and prostate.[1] Urokinase-type plasminogen activator expresses proteolytic activity that facilitates tumor cell invasion and metastases. Selected clones expressing the PAI-1 protein were inoculated into mice with the result that tumor growth was slower, angiogenesis was inhibited, and lung and liver metastases were not found in mice with clones expressing PAI-1. As noted, chemical inhibitors of uPA are known, and gene transfer could be used to hyperexpress PAI-1 in vivo...but with difficulty. This report is of interest because it provides guidelines for a potentially specific pharmacologic approach to controlling prostatic cancer growth in vivo.

J.R. Shapiro, M.D.

Reference

1. Kwaan HC: The plasminogen-plasmin system in malignancy. *Cancer Metastasis Rev* 11:291–311, 1992.

Deletion of the p16 and p15 Genes in Human Bladder Tumors

Orlow I, Lacombe L, Hannon GJ, et al (Mem Sloan-Kettering Cancer Ctr, New York; Howard Hughes Med Inst, Cold Spring Harbor, NY; Cold Spring Harbor Lab, NY)

J Natl Cancer Inst 87:1524–1529, 1995   5–8

Introduction.—Recently, the p16 and p15 genes, located at chromosome 9p21, have been identified as negative cell cycle regulators, functioning as inactivators of certain cyclin-protein kinase complexes required for the progression through the cell cycle. They may therefore function as tumor suppressor genes. This hypothesis has been supported by studies showing that homozygous deletion of these 2 genes is common in certain cancers, including transitional-cell carcinomas of the urinary bladder. The frequency and clinical relevance of alterations in the p16 and p15 genes were studied in primary bladder tumors.

Methods.—Both tumor and normal tissue samples were obtained from 110 patients who had transitional-cell carcinomas of the urinary bladder.

These samples plus 4 melanoma cell lines with known p16 point mutations (for positive controls) were examined with Southern blot analysis to determine p15 and p16 gene status and with polymerase chain reaction with single-strand conformation polymorphism (PCR-SSCP) assays and DNA sequencing of the PCR products to detect point mutations.

Results.—Southern blot analysis revealed homozygous deletion of the p16 gene in 11 tumors, of the p15 gene in 9 tumors, and of both in 8 tumors. In addition, 8 tumors, all invasive, had loss of heterozygosity of p16 and/or p15. Alterations in the p16 and/or p15 genes were significantly associated with lower stage tumors, and p15 alterations were nonsignificantly associated with lower grade tumors. Gene deletion and rearrangement occurred at a rate of 18%. The PCR-SSCP analysis and DNA sequencing revealed no specific point mutations.

Conclusions.—Alterations in the p16 and p15 genes are relatively common in bladder cancer and are associated with lower stage, lower grade tumors, suggesting that determination of p16 and p15 status may have both diagnostic and prognostic significance. The findings suggest a multistep carcinogenesis in bladder cancer, with p16 and p15 gene alterations allowing selective growth enhancement of urothelial tumor cells and mutations in other genes required for overt malignancy.

▶ This article was selected for comment because of 2 features. First, it demonstrates how powerful techniques in molecular biology permit the definition of genetic alterations in complex proteins that are involved in the regulation of cell proliferation. Second, it demonstrates how alterations in gene function are related to malignancy. Using Southern (DNA-based) hybridization gels with gene-specific probes, the authors have sought mutations in the potential tumor suppressor genes, p16 and p15, that normally code for proteins that are negative regulators of the cell cycle. Different patterns of p16 and p15 deletions were found with a frequency of 18% for each gene in this tumor. However, no point mutations were identified by the single-strand conformational polymorphism (SSCP) electrophoretic method, a method that is usually sensitive for this purpose.

The results of this study are important for several reasons. Both genes, normally arrayed in tandem on chromosome 9, were altered in 8 of 11 tumors. These authors have previously identified 2 distinct regions on chromosome 9 that harbor suppressor loci and these, including the p16 and p15 gene loci, may be particularly susceptible to mutation by environmental agents. Also, there was correlation between the p16 mutation and the occurrence of low-grade bladder tumors, a fact that may be of broad diagnostic value in the future.

J.R. Shapiro, M.D.

Cellular Aging, Destabilization, and Cancer
Rubin H, Chow M, Yao A (Univ of California, Berkeley)
Proc Natl Acad Sci USA 93:1825–1830, 1996   5–9

Objective.—Some disease-related chromosomal aberrations become markedly more frequent with age; cells destabilize as the organism ages. Any culture simulation of the in vivo aging process would have to show differences similar in type and magnitude to those noted in recently cultured cells from young and old individuals. In previous studies, the authors found that prolonged confluence of NIH 3T3 cells led to neoplastic transformation, a reduced cell growth rate, and destabilization predisposing to neoplastic transformation. New experiments were done to test the hypothesis that the impairment of proliferation resulting from prolonged confluence simulates these aspects of the aging process.

Findings.—Growth impairment was noted to the same degree in each of 4 parallel NIH 3T3 cell lineages after 1 and 2 rounds of confluence. Proliferative impairment increased progressively with successive rounds of prolonged confluence. The reduced slope of the postconfluent growth curves and the pervasive size reduction in short-term colonies suggested that the growth impairment involved the entire cell population. The effect seemed to be an epigenetic rather than a mutational one. Neoplastic transformation was an infrequent, irregular event, occurring only after the growth impairment. The growth impairment persisted after neoplastic transformation, but the extent of transformation was not correlated with the degree of growth impairment. After prolonged confluence, the cell cytoplasm showed large numbers of residual bodies, analogous to the age pigments known as lipofuscin.

Conclusions.—The responses of NIH 3T3 cells to confluence are similar to those of the cellular aging process in humans, i.e., impaired proliferation and cell destabilization that increases the probability of neoplastic transformation. The NIH 3T3 culture system used permits controlled induction of the effects of aging, coupled with the long-term survival needed to determine the relationship between cellular aging and neoplastic transformation. Cellular aging seems to reflect the accumulation of metabolic damage to cells with resultant cell decline and destabilization, rather than any fixed limit on the number of cell divisions.

▶ In this provocative study, the authors describe a fairly simple model using NIH 3T3 cells that explores the relationship between cell aging and neoplastic transformation. The occurrence of many cancers seems to be age-related, and multiple genetic changes must occur before malignancy ensues. Certain mouse cell strains undergo malignant transformation when grown to confluence. The central hypothesis is that growth to the point of confluence, a lengthy period of quiescence, induces an effect on cell growth similar to that of aging. This involves impaired cell proliferation, characteristic age-related pigmentary changes (lipofuscin) and an increased chance of neoplastic transformation (destabilization). The model lends itself to genetic analysis of alterations that could provide insight into mechanisms of aging. However, the degree of neoplastic transformation was not related to the degree of growth impairment resulting from confluence. Overall, the results suggest an epigenetic mechansim as underlying these changes, rather than the occurrence of specific mutations, although nonmutational chromosomal changes could not be ruled out. The authors suggest that cell aging is not related to the number of cell divisions, but rather to cell damage that leads to destabilization. Obviously, this model is ideal for examining the effects of growth factors on the destabilization process, specifically those that alter proteins regulating the cell cycle.

J.R. Shapiro, M.D.

Disturbances in Immune Function

Interleukin 5 Deficiency Abolishes Eosinophilia, Airways Hyperreactivity, and Lung Damage in a Mouse Asthma Model
Foster PS, Hogan SP, Ramsay AJ, et al (Australian Natl Univ, Canberra, Australia)
J Exp Med 183:195–201, 1996   5–10

Introduction.—Airways inflammation is believed to be a key pathogenetic factor in the development of asthma. However, little is known about the contributions of inflammatory cells and mediators to the development of airways hyperreactivity or about the morphologic changes occurring in the lung during allergic pulmonary inflammation. There is increasing interest in the role played by eosinophils and interleukin-5 (IL-5) in the development of asthma. A mouse model of asthma was used to study the importance of IL-5 and eosinophils in the pathogenesis of asthma.

Methods and Results.—In the mouse asthma model, sensitization and aerosol challenge with ovalbumin produced airways eosinophilia and extensive lung damage, comparable to that occurring with asthma. After allergenic challenge, the mice also showed airways hyperreactivity to challenge with β-methacholine. Further studies were performed in IL-5–deficient mice, which completely lack this cytokine; in these animals, aeroallergen challenge did not result in eosinophilia, lung damage, or airways hyperreactivity. When the IL-5–deficient mice were given recombinant vaccinia viruses to restore IL-5 production, the eosinophilia and airways dysfunction resulting from allergen challenge were restored as well. In mice with and without IL-5, sensitization and aeroallergen challenge produced no increase in mast cells.

Conclusions.—Interleukin-5 and eosinophils seem to play a major role in aeroallergen-induced lung damage and airways hyperreactivity. Eosinophils seem to be the proinflammatory cells involved in altering pulmonary structure and function. The results provide experimental evidence supporting the clinical investigation of IL-5 as a target for asthma therapy.

▶ The classic method of showing the function of a hormone or other intercellular communication molecule is surgical extirpation of the organ followed by observation of the abnormalities created; extracts of the extirpated organ are injected to determine which of the abnormalities can be corrected. Whereas this technique has been useful for organs in which the endocrine function is the sole or dominant function, it clearly is unsuitable for an organ (such as liver, kidney, and brain) that has many other functions in addition to the endocrine function. It also fails when the sites of production are multiple or widely distributed. It is under these circumstances that the modern biological approaches to the deficiency state are especially valuable. Here the authors use animals that lack IL-5, so-called "knockout mice." In this mouse model, allergic lung disease did not develop in the IL-5–deficient animals when challenged. Administration of IL-5 restores their susceptibility, confirming the hypothesis about the role of IL-5 in this disease model. Whether these findings are applicable to asthma in the young or the elderly patient is not yet clear. However, the recognition that 1 or only a small number of intercellular communication molecules may be at the root of the asthmatic process generates optimism that prophylactic or therapeutic techniques that are simpler and more effective will become available.

J. Roth, M.D.

Immune Dysregulation in the Aging Human Lung
Meyer KC, Ershler W, Rosenthal NS, et al (Univ of Wisconsin, Madison)
Am J Respir Crit Care Med 153:1072–1079, 1996   5–11

Objective.—Many different morphologic and physiologic abnormalities have been observed in the lungs of aging adults. The results suggest age-related dysregulation of the humoral immune system along with decreased functional capacity. Few studies have systematically examined the lower respiratory tract immune status of normal, healthy older adults. Such a study was done using bronchoalveolar lavage (BAL) in healthy adult volunteers in various age groups.

Methods.—Bronchoscopy and BAL were done in 3 groups of clinically normal subjects: 15 subjects aged 20–36 years, 9 aged 45–55 years, and 15 aged 65 years or older. The BAL fluid was processed and analyzed for immunoglobulin, albumin, interleukin (IL)-6 and IL-10 concentrations; bronchoalveolar cell profiles; cell surface antigen expression; and superoxide anion production.

Results.—All subjects had normal, age-corrected results on pulmonary function testing. The elderly subjects had significantly higher cell concentrations, neutrophil counts, and BAL immunoglobulin contents than the young adult subjects did. There were no significant differences in serum immunoglobulins, however. A significant increase in the CD4+/CD8+ T-cell ratio was noted with age, whereas the percentage of lymphocytes labeled by anti-CD19 decreased significantly with age. There were no age-related differences in the proportions of cells expressing CD56, natural killer cells, or CD25. Superoxide anion release in response to phorbol myristate acetate was significantly greater in cells from the elderly subjects than in cells from the younger groups, with the results suggesting increased superoxide anion release by alveolar macrophages. Concentrations of IL-6 in BAL fluid were significantly increased in the elderly subjects, and the bioactive IL-6 concentrations were strongly correlated with the neutrophil number and with priming for superoxide anion release. There were no significant differences in IL-10 concentration, however.

Conclusions.—Even in healthy adults who have never smoked, the immunologic cell profile of the epithelial lining fluid increases with age. Elderly subjects also show more indicators of low-grade inflammation than younger adults do. These changes could involve age-related relaxation of cytokine regulation, possibly caused by repetitive antigenic stimulation or environmental irritation. The sustained, low-level inflammation may be associated with the age-related decline in lung function that begins in the fourth to fifth decade of life in normal subjects.

▶ This study addresses a topic that has important therapeutic implications: To what extent does altered immune function contribute to altered pulmonary function in elderly individuals? The authors attempt to answer the question regarding subjects without the confounding factors that have biased earlier studies by altering susceptibility to infection such as pre-existing chronic obstructive pulmonary disease and heart failure. Healthy volunteers in different age groups who never smoked were studied.

The results implicate low-grade inflammation with altered lymphocyte subsets, increased presence of neutrophils, and altered immunglobulin regulation in the setting of diminished elastic recoil in the aging lung. Increased IL-6 production and increased production of destructive superoxide anions that damage alveolar elastin and collagen fibers eventually impair gas exchange.

However, the problem is that these are observational studies; the mechanisms behind these events are unknown, although one could speculate that inflammation is the initial event. It would be interesting to know which are the limiting factors that impair the normal defense mechanisms in pulmonary tissues as one ages.

J.R. Shapiro, M.D.

Ig V_H Hypermutation Is Absent in the Germinal Centers of Aged Mice
Miller C, Kelsoe G (Univ of Maryland, Baltimore)
J Immunol 155:3377–3384, 1995   5–12

Background.—Studies in aged mice indicate that, in some instances, antibodies are encoded by genes different from those involved in young adult animals. There is also evidence that these antibodies produced by older animals are less protective. When immunogenic conjugates of the hapten (4-hydroxy-3-nitrophenyl)acetyl (NP) are injected, 2 B-cell populations are found in the spleen. One of them produces antibodies, and the other—the germinal centers—is the site of immunoglobulin somatic hypermutation.

Objective.—The B cells present within germinal centers of young (1.5–2 months) and aged (22 months and older) female C57BL/6 mice were compared after administration of NP.

Results.—Antibody responses to NP were impaired in aged mice. Analysis of the germinal center B-cell populations specific for NP and sequencing of the immunoglobulin heavy-chain variable region genes demonstrated that somatic hypermutation is not present in the germinal centers of aged animals. Nevertheless, antigen is selected through competition between nonmutated clones of antigen-activated B lymphocytes.

Implication.—A lack of protective antibody responses may relate not exclusively to the amount of serum antibody, but also to its quality. A better understanding of the mechanisms involved in somatic hypermutation and affinity maturation may lead to effective methods of augmenting immunologic responsiveness in aged individuals.

▶ The immune defects associated with aging continue to attract investigators, especially because heightened susceptibility to infections is such a serious, often lethal, hazard for the elderly population. The primary immune response occurs in 2 distinct sites within secondary lymphoid tissues. Initially, antigen-activated B cells proliferate and also produce foci of B cells that produce antibodies. However, these antibodies are of relatively low affinity. Some of the lymphocytes migrate to other regions and form germinal centers, where they undergo a rapid proliferation and rapid mutation of the immunoglobulin V(D)J genes, which leads to the production and selection of higher affinity antibodies.

It appears that in older mice, one of the most striking defects is the presence of antibodies with lower affinity associated with the relative scarcity of antibodies with high affinity in conjunction with a failure to mutate the original antibody templates into high-affinity forms, a normal part of antibody maturation. Given the important role of humoral factors in a whole range of stages of B-cell maturation and other immune cell function, the finding in this study of impaired enhancement of affinity of antibodies over time, if extrapolated to humans, will become the target for therapeutic interventions. One can envision growth factors and other humoral agents introduced to overcome the impaired immunity and immune responses to vaccines in older people.

J. Roth, M.D.

Isolation and Characterization of Cell Lines With Genetically Distinct Mutations Downstream of Protein Kinase C That Result in Defective Activation-Dependent Regulation of T Cell Integrin Function

Mobley JL, Ennis E, Shimizu Y (Univ of Minnesota, Minneapolis)

J Immunol 156:948–956, 1996   5–13

Introduction.—Activation-dependent up-regulation of integrin function is believed to play an important role in the interaction of T cells with their cellular partners in the immune response. This regulation of integrin function may involve a conformational change in the integrin molecule that permits it to bind with its ligand. Protein kinase C (PKC) may play a role because phorbol esters can induce up-regulation of integrin function. Genetic studies were done to find other factors regulating activation-dependent β_1-integrin function on T cells.

Methods and Results.—The study used mutants of the Jurkat T cell line selected for their expression of β_1- and β_2-integrins and lack of increased integrin activity on PMA stimulation or CD3 crosslinking. The cells expressed normal levels of VLA integrins at the cell surface, as well as normal levels of molecules that regulate VLA integrin function. The mutants had apparently normal PKC activity. One mutant had an altered form of ERK1, a mitogen-activated protein kinase, and was unable to produce interleukin-2 (IL-2). Another mutant had intact IL-2 production but defective integrin function. The 2 mutants were genetically distinct on complementation analysis. The defects responsible for impaired activation-dependent regulation in these mutants seemed to be located downstream of PKC. The defects were not apparently related to the integrin molecules per se.

Discussion.—T-cell mutants are identified with mutations downstream of PKC affecting the process of integrin regulation, without affecting T-cell viability or proliferative capacity. The 2 mutants described could be new reagents for the study of integrin regulatory factors. They may help determine sites for pharmacologic intervention that could prevent integrin-dependent migration and localization in the inflammatory process, without affecting other T-cell functions.

▶ This study explores, in an ingenious manner, cellular mechanisms involved in processing information between T-cell adhesion to matrix proteins, intracellular signal-transducing proteins, and gene transcription. Mutations altering T-cell integrin activation were induced by irrradiation and activities distal to the integrin receptor, such as cell viability, proliferation, and IL-2 synthesis, were analyzed.

Integrins, transmembrane $\alpha\beta$ chain glycoprotein receptors, are connected to the cell cytostructure, intracellular transducing phosphoproteins, and ultimately to proteins regulating gene transcription. Integrin receptors bind a series of extracellular matrix proteins such as collagen, laminin, and fibronectin, each containing the RGD sequence (arg-gly-aspartic) as well as extracellular proteins (VCAM-1 and ICAM-1) that are essential to lymphocyte migration and adhesion. T-cell integrin receptors are activated by various agents, including phorbol esters and integrin-specific crosslinking antibodies. After integrin receptors are activated, there ensues a cascade including PKC activation and eventually phosphorylation of the Fos/jun complex leading to IL-2 production. In this study, various mutations of the Jurkat T cell line intefering with fibronectin binding permitted an analysis of relationships between β_1- and β_2-integrin activation and the intracellular signal-transducing phosphoproteins. Different mutations in 2 strains seemed to affect the transducing cascade downstream of PKC. In 1 mutation, this was identified as an altered form of the signal-transducing protein-kinase ERK1 that led to defective IL-2 production. Yet another mutation intefered with binding to activation-dependent integrin ligands but ERK1 expression and IL-2 synthesis were intact. As noted by the authors, the real value of these mutant T-cell strains lies in the ability to dissect the genes capable of restoring normal β_1- and β_2-integrin function in these cells, thus altering cell adhesion in response to extracellular stress such as inflammation.

J.R. Shapiro, M.D.

Prevention of Age-Related T Cell Apoptosis Defect in CD2-*fas*-Transgenic Mice
Zhou T, Edwards CK III, Mountz JD (Univ of Alabama, Birmingham; Marion Merrell Dow Research Inst, Cincinnati, Ohio)
J Exp Med 182:129–137, 1995   5–14

Background.—Involution of the thymus, an age-related form of immune dysfunction, has been ascribed to either defective thymocyte precursors or defective expression of thymic factors or growth factors needed for normal development of T cells. The latter is favored by the finding that replacing growth factors has inhibited the thymic involution as well as several other manifestations of T-cell dysfunction associated with advancing age. Apoptosis may be a critical event in regulating the T-cell responses to various stimuli. The process is mediated in part by *Fas*/apolipoprotein 1 (CD95), a cell surface–signaling molecule.

Objective.—The expression of *Fas* and its effects on T-cell apoptosis were examined in young mice that were 2 months of age and older animals that were 22–26 months of age. Studies were also performed on old CD2-*fas*-transgenic mice.

Findings.—The expression of both *Fas* and ligand-induced apoptosis were less evident in T cells from old mice than in cells from young animals. An age-related increase in CD44+*Fas*− T cells also was observed. The proliferative response of T cells to stimulation with anti-CD3 antibody was markedly less in old mice. Stimulated T cells from young mice produced increased amounts of interleukin (IL)-2 and decreased amounts of IL-10 and interferon-γ, compared with cells of old mice. Total thymocytes were reduced in old animals to levels of approximately 20% of those in the young. No such changes were observed in old CD2-*fas*-transgenic mice.

Interpretation.—It appears that defective intrathymic signaling by *Fas* in aged mice leads to a developmental defect and promotes the apoptosis of thymocytes by a *Fas*-independent pathway. This defect in *Fas* signalling may have a key part in the thymic atrophy associated with aging.

▶ We are witnessing a rapid growth in our understanding of how cell growth and cell death are balanced in normal health and now how these processes are deranged in disease and with aging. Apoptosis is a cellular program that leads to a programmed form of cell death when activated. Apoptosis occurs in a very wide range of cells throughout the lifetime of the organism. Each cell has a threshold for apoptosis, and various signals can lower the threshold for apoptosis, making it a more common event, or it can elevate the threshold for apoptosis so that the rate of programmed cell death is diminished.

Although the potential for increased apoptosis to cause disease seems obvious, the mechanisms by which decreased apoptosis may cause disease are more subtle. A normal cell population requires a normal rate of cell division and a normal rate of cell death, and these need to be closely regulated. In the case of the immune system as well as other systems in the body, programmed cell death is a very important part of the normal physiology of that cell population. Anything that accelerates or diminishes apoptosis will result in abnormal depletion or accumulation of cells. That the apoptosis pathway is subject to so many influences, both positive and negative, suggests that in any given cell type, it may be possible in the future to reset the threshold for apoptosis and, thereby, control cell populations more precisely.

In this study, the authors examine apoptosis during T-cell development to see how it might relate to the defects in immune function in old mice. In aging mice, there are a multiplicity of dysfunctions of T cells, including thymic involution, decreased cell responsiveness to natural and artificial stimuli, and altered cytokine expression. The authors examined *Fas*, a cell surface–signalling molecule (also known as apolipoprotein 1, or CD95) that mediates apoptosis. When the expression of the *Fas* gene was experimentally impaired, self-reactive T cells survived, associated with a loss of self-tolerance, autoimmunity, and lymphoproliferation. Normally, there is a close association between apoptosis and proliferation, both of which are mediated by *Fas* and other apoptosis-related molecules. Apoptosis that follows stimulation and proliferation is thought to be critical for regulating the T cells' response to stimuli by removing cells that are defective or have potential for autoimmunity.

The authors propose that this selective depletion of T cells is necessary throughout the lifespan of the animal to prevent the accumulation of dysfunctional senescent T cells. They show that *Fas* expression and function are both decreased in T cells from old mice and that when the defect was circumvented by reconstituting a new *Fas* gene, the number of thymocytes in aged mice was retained at the same level found in young animals. Furthermore, several tests of lymphocyte function were restored to normal, and cytokine expression after stimulation was also comparable to levels observed in young mice.

J. Roth, M.D.

Chemokines Regulate T Cell Adherence to Recombinant Adhesion Molecules and Extracellular Matrix Proteins
Lloyd AR, Oppenheim JJ, Kelvin DJ, et al (Natl Cancer Inst, Frederick, Md)
J Immunol 156:932–938, 1996   5–15

Objective.—T lymphocytes must migrate through endothelium that has been activated by local release of cytokines, which involves both β_1- and β_2-integrin interactions, to reach sites of inflammation from the bloodstream. The chemotactic process of T-lymphocyte migration is believed to involve sequential adhesion and de-adhesion of the lymphocyte with the matrix components, with passage of the adherent site from the leading edge to the trailing edge of the cell. A number of different chemokines have proved to be potent regulators of T-cell chemotaxis in in vitro studies. The role of chemokines in regulating T-cell migration through the extravascular compartment was analyzed.

Methods.—In vitro studies were performed with the use of the recombinant human chemokines macrophage inflammatory protein (MIP)-1α, MIP-1β, RANTES, interferon-inducible protein-10 (IP-10), and monocyte chemotactic and activating factor. T-cell adhesion studies were based on the binding of ^{51}Cr-labeled T cells to purified substrates.

Results.—Adherence was induced by both unstimulated and anti-CD3-activated T cells. T-cell adhesion was increased by MIP-1α, MIP-1β, the potent chemoattractant cytokine RANTES, and IP-10 but not by monocyte chemotactic and activating factor. Maximal adhesion occurred at chemokine concentrations of 1–10 ng/mL. Adhesion was significantly enhanced in chemokine-treated cells from 15 to 180 minutes; the maximal response occurred at 30–60 minutes. Anti-CD18 significantly inhibited the augmented adhesion to recombinant human intracellular adhesion molecule-1 (ICAM-1), whereas anti-CD29 did not; the opposite was true for adhesion to the lymphocyte adhesion receptor rhVCAM-1 (Fig 4). T-cell adhesion to extracellular matrix proteins was also enhanced by MIP-1α, MIP-1β, RANTES, and IP-10 but not by monocyte chemoattractant. In contrast to RANTES or IP-10, MIP-1α induced significantly greater adhesion of CD8 T cells, whereas MIP-1β had greater effects of CD4 T-cell adhesion.

Conclusions.—Chemokines appear to play a critical role in T-cell adhesion to endothelial adhesion molecules and extracellular matrix proteins. Chemokines rapidly enhanced T-cell adhesion, which suggests a direct signaling pathway between chemokine receptors and integrin adhesion molecules on the T-cell surface. Chemokine ligand–receptor interactions appear to stimulate rapid changes in the affinity of β_1 and β_2 integrin molecules. At the site of an immune response, the nature and timing of

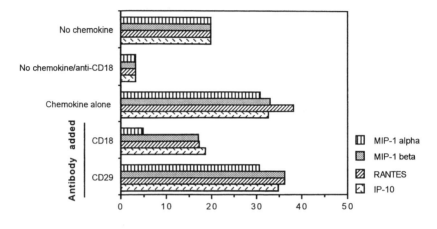

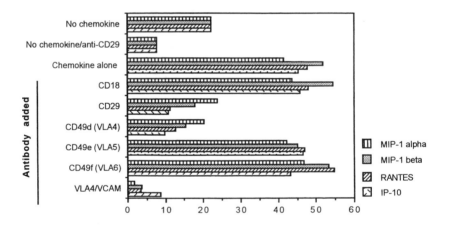

Percentage adhesion

FIGURE 4.—β_1 and β_2 integrins mediate chemokine-induced T-cell adhesion to purified, recombinant human adhesion molecules (rhICAM-1 or rhVCAM-1). Peripheral blood T cells were treated with chemokines, macrophage inflammatory protein (MIP)-1α, MIP-1β, RANTES, or IP-10 for 60 minutes at 37°C before the adhesion assay on rhICAM-1 or rhVCAM-1 in the presence or absence of 10µg/mL of neutralizing monoclonal antibody against leukocyte and/or extracellular adhesion molecules. Results are data means (± standard deviation) of triplicate samples from a single representative experiment of 3 performed. Statistical analysis of the replicate experiments showed that anti-CD18 antibody significantly reduced adhesion in comparison to chemokine treatment alone ($P < 0.01$). (Courtesy of Lloyd AR, Oppenheim JJ, Kelvin DJ, et al: Chemokines regulate T cell adherence to recombinant adhesion molecules and extracellular matrix proteins. *J Immunol* 156:932–938, 1996. Copyright 1996. The American Association of Immunologists.)

chemokine production may determine which specific lymphocyte sub-populations are recruited.

▶ I chose this article not because of its immediate association with aging, but because the subject is of importance in defining the T-cell response to inflammation and infection, one of the major problems in geriatric medicine.

The interaction between the extracellular matrix and the membrane of a cell depends on a series of adhesion proteins that respond to changes in the extracellular environment.[1] The chemokines are a family of proteins and receptors that facilitate cell adhesion and regulate leukocyte migration. In addition to the chemokines, the integrins, a large and diverse family of cell membrane receptors, interact with a wide range of matrix proteins, including collagen, fibronectin, laminin, vitronectin, and the glycosaminoglycan hyaluronan.[2] Integrins are dimers, composed of a series of different α and β chains that connect to the cytoskeleton. Integrins on the T-cell membrane promote cell adhesion and facilitate signal transduction from the matrix to the cell interior and from the inside of the cell back to the extracellular matrix. In the process, cell shape and protein synthesis may be altered. This complex network is also subject to the influence of inflammatory cytokines, such as interleukin-1 and tumor necrosis factor-α. The study suggests that chemokines and their receptors upregulate the T-cell β_1 and β_2-integrin receptor chains and, thus, promote adhesion to vascular endothelium and transendothelial migration. The question of how this highly integrated process is affected by age, illness, and drugs remains.

J.R. Shapiro, M.D.

References

1. Shimuzu Y, Shaw S: Lymphocyte interactions with extracellular matrix. *FASEB J* 5:2292, 1991.
2. Horton MA: Interactions of connective tissue cells with the extracellular matrix. *Bone* 17:51S–53S, 1995.

TRH Receptor on Immune Cells: In Vitro and In Vivo Stimulation of Human Lymphocyte and Rat Splenocyte DNA Synthesis by TRH

Raiden S, Polack E, Nahmod V, et al (Universidad de Buenos Aires, Argentina; Consejo Nacional de Investigaciones Científicas y Técnicas, Buenos Aires, Argentina; Max-Planck Inst, Munich)
J Clin Immunol 15:242–249, 1995

5–16

Introduction.—Immune cells may be affected by hormones, neurotransmitters, and neuropeptides in addition to changes in brain function. Various regulatory peptides and receptors are also known to be expressed by both the brain and the immune system. These interactions are apparent in the immune activities of the hypothalamic-pituitary-thyroid axis (HPTA). Thyrotropin-releasing hormone (TRH) may also be involved in regulating the function of the cells of the immune system. Although receptors for

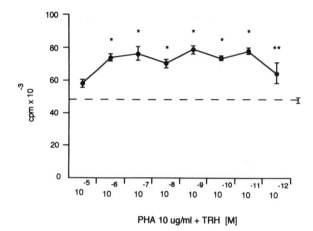

PHA 10 ug/ml + TRH [M]

FIGURE 2.—Dose-response curve of thyrotropin-releasing hormone (*TRH*) stimulation of human peripheral blood mononuclear cells (*PBMC*) cultured in vitro. A total of 1×10^6 cells/mL were cultured and stimulated with phytohemagglutinin (*PHA*), 10μg/mL, in the presence of decreasing doses of TRH (10^{-5} to 10^{-12} M). Incorporation of [³H]-thymidine was determined at 48 hours (after a 10-hour [³H-thymidine pulse). The results (mean value ± standard error) show 1 of 9 representative experiments. Each experimental condition was performed in triplicate. *Dotted line*, PBMC stimulated with PHA. Basal values, without any stimulus: 2,049 ± 223 cpm. *Asterisk*, $P < 0.01$; *double asterisk*, $P < 0.05$ with respect to PBMC stimulated with PHA. Statistics were performed with the use of Student's *t*-test. (Courtesy of Raiden S, Polack E, Nahmod V, et al: TRH receptor on immune cells: In vitro and in vivo stimulation of human lymphocyte and rat splenocyte DNA synthesis by TRH. *J Clin Immunol* 15:242–249, 1995.)

TRH and other HPTA hormones have been found on immune cells, their synthesis remains unknown. Whether TRH receptor genes are expressed in peripheral or lymphoid immune cells was determined in rats.

Methods.—Four groups of female Wistar rats were studied. One group was injected intraperitoneally with TRH, 6 μg/kg; 1 group received simultaneous treatment with rabbit anti-rat thyroid-stimulating hormone (TSH) antibody; 1 group received only anti-rat TSH; and 1 group received saline solution. The animals were killed after 5–180 minutes or at 24 hours to determine the effects of TRH administration on splenocyte proliferation. Rat splenocytes and human peripheral blood mononuclear cells were cultured and stimulated for DNA synthesis assay and RNA analysis. Expression of TRH receptor messenger RNA was determined in each cell type, and the direct effect of TRH was noted for functional correlation.

Results.—On Northern blot analysis of RNA extracted from peripheral blood mononuclear cells, TRH receptor messenger RNA appeared as a single band of 3.8 kb, when hybridizing with a 0.18-kb TRH receptor complementary RNA. Although this band was the same as that observed in human prolactinoma cells, its level of expression was lower. The band was present in both stimulated and basal conditions. Lymphocytes stimulated with phytohemagglutinin showed a significant increase in DNA synthesis (Fig 2). Stimulated splenocytes showed a significant increase in DNA synthesis after the addition of TRH. Proliferation of rat splenocytes in response to concanavalin A was observed at all intervals after in vivo administration of TRH. After 30 minutes, this response was blocked in animals that received anti-rat TSH antibody.

Conclusions.—Both human lymphocytes and rat splenocytes express TRH receptor messenger RNA. The findings suggest that TRH has direct immunostimulatory function through its receptor, as well as indirect immunologic effects through thyrotropin and other immunostimulatory factors. The nature of the stimulatory effect of TRH on lymphocyte proliferation suggests that these effects could be mediated by interleukin-2.

▶ There is extensive literature describing the role of thyroid hormones, including TRH, in the immune processes. This paper demonstrates the presence of TRH receptors on peripheral blood mononuclear cells in the basal and activated state and on activated splenocytes with a direct immunoregulatory effect on these cells. Moreover, an in vivo correlate of these responses was demonstrated, because administration of TRH led to prompt increase in splenocyte proliferation. This finding would be associated with an increase in secretion of TSH, and TSH may independently increase antibody responses.[1] Several important issues relate to these findings.

First is the question of the mediators of the TRH immunostimulatory effect on the peripheral blood cells: both interleukin-1 and interleukin-2 alter immune reponses and could play a role in stress-related immunoregulatory dysfunction. Second, there is the question of altered immune responsiveness in residents of geriatric units, 2% to 5% of whom are found to have hypothyroidism.

J.R. Shapiro, M.D.

Reference

1. Kruger TE, Blalock JE: Cellular requirements for thyrotropin enhancement of in vitro antibody production. *J Immunol* 137:197–200, 1986.

Cardiovascular Disturbances

Hormonal Responses to Maximal and Submaximal Exercise in Trained and Untrained Men of Various Ages
Silverman HG, Mazzeo RS (Univ of Colorado, Denver)
J Gerontol 51A:B30–B37, 1996   5–17

Purpose.—Neuroendocrine responsiveness to acute stressors in old age—and whether exercise training can improve responsiveness—is not well understood. Although hormonal and metabolic changes occur with aging, the exercise responses of trained older and younger men are similar. The effects of age and training on the responsiveness of hormones that affect the metabolic and physiologic adjustments in response to acute exercise were studied.

Methods.—Twenty-three sedentary men and 24 trained cyclists participated. Each group was divided by age—young, middle-aged, and old—for a total of 6 groups. The men performed an initial graded exercise cycle ergometer test to determine their maximal workload. Within 1 week, they returned for a submaximal exercise test performed at the workload that corresponded to their individual lactate threshold. Frequent blood samples were obtained for analysis. Whether the hormonal exercise responses of trained men would be positively altered to provide optimal maintenance of homeostasis and responsiveness to the stress of exercise was determined.

Results.—Peak oxygen consumption decreased with advancing age and was higher in all trained vs. sedentary groups of similar age. The $\dot{V}O_2$ eliciting the lactate threshold decreased with advancing age and was lower in all trained groups than in their age-matched sedentary group. The 2 older groups of sedentary men had higher plasma levels of norepinephrine than did the younger men. Among the trained groups, levels of norepinephrine were similar in the young and middle-aged men but higher in the old men. Pre-exercise plasma levels of cortisol were higher in the trained groups than in their sedentary counterparts. In response to maximal exercise, the groups of older individuals had lower maximal lactate concentrations than did their young counterparts, and the trained groups had higher maximal catecholamine concentrations than did their sedentary counterparts. Aging and training effects were apparent in the maximal concentrations of growth hormone and cortisol.

In response to submaximal exercise, the mean concentration of lactate was higher in the old sedentary men than in the 2 younger groups and lower in the trained groups than in their sedentary counterparts. Concentrations of norepinephrine and epinephrine were higher in the middle-aged and old sedentary men than in the young sedentary men. Also, these concentrations were higher in the trained men than in their sedentary counterparts. Growth hormone concentration showed no aging effect. Growth hormone concentration, however, was higher in all groups of trained men than in their sedentary counterparts. The mean concentration of cortisol was higher in the middle-aged trained men compared with the sedentary men but was higher in the sedentary men than in the old trained men.

Conclusions.—Hormonal responses to maximal and submaximal exercise are increased in men trained for chronic endurance at all ages. The responses of old trained men to submaximal exercise are comparable to those of younger trained men and greater than those of young and middle-aged sedentary men. Exercise training appears to enhance neuroendocrine responsiveness, and continued training throughout life may be able to diminish the age-related decrease in responsiveness. The exception may be cortisol response to submaximal exercise, which shows a training effect only in young and middle-aged men.

▶ There is a high level of interest in the effects of training on the physiology of aging as well as the effects of certain interventions, such as growth hormone replacement, on the preservation of muscle mass. The hypothesis of this study was that chronic endurance training (i.e., trained cyclists) would condition the age-related hormonal response to maximal and submaximal exercise to buffer the stress of exercise effectively. The results support this hypothesis: Chronic endurance training improved the hormone profile at all ages. Although age-related decreases were seen in lactate, growth hormone, and cortisol peaks during maximal exercise, the hormonal responses of old vs. young men were similar at a submaximal workload. Interestingly, the cortisol response to training was not seen in the older group of men. This finding is unexpected, because aging is associated with an overshoot rather than a decrease in the plasma cortisol response to stress. The results of this study (and previous studies) indicate that fitness training may be a better solution to age-related changes in hormone secretion and body composition (less muscle/more fat) than are pharmacologic interventions, such as growth hormone treatment of elderly individuals.

J.R. Shapiro, M.D.

H_1- and H_2-Histamine Receptor-Mediated Vasodilation Varies With Aging in Humans
Bedarida G, Bushell E, Blaschke TF, et al (Stanford Univ, Calif; Veterans Affairs Med Ctr, Palo Alto, Calif)
Clin Pharmacol Ther 58:73–80, 1995   5–18

Introduction.—Both structural and functional aging-associated alterations have been noted in the cardiovascular system, including vasodilation. Two major pathways are involved in vasodilation: the cyclic adenosine monophosphate (cAMP)–dependent and the cyclic guanosine monophosphate (cGMP)–dependent pathways. Studies have suggested that the β-receptor–mediated cAMP pathway is impaired by aging, which may affect responses to vasoactive drugs. To investigate vascular responses to vasoactive drugs in aging, responses to histamine in hand veins were evaluated in subjects of varying ages.

Methods.—Sixteen subjects, ranging in age from 21 to 80 years, were studied. The dorsal hand vein was preconstricted with phenylephrine, then injected with histamine in various doses. Responses of the vein were measured with a linear variable differential transformer. The dose-response curves were assessed with histamine alone and with histamine after infusions of either the H_2-receptor blocker cimetidine or the H_1-receptor blockers brompheniramine or methylene blue.

Results.—Effective vasodilation occurred with histamine in subjects of all ages, without statistically significant age-related variations in response. The infusion of cimetidine had less inhibitory effects in the elderly than in the younger subjects. In the presence of cimetidine, the maximal response to histamine, but not the dose-producing half-maximal response, was significantly correlated with age. The residual histamine response was nearly completely abolished with either brompheniramine or methylene blue.

Conclusions.—There is no change in the efficacy or potency of histamine-mediated vasodilation with aging. However, elderly subjects demonstrate diminished functioning of the response mediated by the H_2-receptor signal-transduction pathway, whereas the H_1-receptor–mediated pathway is preserved. Aging appears to produce a shift in the balance between the cAMP pathway, which predominates in youth and is blunted in the elderly, and the cGMP pathway, which predominates in the elderly.

▶ This paper illustrates the type of significant alterations in receptor function related to aging that may modify the response to endogenous vasoactive agents such as histamine.

Vasodilation can be accomplished by a variety of mechanisms including via a cAMP-dependent pathway as well as a cGMP-dependent pathway. Histamine is a vasodilator: 2 receptors, H_1 and H_2, are involved. The H_1 receptor is activated by an endothelial relaxation factor, now identified as nitric oxide. This vasodilatory response appears to be intact with age except where reactivity is compromised by blood vessel disease. Activation of the H_2 receptor is cAMP-dependent. β-Adrenergic cAMP-dependent (i.e., isoproterenol activated) vein dilation was previously recognized to decrease with age, and this finding is supported by the fact that an H_2 blocker, cimetidine, did not alter histamine-induced vasodilation in the older subjects.

Unexplained is the mechanism involved: Altered receptor affinity is not usually considered a feature of aging. Similarly, age-dependent alterations in intracellular signal transduction appear to be uncommon. This model provides an excellent opportunity to dissect the process from the point of H_2 receptor to second messenger to the activation of protein kinase pathways. Understanding these relationships is important when considering the age effect on the response to vasoactive substances.

J.R. Shapiro, M.D.

Age-Related Alterations in the Morphology of Femoral Artery Vasa Vasorum in the Rat

Phillips GD, Stone AM, Schultz JC, et al (Univ of Minnesota, Minneapolis; Macalester College, St Paul, Minn)
Mech Ageing Dev 82:149–154, 1995   5–19

Objective.—In a study designed to identify the mechanisms behind the age-related changes in the vasa vasorum architecture, investigators examined the femoral arteries of young and aged rats. Age-related alterations in the morphology and density of the vasa vasorum were hypothesized to increase the risk of formation of atherosclerotic lesions.

Methods.—The rats used in the study were 2, 12, and 24 months old. Vascular corrosion casts of the femoral arteries were prepared, and replicas of the vasa vasorum lumina were examined for morphological changes with the scanning electron microscope.

Results.—The casts prepared from 2-month-old rats exhibited a dense, elaborate network of capillaries surrounding the femoral arteries. Many capillaries formed anastomoses between the longitudinal vessels, and the vasa vasorum were not seen to originate from the lumina of the femoral arteries. By 12 months of age, the bridging capillaries were markedly reduced in number. Capillaries connecting the longitudinal vasa vasorum were slightly larger in diameter than those in 2-month-old rats, and they appeared perpendicular to the femoral artery. At 24 months of age, even greater reductions were observed in vasa vasorum number, perpendicular capillaries, and the diameter of the connecting capillaries.

Conclusions.—The reduction in capillary density observed in the aging rat is consistent with age-related changes in oxygen tension. A decrease in oxygen tension may tip the balance toward hypoxia and initiate the formation of age-associated atherosclerotic lesions.

▶ The authors provide evidence that the vasa vasorum of the femoral artery, as has been reported elsewhere for other vessels, decrease with age. They suggest that the decrement in vascularity makes the vessel more susceptible to hypoxia, hypoxic damage, and atherosclerosis.

J. Roth, M.D.

Activated Platelets Signal Chemokine Synthesis by Human Monocytes
Weyrich AS, Elstad MR, McEver RP, et al (Nora Eccles Harrison Cardiovascular Research and Training Inst, Salt Lake City, Utah; Veterans Affairs Med Ctr, Salt Lake City, Utah; Univ of Utah, Salt Lake City; et al)
J Clin Invest 97:1525–1534, 1996   5–20

Purpose.—The adhesion protein P-selectin recognizes a specific ligand on leukocytes, P-selectin glycoprotein-1. Human monocytes show rapid and prolonged adhesion to activated platelets expressing P-selectin. When presented in a purified, immobilized form or by transfected cells, P-selectin regulates cytokine expression and secretion by stimulated monocytes. The role of platelet activation and adhesion by means of P-selectin in chemokine synthesis by monocytes was examined.

Findings.—Experiments showed that monocyte chemotactic protein-1 and interleukin-8 were expressed and secreted by activated monocytes, and these responses were dependent on adhesion of monocyte to platelet by means of P-selection. However, chemokine secretion was not signaled by P-selectin directly. Instead, the monocytes had to be tethered by P-selectin before being activated by the platelet chemokine RANTES (regulated upon activation normal T cell expressed presumed secreted). Monocyte adhesion to activated platelets led to nuclear translocation of p65, or RelA, an NF-κB transcription factor that binds κB sequences in the regulatory regions of immediate-early genes, including monocyte chemotactic protein-1 and interleukin-8. Monocytes adherent to activated platelets did not induce expression of the coagulation protein tissue factor, which has a κB sequence in the 5' regulatory region of its gene.

Discussion.—Contact between human monocytes and activated platelets influences which monocyte products are expressed. In inflammatory lesions, chemokine secretion by monocytes may be regulated by activated platelets. The model used in this study will be useful in examining gene regulation in cell-cell interactions.

▶ I selected this article because it shows an increasing understanding of the richness of cell–cell communication as part of the response to injury or the inflammatory process. Thrombin, whose best known role is as a proteolytic enzyme in the clotting cascade, also can act as a signal by binding to specific cell surface receptors on platelets and thereby activating them. The platelets, when activated, become communicators. In particular, P-selectin, an adhesion protein contained in cytoplasmic granules, is translocated to the cell surface. P-selectin on the surface of the platelet binds to P-selectin glycoprotein-1 on monocytes and other leukocytes. The prolonged display of P-selectin on the platelet surface allows the tethering of the monocyte to the activated platelet and thereby makes it a highly selected target for other secretory products released by the activated platelet. The authors of this article showed some of the further steps that are carried out by specific signals released from the platelets and that act at close proximity to the monocyte tethered to that platelet.

The timed programmed expression of adhesion molecules on the surface of platelets (and endothelial cells) is a major mechanism for the recruitment of leukocytes to a particular location such as the site of a thrombus. The cell–cell interaction, mediated by these 2 cell surface complementary proteins, provides for specificity of cell recognition and in addition may serve signaling purposes. The authors in this case showed that the signaling provided directly by the 2 adhesion proteins is overshadowed by the release of other signaling molecules. Most important, the richness of the cell signaling that goes on between platelets and monocytes or other cells in similar disease processes opens up a wide range of venues for specific interventions; it is clear that a whole series of intercellular communication events must take place and that interference with 1 or more of these may be effective in preventing the full program from being carried out.

In summary, we are increasingly witnessing that anatomical events such as thrombus formation have fundamental cellular biological events going on that involve intercellular communication using cell surface receptors and intercellular communication molecules. Understanding the details of these interactions permits plans for specific interventions that can be expected in the near future.

J. Roth, M.D.

Shear Stress Modulates Expression of Cu/Zn Superoxide Dismutase in Human Aortic Endothelial Cells

Inoue N, Ramasamy S, Fukai T, et al (Emory Univ, Atlanta, Ga; VA Hosp, Atlanta, Ga; Georgia Inst of Technology, Atlanta)
Circ Res 79:32–37, 1996   5–21

Objective.—Dismutation of superoxide anion ($O_2^{-\cdot}$) by superoxide dismutase (SOD) is a major factor affecting the level of cellular $O_2^{-\cdot}$. Although there are 3 different types of SOD, the primary form outside the mitochondria in endothelial cells is the cytosolic copper/zinc-containing (Cu/Zn) type. Fluid shear stress has important effects on the structure and function of epithelial cells. A cultured human aortic endothelial cell system was used to assess the effects of laminar shear stress on Cu/Zn SOD expression.

Findings.—Levels of Cu/Zn SOD messenger RNA in endothelial cells increased in time- and dose-dependent fashion as laminar shear stress increased from 0.6 to 15.0 dyne/cm². Concomitant increases in Cu/Zn SOD protein content and enzyme activity were noted as well. Exposure to laminar shear stress significantly expressed transcriptional activity of the Cu/Zn SOD gene in the nuclei of aortic endothelial cells. Levels of Cu/Zn SOD in human aortic smooth muscle cells were unaffected by shear stress.

Conclusions.—Shear stress increases endothelial expression of Cu/Zn SOD in a way that is at least partly mediated by transcriptional activation of the Cu/Zn SOD gene. This effect could enhance the impact of locally produced NO$^{\cdot}$, thus contributing to the anti-atherogenic and anti-inflammatory properties of endothelial cells. The impact of Cu/Zn SOD on $O_2^{-\cdot}$ levels could offer new insight into how hemodynamic factors affect various vascular diseases.

▶ The authors remind readers that shear stress modulates endothelial cell function acutely and over the long term by both immediate and late signaling events. In addition, it modulates endothelial cell morphology and alters gene expression. In vivo, levels of high shear are associated with diminished amounts of atherosclerosis, whereas regions chronically exposed to low shear show heightened susceptibility to atherosclerosis. The authors point out some of the molecular signaling consequences of high shear in terms of increasing NO production and vascular relaxation. The molecular and cellular events associated with shear and with atherosclerosis are becoming increasingly clear and lend themselves to therapeutic interventions. They also provide a cellular and molecular basis for the beneficial effects of training and exercise.

J. Roth, M.D.

Food Restriction Increases the Protection of Erythrocytes Against the Hemolysis Induced by Peroxyl Radicals

Pieri C, Moroni F, Marra M (Cytology Ctr, Ancona, Italy)

Mech Ageing Dev 87:15–23, 1996   5–22

Background.—Experimental animals whose food intake is restricted live longer, although the biochemical mechanisms of this effect are unclear. Previous studies have suggested that the plasma membranes of food-restricted rats are better protected against oxidative stress. Peroxidative hemolysis in erythrocytes, an indicator of peroxidative damage to biomembranes, was evaluated in young and old food-restricted rats and rats fed ad libitum (AL).

Methods.—Female rats were assigned to either food-restricted or AL feeding groups. The food-restricted animals were fed on an every-other-day basis, starting at 3.5 months of age. Radical-mediated hemolysis in erythrocytes was determined using the azo-compound 2-2'-azo-bis-(2-amidinopropane)hydrochloride (AAPH) as the free radical initiator. The time-dependent curve of AAPH-induced hemolysis was analyzed to determine differences in erythrocyte peroxidation between young, adult, and old AL-fed rats and adult and old food-restricted rats.

Results.—As the animals aged, the time needed to achieve 50% erythrocyte hemolysis decreased. This decline was prevented by food restriction. Lag time, as an indicator of the cell's ability to buffer free radicals, was longer in young vs. old animals after an AL diet. Again, this effect was virtually prevented by food restriction. The peak level of hemolysis achieved per dose of AAPH given and the time needed to reach this level also were favorably affected by food restriction.

Conclusions.—Erythrocyte membranes from food-restricted rats are better protected from peroxyl-radical induced hemolysis than those from rats fed AL. Food restriction can prevent the increased erythrocyte susceptibility to peroxidation damage that is seen in aged animals. The protective effect of food restriction may result from differences in the chemical composition of the erythrocyte membranes.

▶ The effectiveness of food restriction as a buffer against aging has been intriguing scientists during the past several years. The mechanisms by which food restriction works is under intense study, and multiple mechanisms are probably responsible. In this article, the authors show that free radical damage to red blood cells increases with age and that food restriction undoes the effect of age. Because peroxidized lipids are an important part of the free radical pool capable of causing damage, the composition of the plasma membrane lipids would be an interesting further study.

J. Roth, M.D.

Calorie Restriction Lowers Body Temperature in Rhesus Monkeys Consistent With a Postulated Anti-aging Mechanism in Rodents
Lane MA, Baer DJ, Rumpler WV, et al (NIH, Baltimore, Md; US Dept of Agriculture, Beltsville, Md; Univ of Wisconsin, Madison; et al)
Proc Natl Acad Sci USA 93:4159–4164, 1996   5–23

Introduction.—Caloric restriction in rodents extends life, reduces disease, and maintains more youthful physiologic function. These age-retarding effects are thought to be at least partly related to the influence of caloric restriction on energy metabolism. Core body temperature is reduced in rodents with caloric restriction, and this may influence the mechanism of the anti-aging effects of caloric restriction. The effects of caloric restriction on body temperature were evaluated in nonhuman primates.

Methods.—Two separate studies were performed to evaluate the effects of caloric restriction on rhesus monkeys. One experiment assessed the effects of 6 years of caloric restriction on rectal temperature in monkeys whose ages ranged from juvenile to old age at the start of the study. The other experiment evaluated the effects of 30 days of 30% caloric restriction in young monkeys. This experiment used radiotelemetry implants to evaluate circadian patterns of subcutaneous body temperature, locomotor activity, and heart rate, as well as indirect calorimetry to measure 24-hour oxygen expenditure.

Results.—In control monkeys fed ad libitum, core body temperature fell progressively from the ages of 2 to 30 years. Monkeys receiving long-term caloric restriction had approximately a 0.5°C reduction in body temperature compared with age-matched controls. Short-term caloric restriction led to a 1.0°C reduction in subcutaneous body temperature, compared with animals fed ad libitum. Short-term caloric restriction also was associated with a 24% decline in 24-hour energy expenditure. Short-term caloric restriction had no significant impact on overall activity level.

Conclusions.—Calorie restriction in monkeys is associated with reductions in body temperature and energy expenditure. Caloric restriction may induce some type of energy-conservation method. Calorie restriction in primates may have anti-aging effects similar to those observed in rodents. The metabolic processes occurring during caloric restriction need to be studied further.

▶ These authors extend the calorie-restriction model of enhanced longevity from rodents to rhesus monkeys and find that there is a drop in body temperature and a substantial diminution in 24-hour energy expenditure associated with calorie restriction. The authors try to relate the beneficial effects of calorie restriction to the reduced calorie expenditure.

J. Roth, M.D.

Reduced Immune Responses in Rhesus Monkeys Subjected to Dietary Restriction

Roecker EB, Kemnitz JW, Ershler WB, et al (Univ of Wisconsin, Madison; Wm S Middleton VA Med Ctr, Madison, Wis)
J Gerontol 51A:B276–B279, 1996   5–24

Background.—Dietary restriction, which involves restricting calories without restricting nutritional content, has been the only intervention that has consistently and significantly increased life span and retarded aging in rodent studies. It has been hypothesized that these effects may be related to improved immunologic function induced by dietary restriction. The effects of 4 years of dietary restriction on several markers of immune function were evaluated.

Methods.—A group of 30 male rhesus monkeys were randomly assigned to either a restricted diet (R) group or the control (C) group during young adulthood. The animals were followed for 2–4 years. Heparinized blood samples were obtained regularly to evaluate peripheral blood lymphocyte counts; the proliferative responses of peripheral blood mononuclear cells (PBMCs) to concanavalin A, phytohemagglutinin, or pokeweed mitogen; natural killer cell lysis of human K562 leukemia cells; PBMC expression of cell surface antigens (CD2, CD4, CD8, and CD45RA); and the plasma antibody response to influenza vaccine.

Results.—Compared with the C group, the R group was significantly thinner and demonstrated better glucoregulation. The 2 groups had comparable peripheral blood lymphocyte counts and PBMC expression of cell surface antigens. However, the R group had a 37% lower proliferative response of PBMC to pokeweed mitogen and a 24% lower proliferative response to concanavalin A than the C group, although the response to phytohemagglutinin was similar in the 2 groups. Natural killer cell activity against the leukemia cells was also reduced by 25% in the R group. Between 2 and 4 years of dietary restriction, the R group demonstrated an 18% lower plasma antibody response to influenza vaccine compared with the C group.

Conclusions.—After 2–4 years of dietary restriction, rhesus monkeys demonstrated specific reductions of immunologic function associated with increased age, which is inconsistent with the hypothesized deceleration of immunologic aging in animals fed restricted diets. Additional study of the immunologic function in older monkeys fed restricted diets and in monkeys fed restricted diets for more prolonged periods is needed.

▶ Dietary restriction has proved to be successful in extending the life span of primates and rodents and is of broad scientific interest. If we can determine and then mimic body changes associated with the extended longevity of caloric restriction, we may be able to achieve the extended longevity without extreme caloric deprivation. In essence, we could get the benefits of calorie restriction by co-opting the cellular mechanisms that carry out this effect. In this study, contrary to some expectations, it was found that dietary restriction, although it extended life span, reduced immunologic responses. This suggests that other pathways are responsible for the enhanced longevity. An additional point is that starvation enhances infectious diseases and the mechanism of death (i.e., modus moriendi) of patients with starvation is often infectious. The findings in this study suggest that some of the parts of the immune system may be impaired by calorie restriction.

J. Roth, M.D.

The Effect of Reduced Physical Activity on Longevity of Mice
Mlekusch W, Tillian H, Lamprecht M, et al (Karl Franzens Universität, Graz, Austria)
Mech Ageing Dev 88:159–168, 1996   5–25

Background.—Food restriction has been shown to increase survival in mice in several studies. Several studies have also demonstrated the survival benefits of exercise in mice. The effects of exercise restriction on the growth, food intake, and survival of mice was investigated.

Methods.—Young (8 weeks old) female mice were randomly assigned to an active control group (80 mice) or an inactive experimental group (80 mice). The active group was housed in groups of 5 animals in polycarbonate cages with a bottom area of 1,820 cm², which had a metal grid for climbing and running wheels. The inactive group was housed in groups of 5 animals in polycarbonate cages with a bottom area of 400 cm², which had a special plastic grid that prevented climbing and no running wheels. The mice were weighed weekly. Both groups had free access to food, and food intake was calculated weekly. The mice were allowed to die of natural causes, and survival in the 2 groups was compared.

Results.—The inactive group gained weight more quickly than the control group after the 20th week, reaching a steady state at a younger age. However, the mean food consumption was consistently significantly lower in the inactive group. Compared with the control group, the inactive group had a decrease in average life span of approximately 10% and in maximal life span of approximately 20%. The average age of death was 497 days in the inactive group and 557 days in the control group.

Conclusions.—Activity restriction significantly reduces longevity. The inactive animals demonstrated increased growth even though their food intake was lower compared with the active animals. Therefore, the effect of exercise on longevity appears to be independent of the effect of food restriction. Because the active animals had a survival that was in the upper range of normal and not prolonged, the effect of exercise is likely to be largely protective.

▶ Food restriction extends the lifespan. Exercised animals share many features with food restricted animals. Exercised animals do not increase their food intake enough to compensate for the increased energy expenditure. Similarly, food restricted animals show a high level of spontaneous motor activity. Chronic exercise prevents many age-related changes and enhances survival.

In this study, 2 sets of mice, both having free access to a balanced diet, were put into cages where exercise was either encouraged or discouraged. The unexercised animals had a higher growth rate and a higher body weight, which was associated with a significant decrease in food intake. Overall, the sedentary animals had more than a 10% shorter lifespan.

J. Roth, M.D.

Caloric Restriction Decreases Age-Dependent Accumulation of the Glycoxidation Products Nε-(Carboxymethyl)lysine and Pentosidine, in Rat Skin Collagen
Cefalu WT, Bell-Farrow AD, Wang ZQ, et al (Bowman Gray School of Medicine, Winston-Salem, NC; Univ of South Carolina)
J Gerontol 50A:B337–B341, 1995   5–26

Background.—The formation of advanced glycosylation end products (AGEs) is implicated in the aging process and in the development of certain age-associated pathology. Two AGEs that accumulate in tissue protein with age are N^ϵ-(carboxymethyl)lysine (CML) and pentosidine, compounds that are products of both glycation and oxidation reactions. Because caloric restriction is known to retard the aging process in the rodent model, it might be expected to reduce tissue protein glycation and accumulation of AGEs. The effects of chronic caloric restriction on glycation of blood proteins and accumulation of CML and pentosidine in rat skin collagen were evaluated.

Methods.—Female Brown-Norway rats fed ad libitum from birth were allocated to follow ad libitum or caloric-restriction diets at 4 months of age. Those in the caloric-restriction group received essential nutrients but were allowed only 60% of ad libitum food. Animals continued receiving the respective diets until sacrifice at 11, 17, or 29 months of age. Glycated hemoglobin was measured by affinity high-pressure liquid chromatography and glycated plasma protein by the fructosamine assay at necropsy. Extracts of skin collagen were analyzed for CML by gas chromatography-mass spectrometry and for pentosidine by reversed-phase high-pressure liquid chromatography.

Results.—At the end of the study, rats in the caloric-restriction group weighed approximately 50% less than rats fed ad libitum. Glycation of hemoglobin, plasma proteins, and skin collagen was significantly lower in the caloric-restriction group at 17 months of age, a difference maintained for the duration of the study. Between 11 and 29 months of age, the rats fed ad libitum had a twofold increase in CML and a threefold increase in fluorescence content of the skin. These increases were all lower in the rats with caloric restriction; the levels of CML were reduced by 25%, pentosidine by 50%, and fluorescence by 15% in collagen of the oldest rats in the caloric-restriction group.

Conclusion.—Caloric restriction in the rat reduces the extent of glycation of blood and tissue protein and the age-related accumulation of glycoxidation products in skin collagen. Advanced glycosylation end products appear to be useful biomarkers of aging, and the decrease in AGEs in animals fed a restricted-calorie diet may be an effect of the decrease in the rate of aging produced by caloric restriction.

▶ The prolongation of life with caloric restriction in rodents has stimulated interest in this experimental model. Multiple mechanisms have been proposed to account for the decreased mortality. This paper takes one of the more interesting leads on the biochemical basis of aging and shows its correlation with caloric restriction, i.e., proteins regularly react nonenzymatically with glucose and other sugars to form reversible but, later, irreversible covalently linked fusion products.

Glycated hemoglobin is the best studied example. The sugar adducts can alter the function of the proteins to which they are linked. Also, some of the end products formed from the sugar moiety can react with receptors present on the surface of many cells, thereby activating them. Receptor activation on macrophages, endothelial cells, and kidney mesangium may be the mechanistic basis for pathologic change, especially in patients who have chronic hyperglycemia but possibly in subjects who have normoglycemia as well, albeit at a slower rate. In this paper, the authors link caloric restriction and a reduced accumulation of sugar adducts, referred to as glycoxidation products, in both short-lived proteins (such as those found in blood) and long-lived proteins (such as those found in skin collagen), making it tempting to suggest that 1 mechanism by which caloric restriction prolongs life is by slowing and reducing glycoxidation of proteins, especially those that have a slow turnover.

J. Roth, M.D.

Longevity and the Genetic Determination of Collagen Glycoxidation Kinetics in Mammalian Senescence
Sell DR, Lane MA, Johnson WA, et al (Case Western Reserve Univ, Cleveland, Ohio; NIH, Baltimore, Md; Food and Drug Administration, Laurel, Md; et al)
Proc Natl Acad Sci USA 93:485–490, 1996   5–27

Objective.—Life spans vary significantly among animals, prompting the question of whether there is a universal aging process. If there is, this process would probably develop at a faster rate among short-lived species than among long-lived ones. Pentosidine has been identified as a biomarker for carbohydrate-dependent protein damage and as an indicator of the extent of underlying chemical modification, oxidation, and crosslinking of tissue protein caused by reducing sugars ("glycoxidation"). Pentosidine concentrations in human tissues increase progressively with age. Pentosidine was studied as a potential marker of the fundamental aging process.

Methods.—Concentrations of pentosidine were measured in skin specimens from 8 mammalian species representing a wide range of life spans: rat, least shrew, dog, cow, miniature pig, squirrel monkey, rhesus monkey, and human. The effects of dietary restriction, which has been shown to increase life span significantly, on pentosidine levels in rats were studied as well.

Results.—Pentosidine concentrations increased significantly with age, with a curvilinear increase modeled for all species. The relationship was not absolute because maximum pentosidine concentrations varied among species with approximately equal life spans, i.e., dog, pig, and cow. The shrew and rat had the highest rates of pentosidine formation, although the absolute concentrations at the end of the life span were small. Dietary restriction in rats was associated with marked inhibition of the glycoxidation rate.

Conclusions.—The longevity of mammalian species seems to be inversely related to collagen glycoxidation rate. As animals age, there may be a progressive deterioration of the process controlling collagen glycoxidation. Thus, genetic factors may control the ability to withstand damage caused by the Malliard reaction. It is still unknown whether interventions that decrease glycoxidation rates can also increase longevity.

▶ Studies to determine the biochemical basis of aging have focused on glycation and oxidation (referred to as glycoxidation), which occurs when sugars and proteins interact nonenzymatically over time. In this study, the authors used one of the intermediates, pentosidine, as a marker of glycoxidation in skin collagen from 8 mammalian species. They showed that the slope describing the rate of pentosidine accumulation is steep in short-lived species and shallow in long-lived species. Furthermore, in long-lived species they showed that with time the curve accelerates upward, suggesting that protections against glycoxidation may fail with aging. They also showed that calorie restricted rodents have a slowed accumulation of glycoxidation products, which they note is associated with the prolongation of life that occurs in these animals when their calories are restricted. Whether the glycoxidation rate is a marker for aging or the etiology of aging is not yet known, but this continues to be a fruitful area for investigation, especially because agents have now been developed that can alter glycoxidation reactions in vivo. Such a pharmacologic approach may be more acceptable in humans than strict calorie restriction lifelong.

J. Roth, M.D.

Prevention of Cardiovascular and Renal Pathology of Aging by the Advanced Glycation Inhibitor Aminoguanidine
Li YM, Steffes M, Donnelly T, et al (Picower Inst for Med Research, Manhasset, NY; Univ of Minnesota, Minneapolis)
Proc Natl Acad Sci U S A 93:3902–3907, 1996   5–28

Purpose.—Cardiovascular disease and reduced renal function are characteristic of aging in humans. Diabetes- and aging-related tissue damage are associated with advanced glycation end products (AGEs). Studies in diabetic animals have suggested that aminoguanidine (AG), an AGE inhibitor, can inhibit the development of renal and vascular pathologic changes. The ability of AG to prevent AGE accumulation and aging-related vascular and renal impairment was studied in rats.

Methods and Results.—Nondiabetic female rats received AG, 0.1% in drinking water, for 18 months. This treatment prevented increases of AGE content in the cardiac, aortic, and renal tissues of aged animals. In addition, AG treatment prevented aging-related vasodilatory impairment in response to acetylcholine and nitroglycerine and aging-related cardiac hypertrophy. The AGE/creatinine clearance ratio decreased by threefold in old vs. young rats; this change was significantly less pronounced in aged animals treated with AG. Sprague-Dawley rats treated with AG showed complete prevention of an age-linked nephron loss, and considerable reduction in glomerular sclerosis; these effects were not seen in F344 rats, however. Both species showed significant inhibition of age-related albuminuria and proteinuria with AG treatment. The AG-treated rats in general seemed significantly healthier than untreated controls matched for age and weight.

Conclusions.—Treatment with the AGE-inhibitor AG can inhibit the progressive, age-related cardiovascular and renal changes occurring in aged rats. The lessening of age-related albuminuria and proteinuria in AG-treated rats is a particularly striking effect. Further study is needed to see whether AG treatment and reduction of AGE-related toxicity lead to improved survival.

▶ The medical problems of diabetes and aging have been linked to a complex process, the covalent bonding of glucose to amino groups on proteins and the further evolution of the glucose into biologically active AGEs. Aminoguanidine is a simple organic compound that decreases AGEs and favors the conversion of the protein-linked glucose to other end products that are biologically inert. In these studies, some of the age-related changes in the kidney and the heart have been diminished along with a decrease in AGEs. This provides support for the idea that the production of AGEs contributes significantly to the aging process and that, by interfering with their production, the aging process can be slowed. This drug, or others that function the same way, may prove to be powerful agents in slowing the complications of diabetes and possibly slowing the aging process itself.

J. Roth, M.D.

Biology of Aging

Positional Cloning of the Werner's Syndrome Gene

Yu C-E, Oshima J, Fu Y-H, et al (Veterans Affairs Puget Sound Health Care System, Seattle; Univ of Washington, Seattle; Darwin Molecular Corp, Bothell, Wash; et al)

Science 272:258–262, 1996

5–29

Background.—Werner's syndrome (WS), an inherited disease, is characterized by clinical symptoms similar to premature aging. A key feature of this disorder is early susceptibility to several major age-related illnesses. Initially, the WS locus (*WRN*) was localized to 8p12 by linkage analysis, and its genetic position was refined by meiotic and homozygosity mapping. The locus was originally mapped to an 8.3-cM interval flanked by markers D8S137 and D8S87. The closest marker was D8S339. Short tandem repeat polymorphism markers at the glutathione reductase gene and D8S339 were later found to be in linkage disequilibrium with WS in Japanese patients with WS. This indicates that these markers are most likely close to *WRN*. The positional cloning of *WRN* was described.

Methods and Findings.—Four mutations were identified in patients with WS. Two were splice-junction mutations. The predicted result was exclusion of exons from the final messenger RNA. One mutation, resulting in a frameshift and predicted truncated protein, was detected in the homozy-

TABLE 1.—Werner's Syndrome (*WS*) Mutations

Mutation	Individual	Nucleotide sequence	Predicted protein length (aa)
1	Normal	LeuGluArgAla TTGGAGCGAGCA ↓ TGA	1,304
2	WS Normal	AlaArgGlnLys GCTAGGCAGAAA ↓ TAG	1,164
3	WS Normal	ThrAspLeuPhe ctgtag ↔ ACAGACCTCTTT ↓ ctgt- - ↔ - - AGACCTCTTT	1,392
4	WS Normal	GlyArgAsn ttttaatag ↔ GGTAGAAAT ↓ c	1,060
	WS		

Note: Splice junctions are denoted by a *double-headed arrow* and deleted bases with a *hyphen*. Mutated or deleted bases are in *bold*. Intronic sequence is in *small letters*, and exonic sequence in *capital letters*.

Abbreviation: aa, amino acids.

(Reprinted with permission from Yu C-E, Oshima J, Fu Y-H, et al: Positional cloning of the Werner's syndrome gene. *Science* 272:258–262, 1996. Copyright 1996 American Association for the Advancement of Science.)

gous state in 60% of the Japanese patients studied. The other 2 mutations are nonsense mutations (Table 1).

Conclusions.—The finding of a mutated putative helicase as the gene product of the WS gene suggests that defective DNA metabolism is involved in the disease process. Indicators of defective DNA metabolism in WS include chromosomal instability, increased mutation rate at specific genes, increased rates of nonhomologous recombination, reduced accuracy of ligation of disrupted plasmids, decreased telomere repair rate, rapid decrease in telomere length, and possibly altered DNA replication. These features distinguish WS from other disorders in which inherited defects have been found in helicases potentially involved in DNA repair and/or chromosome exchange events.

▶ This is an exciting paper because it demonstrates that certain components of aging and disease susceptibility may be secondary to a defect in DNA metabolism. Werner's syndrome is an inherited disease resembling premature aging. Patients with this disorder are susceptible to a number of age-related diseases. This article demonstrates the power of positional cloning methodology in zeroing in on the gene responsible for the disorder.[1] Positional cloning requires no functional information about a gene. Rather, it depends on pedigree analysis and linkage analysis to generate a genome map, with identification based solely on map position. In the context of WS, this methodology opens the potential for defining other mutations that may be responsible for the premature development of type II diabetes, osteoporosis, arteriosclerosis, and other features of premature aging.

The WS protein predicted from the cDNA sequence is 1,432 amino acids in length, and is similar to DNA helicases from a wide range of organisms. Helicase proteins are enzymes that catalyze the unwinding of 2 strands of DNA as a cycle of replication is initiated. A mutated helicase enzyme associated with WS (see Table 1) could be predicted to affect several steps in normal DNA processing dependent on normal unwinding, and in turn lead to chromosome instability, the occurrence of other mutations, and altered DNA replication. It is this secondary process that may underlie the appearance of age-related diseases in patients with WS.

J.R. Shapiro, M.D.

Reference

1. Collins FS: Positional cloning moves from perditional to traditional. *Nature Genetics* 9:347–350, 1995.

▶ Werner's syndrome is a rare genetic disease that has long intrigued students of human aging because patients with WS have many age-related diseases, including cardiovascular diseases, malignancies, diabetes, osteoporosis, and cataracts, develop very prematurely and also have early graying and thinning of the hair, skin atrophy, and an aged appearance. (However, the similarity to normal aging is imperfect.) Further stimulating the interest of the biologist is the finding that fibroblasts from patients with WS, when cultured, undergo a reduced number of replications before they stop dividing, as one would expect from donors of substantially older age; in essence, the fibroblast is also prematurely aged.

This study of the gene that harbors the mutations responsible for WS suggests that it codes for a protein with a structure, inferred from the DNA coding sequence, of a helicase-like protein (helicases are enzymes that unwind the double helix of DNA). Recall that DNA is not only a coiled double helix but undergoes further systematic tight packing to keep the very long polymer neatly stored in the nucleus. When DNA needs to be replicated or when a portion of DNA needs to be exposed to make an RNA copy, that portion of the DNA must be retrieved from the highly coiled storage file. A series of enzymes and other proteins are needed to carry out this process; a helicase is among them. The putative helicase, presumed to be defective in patients with WS, could be involved in DNA replication, recombination, chromosome segregation, DNA repair, transcription, or other functions that require DNA unwinding. Some defects in DNA metabolism that have been detected in WS include chromosomal instability, an elevated mutation rate in specific genes, elevated rates of nonhomologous recombination, decreased repair rate of telomeres, rapid decrease in telomere length, and, possibly, altered DNA replication. Telomere shortening typically occurs with each cell division and may be the fundamental mechanism by which dividing cells keep track of how many divisions they have undergone previously. This accelerated shortening of telomeres would go along with the finding of the limited number of cell divisions of fibroblasts in culture of patients with WS. Much more study will be needed to discover the exact role of the particular helicase-like protein and consequences of the mutations in vivo. Other disorders associated with inherited defects in helicases have been found in patients with xeroderma pigmentosum, Cockayne's syndrome, and Bloom's syndrome. Defining the precise function of the helicase-like protein that is defective in Werner's syndrome and relating it to the clinical syndrome is likely to provide interesting insights into the syndrome and mechanisms of aging.

J. Roth, M.D.

Requirement for Ceramide-Initiated SAPK/JNK Signalling in Stress-Induced Apoptosis

Verheij M, Bose R, Lin XH, et al (Mem Sloan-Kettering Cancer Ctr, New York; Med College of Virginia, Richmond; Natl Cancer Inst, Rockville, Md; et al)
Nature 380:75–79, 1996   5–30

Introduction.—Many elements of the signaling system that lead to apoptosis are not known. The sphingomyelin and stress-activated protein kinase (SAPK/JNK) intracellular signaling systems may play a role because environmental stresses stimulate a SAPK/JNK. The role of ceramide-initiated SAPK/JNK signaling in stress-induced apoptosis is reported and evi-

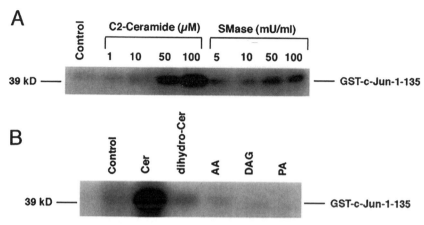

FIGURE 3.—Ceramide induces stress-activated protein kinase activation in U937 cells. Autoradiograph after SDS-PAGE showing the effect of C2-ceramide and sphingomyelinase (**A**) and of other lipid second messengers (**B**) on stress-activated protein kinase activation. The phosphorylated GST-c-Jun-1-135 band is indicated. (Reprinted with permission from *Nature*. Verheij M, Bose R, Lin XH, et al: Requirement for ceramide-initiated SAPK/JNK signalling in stress-induced apoptosis. *Nature* 380:75–79, 1996. Copyright 1996 Macmillan Magazines Limited.)

dence is provided for a transducing mechanism that integrates cytokine- and stress-activated apoptosis.

Methods and Findings.—In U937 human monoblastic leukemia cells, ionizing radiation caused a significant increase in ceramide concentration, along with a quantitative reduction in sphingomyelin. The typical morphologic and biochemical features of apoptosis occurred on exposure to stress or C2-ceramide, and this apoptosis was specific to ceramide. Addition of C2-ceramide and sphingomyelinase caused activation of the SAPK/JNK pathway to concentrations as high as 40 times control (Fig 3). Similarly high levels of SAPK activation were noted in response to environmental stress.

Studies using TAM-67, a c-Jun mutant lacking the N-terminus, found that the apoptosis-inducing effects of stress and C2-ceramide were inhibited in U937/TAM-67 cells. Apoptosis was also inhibited by transient TAM-67 expression, suggesting that inhibition of the apoptotic response to environmental stress occurred downstream of SAPK. Studies in cells overexpressing the dominant-negative kinase-inactive SEK1(K → R) construct found a 50% reduction in activation of endogenous SAPK in response to C2-ceramide, with a corresponding reduction in C2-ceramide–induced apoptosis. Thus, stress-induced apoptosis seemed to be signalled by ceramide and to require a functional SAPK/JNK cascade.

Conclusions.—Stress-induced apoptosis seems to be signaled through SAPK, without involvement of the MAPK pathway. It is unknown whether ceramide signaling through the MAPK and SAPK cascades is cell-specific, although distinct tumor necrosis factor (TNF) receptor domains link acid and neutral sphingomyelinases to different downstream signaling pathways. The sphingomyelin and SAPK pathway is not necessarily the only system that mediates apoptosis, and SAPK activation does not necessarily always lead to apoptosis. The microenvironment in which the ceramide increase occurs may determine its end point.

▶ This is a significant study because it demonstrates the role of the SAPK/JNK transducing enzymes in mediating apoptosis, which is the process of programmed cell death. The authors have ingeniously used specific mutants as well as transfected cell strains to demonstrate both the role of SAPK/JNK in apoptosis as well as the role of a cytokine (TNF-α) in this process.

Although several elements regulating apoptosis are known, other components of the signaling system that determine when cell death occurs are not defined. Complex intracellular pathways involving multiple protein kinases conduct information from the cell exterior to the nucleus, and from the interior of the cell back to the membrane and ultimately to the extracellular space. Signal transduction via these proteins and related pathways ultimately lead to the synthesis of proteins that modulate gene function such as c-jun and fos. Hydrolysis of sphingomyelin, a cell membrane phospholipid, generates a second messenger, ceramide. Ceramide is thought to activate apoptosis in response to a variety of cell stresses, including TNF-α, heat shock, and X rays. This study indicates that ceramide activates the SAPK/JNK kinase pathway and that sequential activation of related signal-transducing proteins and gene transcription factors mediates induction of apoptosis. Interestingly, in other cell strains ceramide links the TNF-α receptor to an inflammatory response through another intracellular pathway, the MAPK (kinase) cascade.

Of interest is that the role of SAPK/JNK in mediating apoptosis that resulted from nerve growth factor deprivation has also been demonstrated recently.[1]

J.R. Shapiro, M.D.

Reference

1. Xia X, Dickens M, Raingeaud J, et al: Opposing effects of ERK and JNK-p38 MAP kinases on apoptosis. *Science* 270:1326–1331, 1995.

A Human Telomeric Protein

Chong L, van Steensel B, Broccoli D, et al (Rockefeller Univ, New York; Mem Sloan-Kettering Cancer Ctr, New York)
Science 270:1663–1667, 1995
                                                                    5–31

Introduction.—The telomeric DNA found on human chromosomes is believed to form a protective nucleoprotein cap through its association with telomere-specific proteins. When telomere function is lost, cell cycle arrest and genome instability can result. The proteins involved in the telomeric complex in vertebrates have not been identified. A protein known as telomeric repeat binding factor (TRF) has been found to be strongly specific for vertebrate telomeric DNA. This factor was shown to be a protein component of human telomeres.

Methods and Findings.—An assay was used in which human TRF (hTRF) activity can be detected in HeLa cell nuclear extracts on the basis of its ability to alter the mobility of a double-stranded DNA segment containing the sequence TTAGGG. Purified preparations of HeLa TRF were found to contain a protein that had an apparent molecular mass of 60 kd, which co-purified with hTRF activity. This 60-kd polypeptide proved sufficient to form an hTRF complex with TTAGGG probes. One amino acid sequencing study performed on the tryptic peptides derived from the 60-kd band showed sequence identity to an anonymous partial complementary DNA (cDNA) sequence. After isolation from a HeLa library and sequencing, cDNA sequences were found to contain an open reading frame that encoded all the sequenced peptides.

The open reading frame encoded a 439–amino acid protein that had a predicted molecular mass of 50,341 d. Mobility shift assays and competition experiments indicated that hTRF was encoded by the cloned cDNA. The novel hTRF protein had 3 previously recognized sequence motifs, one of which was a COOH-terminal region with strong homology to the DNA-binding repeats found in *myb* proto-oncogenes. Immunofluorescent microscopic studies showed that epitope-tagged mouse TRF (mTRF) had a punctate pattern in interphase nuclei. This speckled distribution pattern was consistent with the pattern of telomeric DNA detected by TTAGGG repeat-specfic fluorescent in situ hybridization: All telomeric loci contained mTRF, and all mTRF speckles were associated with telomeric DNA. The tagged mTRF was found mainly at the chromosome ends; no discrete internal loci of mTRF were observed.

Discussion.—Telomeric repeat binding factor is a double-stranded telomeric DNA-binding factor that forms complexes with human telomeres. Telomere maintenance in mammals appears to be subject to homeostasis, which may be explained by some factor, such as TRF, that binds along the length of the telomeric repeat array. The adverse effects of telomere attrition might be caused by the failure of chromosome ends to bind hTRF and other protective telomeric proteins.

▶ This elegant study defines for the first time TRF, which may be a key cellular protein. Telomeres, which are DNA-protein complexes at the end of chromosomes, have several functions.[1] One is protecting choromosomes from end-to-end fusion, as might occur after radiation damage. Also, a chromosome end without a telomere is progressively lost as a consequence of both repeated cell replication and degradation in the absence of replication. As shown in yeast, chromosomes without a telomere can induce transient cell arrest.[2] Telomere replication usually requires telomerase, a specialized reverse transcriptase. Telomere length, however, has been found to increase in some human cell lines, even in the absence of telomerase.[3]

In humans, telomerase activity is not found in most somatic tissues but is present in human tumors. The protein component of the telomere (hTRF) associated with the telomeric nucleotides had not been described in humans. In this report, hTRF was purified from HeLa cell nuclei and a cDNA clone that encoded hTRF and was subsequently bound to the telomeric TTAGGG DNA sequence. Telomeric repeat binding factor may serve to protect the chromosome end from the programmed shortening that occurs with senesence and to limit chromosome instability that could precede malignant transformation. This is an important chapter in a fascinating story.

J.R. Shapiro, M.D.

References

1. Zakin VA: Telomeres: Beginning to understand the end. *Science* 270:1601–1606, 1995.
2. Sandell LL, Zakian VA: Loss of a yeast telomere: Arrest, recovery, and chromosome loss. *Cell* 75:729–739, 1993.
3. Rogan EM, Bryan TM, Hukku B, et al: Alterations in p53 and p16$_{INKA4}$ expression and telomere length during spontaneous immortalization of Li-Fraumeni syndrome fibroblasts. *Mol Cell Biol* 15:4745–4753, 1995.

Effect of Age on Marrow Macrophage Number and Function
Wang CQ, Udupa KB, Xiao H, et al (John L McClellan Mem Veterans Hosp, Little Rock, Ark; Univ of Arkansas, Little Rock)
Aging Clin Exp Res 7:379–384, 1995   5–32

Introduction.—Declines in immune function are related to age, induced by cell–cell interaction and via the release of cytokines, such as interleukin 1α, tumor necrosis factor, and colony stimulating factor. Hematopoietic function is affected both positively and negatively by the macrophages and the cytokines that are produced. A cardinal feature of aging in animals is the impaired ability of the hematopoietic system to respond to increased stimulation. The effects of age on marrow macrophage number and function were examined.

Methods.—Female mice, aged 4–6 months (young) and 22 months (old), were used. The size of bone marrow cell pools of these mice were measured using fluorescence-activated flow cytometry and the isolation of cell types by their formation of colony-forming units in tissue culture. A monoclonal antibody was used against the murine macrophage antigen, Mac-1. Tumor necrosis factor concentrations in the marrow macrophage culture were measured.

Results.—There was a significant increase in the number of marrow macrophages in the old mice. The number of colony forming unit macrophage progenitor cells and the number of α-naphthyl acetate esterase positive cells increased significantly with age (Table 1). In old mice, the frequency of colony-forming unit macrophage progenitor cells averaged 33.8±2.2/5 × 10⁴ bone marrow cells, whereas the younger mass had an average of 27.9±0.6/5 × 10⁴ bone marrow cells. Significantly less tumor necrosis factor was generated in the macrophages from the marrow of old mice than from young mice. Less suppression of burst forming unit-

TABLE 1.—Mac-1 Positive Cells, Esterase Positive Cells, CFU-M and CFU-GM
Progenitor Cell Number in Bone Marrow of Young and Old Mice

Measurements	Young	Old
Mac-1 Positive Cells (% of total marrow cells)	$16.2 \pm 1.4\%$	$29.5 \pm 2.3\%*$
Esterase Positive Cells (% of total marrow cells)	$19.8 \pm 0.9\%$	$31.4 \pm 1.4\%*$
CFU-M Progenitors/ 5×10^4 marrow cells	27.9 ± 0.6	$33.8 \pm 2.2†$
CFU-GM Progenitors/ 5×10^4 marrow cells	60.1 ± 2.9	63.7 ± 3.5

Note: Values are Mean ± SEM of 6 mice studied simultaneously in each group and cultured in triplicate.
*$P < 0.01$.
†$P < 0.05$.
Abbreviations: CFU-M, colony-forming unit-macrophage; CFU-GM, colon-forming unit granulocyte-macrophage.
(Courtesy of Wang CQ, Udupa KB, Xiao H, et al: Effect of age on marrow macrophage number and function. *Aging Clin Exp Res* 7:379–384, 1995.)

erythroid (BFU-E) colony growth was seen in the conditioned medium derived from the marrow or peritoneal macrophages of the old mice than from the young mice.

Conclusion.—An increase in the number of marrow macrophages that have an impaired ability to release or generate cytokines is associated with aging. The increase in the number of macrophages may be the result of compensation for the reduced function of the macrophages. The age-related decline in hematopoietic reserve capacity may be related to the altered macrophage number and function.

▶ This study is of particular interest because it explores important relationships among specific bone marrow cells that are affected by aging. Two methods frequently used to study the size of bone marrow cell pools, particularly that of progenitor cells, are fluorescence-activated flow cytometry and the isolation of cell types by their formation of colony-forming units in tissue culture. Applying these techniques, the authors report that in the mouse, aging is associated with an overall *increase* in marrow macrophages. These, however, demonstrate less production of tumor necrosis factor–α and less activity of conditioned medium from older mice towards suppression of BFU-E than seen in younger animals. The authors' previous work[1] attributes a decrease in marrow macrophage number to an increase in BFU-E. (But here, BFU-E numbers were equal in young and old.) However, BFU-E were more sensitive to suppression than were those from younger animals. Is it likely that the increased numbers of marrow macrophages simply compensate for impaired cell function? If true, what signals the marrow macrophage to increase numbers? How large is the progenitor pool and is it also increased in size? Also, if functionally deficient, is the decrease in cytokine production (also noted by others) related to the increased susceptibility of the aged to infections? Understanding these mechanisms may permit a protective bolstering of normal macrophage function with age.

J.R. Shapiro, M.D.

Reference

1. Wang CQ, Udpa KB, Lipshitz DA: The role of the macrophage in the regulation of erythroid colony growth in vitro. *Blood* 80:1702–1709, 1992.

Infectious Disease

Decreased Capacity of Aged Mice to Produce Interferon-Gamma in *Legionella Pneumophila* Infection

Fujio H, Kawamura I, Miyamoto H, et al (Univ of Occupational and Environmental Health, Kitakyushu, Japan; Niigata Univ, Japan)
Mech Ageing Dev 81:97–106, 1995   5–33

Background.—Elderly individuals are unusually susceptible to infectious disease, and aging may be a risk factor for infection by the facultative intracellular bacterium *Legionella pneumophila*. The endogenous production of interferon-γ (IFN-γ) at an early phase appears to be a key factor in resistance to *L. pneumophila* infection in mice.

Methods.—Resistance to *L. pneumophila* was contrasted in young and aged mice and related to both macrophage bactericidal activity and the production of IFN-γ. Studies were performed in groups of mice 3 months and 18–20 months of age. Bacterial growth was measured in peritoneal macrophages collected after injecting 3% thioglycolate medium. Production of IFN-γ by spleen cells was measured in vitro. The mice were injected intravenously with a sublethal dose of bacteria and then were given a single injection of either normal rat globulin or monoclonal antibody against natural murine IFN-γ; afterward, the numbers of viable organisms in the liver were determined.

Results.—Aged mice were significantly more susceptible to intraperitoneally injected *L. pneumophila* than were young mice. Intracellular killing of the organism took place significantly more rapidly in aged mice. Splenocytes from aged mice produced much less IFN-γ than did cells from young animals. The hepatic content of *L. pneumophila* was significantly increased after pretreatment with antibody against IFN-γ in young mice, but not in aged animals.

Conclusion.—The relative inability of aged mice to produce IFN-γ in response to *L. pneumophila* infection may help explain why older individuals are particularly susceptible to the infection.

▶ The heightened susceptibility of elderly individuals to infection is well known and is a continuous and serious threat to health and life. The authors of this paper were able to show in mice that a single humoral agent, IFN-γ, plays a key role in the heightened susceptibility to legionella infection. Although this finding per se in its precise form may have limited applicability, it reminds us of the importance of host factors in fighting infections and how host factors are weakened in the elderly population.

By taking the concept of host factors and redefining it in precise terms of specific molecules, we have an opportunity for therapeutic intervention of high specificity. In particular, the humoral agents of the body that are being discovered at a rapid rate—including the interleukins, other cytokines, lymphokines, and other endocrine-like agents—will enable us to replace deficiencies in these agents and, thereby, make up the defects in the host. One can envision that in the future, the therapy of infectious diseases will include not only the use of traditional vaccinations for prevention and antibiotics for treatment, but also the use of cytokines to assist in both the immunization and the therapy of infections, especially in elderly individuals.

J. Roth, M.D.

Endocrine and Metabolic Disease

Amplified Nocturnal Luteinizing Hormone (LH) Secretory Burst Frequency With Selective Attenuation of Pulsatile (But Not Basal) Testosterone Secretion in Healthy Aged Men: Possible Leydig Cell Desensitization to Endogenous LH Signaling. A Clinical Research Center Study
Mulligan T, Iranmanesh A, Gheorghiu S, et al (Med College of Virginia, Richmond; Salem Veterans Affairs Med Ctr, Va)
J Clin Endocrinol Metab 80:3025–3031, 1995   5–34

Objective.—Although 24-hour testosterone secretion is known to be decreased in older men, the mechanisms of this relative hypogonadism of aging remain unclear. The decreasing level of luteinizing hormone (LH) and testosterone pulse amplitudes observed with aging could result from a relative deficiency of gonadotropin-releasing hormone (GnRH) or decreased pituitary responsiveness to this hormone. The nature of the changes in LH and testosterone secretion in healthy older men were studied with the use of frequent venous sampling and deconvolution analysis of the endocrine time series.

Methods.—Ten healthy young men, aged 21–34 years, and 8 healthy older men, aged 62–74 years, were evaluated. Sensitive and specific assays were used to analyze overnight venous samples of LH and testosterone, obtained every 2.5 minutes. A validated multiparameter deconvolution analytic technique was used to estimate the rates of LH and testosterone secretion in the 2 groups.

Results.—Bursts of nocturnal secretion of LH were more frequent in the older men. In this group only, the frequency of the LH and testosterone secretory bursts was inversely related. The older men had a lower amplitude of nocturnal testosterone secretory bursts and a lower mass of testosterone secreted per burst. In men older than 60 years of age, the hourly nocturnal production rate of testosterone shifted downward.

Conclusions.—Older men show a reduced mean amplitude of the testosterone secretory pulse and a lower mass of testosterone secreted per burst. The pulsatile component of testosterone secretion, in particular, appears to be decreased in elderly men, with preservation of basal testosterone release. It is more likely that pulsatile and basal testosterone secretion differ in their sensitivity to the LH pulse signal than that an effective LH stimulus is simply lost. The increased LH pulse frequency noted in older men is consistent with their mild Leydig cell desensitization. With aging, the hypothalamo-pituitary-testicular axis may increase the frequency of hypothalamic GnRH secretion, decrease pituitary responsiveness to GnRH stimulation, and decrease testicular responsiveness to LH stimulation.

▶ This important study uses advanced methods to define the secretory profile of LH from the pituitary gland and testosterone from the testis in young and aging men. Inconsistent age-related alterations in secretory profiles of LH and testosterone secretion by the testis have been reported. Pituitary LH pulse amplitude has been observed to either decrease or increase with age. Whether this event is primary or secondary to peripheral changes in hormone secretion is unclear.

To study secretion of LH in young vs. elderly men in detail, the authors conducted nocturnal venous sampling every 2.5 minutes, which was a significant departure from previous methods that sampled less frequently. Coupled with highly sensitive LH and testosterone assays and deconvolution analysis of timed endocrine data, the authors could define LH pulse frequency and amplitude as well as profile the secretion of testosterone by testicular Leydig cells. Contrary to the results of previous studies, these results establish that nocturnal LH pulse frequency increases in elderly men at the same time that testosterone output decreases. One question remains: Which is the initiating event?

Testicular fibrosis and Leydig cell atrophy occur in elderly men, which suggests that a decrease in testosterone secretion may be the initiating event. This study shows that although basal levels of testosterone are similar for young and elderly men, pulsatile testosterone secretion decreases with increasing age.

In the same manner, mean serum levels of LH do not differ between healthy young and older men. That LH pulse frequency is increased in older men suggests 2 mechanisms that may be at fault. One is that with aging, increased frequency of hypothalamic secretion of GRH downregulates the pituitary response to GnRH. The second mechanism is the testicular response to LH. Alternatively, a primary decrease in testosterone secretion per pusatile burst may augment hypothalamic output of GnRH and increase LH pulse frequency. This may be an inadequate pituitary response, however, because of testicular involvement, and the increase in LH may act to desensitize the Leydig cells partially, thus decreasing the pulsatile secretion of testosterone.

J.R. Shapiro, M.D.

A Prostaglandin J$_2$ Metabolite Binds Peroxisome Proliferator-activated Receptor γ and Promotes Adipocyte Differentiation

Kliewer SA, Lenhard JM, Willson TM, et al (Glaxo Research Inst, Research Triangle Park, NC)

Cell 83:813–819, 1995

5–35

Introduction.—The J$_2$ series prostaglandins (PGs) influence a number of different biological processes. Most PGs act through G protein–coupled receptors, whereas the mechanism of action of the J$_2$ series PGs is unknown. Previous studies have been unable to identify naturally occurring ligands for the peroxisome proliferator–activated receptors (PPARs). These receptors are members of the nuclear receptor superfamily of ligand-activated transcription factors and are thought to modulate lipid metabolism. Whether the J$_2$ series of PGs act partly by activation of PPAR signaling pathways was determined.

Methods and Results.—A transient transfection assay was performed with the use of expression plasmids for GAL4-PPAR chimeras. Analysis of cyclo-oxygenase metabolites of arachidonic acid suggested that PGD$_2$ activated the PPARα and PPARγ chimeras at a concentration of 1×10^{-5} mmol/L. Prostaglandin$_2$ was relatively impotent in activating the PPAR chimeras, however, which suggested that CV-1 cells might metabolize it into more potent activators. Cotransfection assays showed that the 3 J-ring PGs were effective activators of PPARα and PPARγ chimeras. The 2 PPAR chimeras responded differently to PGD$_2$ and its PGJ$_2$ metabolites, which suggested that they were suggesting that they were pharmacologically distinct.

Direct interaction between a PGJ$_2$ derivative and PPARγ was demonstrated, along with weaker but reproducible competition with PGJ$_2$ and Δ^{12}-PGJ$_2$. The competition binding assay suggested that activation of PPAR by a fatty acid metabolite occurs through direct interactions with the ligand-binding domain of the receptor. Further studies provided strong evidence that 15-deoxy-$\Delta^{12,\ 14}$-PGJ$_2$, an arachidonic acid derivative, promoted adipocyte differentiation through PPARγ.

Conclusions.—The PGJ$_2$ metabolites of PGD$_2$ effectively activate PPARα and PPARγ, and evidence suggests that their effects are mediated at least partly by activation of nuclear receptor–signaling cascades. Prostaglandin$_2$ metabolites may also play a role in adipocyte differentiation. In addition to demonstrating a new PG signaling pathway, the results suggest that other eicosanoids could be ligands for other orphan receptors of the nuclear receptor superfamily.

▶ This article was selected for 2 reasons. First, it relates to an all-too-familiar feature of aging, i.e., the mechanism by which multipotential cells, such as stem cells or fibroblasts, differentiate into adipocytes. The formation of increasing amounts of fat with age in bone marrow is a good example of this process. Second, the article describes a novel pathway for PG action that apparently circumvents the usual cell surface receptor–intracellular signaling cascade by interacting directly with nuclear receptors to influence gene transcription. Peroxisome proliferator–activated nuclear receptors PPARα and PPARγ appear to play a large role in the regulation of lipid homeostasis, which is in part related to activating lipid-related genes. In addition, PPARγ is expressed in adipocytes and has been shown to play a role in adipocyte differentiation.

Several PGs, including PGE_2 and prostacyclin, are synthesized by isolated adipocytes and exert effects on adipocyte differentiation. Prostaglandin D_2, the major PG in bone marrow homogenates, is also found most abundantly in spleen. Prostaglandins of the J_2 series are formed from PGD_2 and exhibit a spectrum of functions including inhibition of cell cycle progression and induction of osteogenesis. This study shows that the nuclear PPARγ receptors in fibroblasts are activated by a PGJ_2 metabolite and that these fibroblasts differentiate into adipocytes. These results are significant because they describe an important mechanism for promoting cell differentiation. They also suggest a mechanism that, when altered, could limit the age-related fatty replacement of bone marrow. This result might permit continued function of both hemopoetic cells and the osteogenic precursor stromal cells that ultimately mature to bone forming osteoblasts.

J.R. Shapiro, M.D.

Components of the Renin-Angiotensin System in Adipose Tissue: Changes With Maturation and Adipose Mass Enlargement
Harp JB, DiGirolamo M (Emory Univ, Atlanta, Ga)
J Gerontol 50A:B270–B276, 1995   5–36

Background.—Angiotensinogen protein and messenger RNA (mRNA) are present in white adipose tissue. Evidence from in vitro studies suggests that angiotensinogen and angiotensin II, its cleavage product, play a role in preadipocyte differentiation into mature fat cells. The role of angiotensinogen in the development of adipose tissue in vivo, however, remains unclear. Male Wistar rats were studied at different developmental stages to determine alterations in angiotensinogen during the age-related process of adipose tissue growth.

Methods.—Rats were studied at 8 weeks of age, when they were lean and growing rapidly, and at 26 weeks of age, when they were fatter but had less rapid growth of adipose tissue. Angiotensinogen protein and mRNA were measured in the retroperitoneal adipose tissue deposit, which accounts for approximately 10% of total body fat and parallels total body lipid.

Results.—Levels of angiotensinogen mRNA were twice as high in the retroperitoneal adipocytes of young rats as in older rats. Angiotensinogen protein levels were 3 times as high in the young rats. There was no difference in angiotensinogen levels when the entire retroperitoneal fat depot was considered. Angiotensin I–generating activity was easily detectable in the adipose tissue, reaching its highest level at acid pH. Although angiotensin-converting enzyme activity was found in whole adipose tissue, it was absent from isolated fat cells.

Conclusions.—Studies in rats show an age-related decrease in angiotensinogen protein and mRNA in adipose tissue. These changes indicate that the local renin-angiotensin system could play a major role in adipose tissue growth. Furthermore, this system could be involved in the adipose mass and cellularity changes observed in old and senescent animals.

▶ This article highlights a hormonal system related to adipogenesis that is usually associated with the renovascular system. White retroperitoneal adipose tissue contains abundant amounts of angiotensinogen protein and mRNA.[1] What is particularly intriguing is that fasting and several hormones, including thyroid hormone, estradiol, and dexamethasone, modulate the levels of angiotensinogen in white adipose tissue. Levels of adipose tissue and isolated fat cell angiotensinogen protein were higher in animals aged 8 weeks than in those aged 26 weeks. However, less angiotensinogen per cell was observed in the older vs. the younger animals, even though the mass of adipose tissue volume was greater in older rats. Thus, increased angiotensinogen expression may be related to rapid growth of white adipose cells in the young rat rather than hyperplasia of adipose tissue, which occurs in the older animals. The total amount of angiotensinogen protein per fat pad was similar in young and old animals. Angiotensin-converting enzyme activity in adipose tissue was demonstrated by a captopril inhibition assay, but renin synthesis was not found. Does angiotensinogen play a role in fat deposition in younger obese individuals, and is it important in humans as intra-abdominal fat deposition occurs with age? That its levels vary depending on several stimuli suggests that it may contribute to changes in adipose tissue mass.

J.R. Shapiro, M.D.

Reference

1. Harp JB, DiGirolamo M: Local renin-angiotensin system in adipose tissue from lean and obese rats. *Int J Obes* 15:175, 1991.

Effects of Droloxifene on Prevention of Cancellous Bone Loss and Bone Turnover in the Axial Skeleton of Aged, Ovariectomized Rats

Ke HZ, Chen HK, Qi H, et al (Pfizer Inc, Groton, Conn; Univ of Utah, Salt Lake City)
Bone 17:491–496, 1995   5–37

Background.—Estrogen can help prevent bone loss and vertebral fractures in postmenopausal women. The tissue-specific estrogen antagonist/agonists are a class of nonsteroidal estrogen analogues with the same bone protective and lipid-reducing effects as estrogen but without the side effects on reproductive tissues. One of these drugs, droloxifene (DRO), was studied for its ability to prevent cancellous bone loss and bone turnover in aged female rats.

Methods.—Nineteen-month-old female Sprague-Dawley rats underwent ovariectomy or sham operation and were then assigned to receive: no treatment; placebo; 17β-estradiol (E_2), 30 µg/kg/day; or DRO at a dose of 2.5, 5.0, or 10.0 mg/kg orally daily. Treatment continued for 8 weeks.

Results.—17β-Estradiol treatment prevented the ovariectomy-related cancellous bone loss and led to lower bone resorption, bone formation, and bone turnover than in sham-operated controls. At all 3 doses, DRO treatment prevented bone loss and bone turnover completely. Treatment with DRO also reduced osteoclast number and perimeter, and the histomorphometric findings were similar to those noted in E_2-treated rats. With DRO treatment, body weight decreased in dose-dependent fashion and total serum cholesterol decreased by 65% to 70%. Whereas E_2 treatment significantly increased uterine weight, DRO treatment produced no uterine weight gain at most doses.

Conclusions.—Droloxifene seems to act as an estrogen agonist on the cancellous bone of aged, ovariectomized female rats. It effectively prevents cancellous bone loss from the lumbar vertebrae and decreases cholesterol as E_2 does, but without increasing uterine weight. This estrogen antagonist/agonist may be a useful treatment for the prevention of vertebral bone loss and spinal fractures in postmenopausal women.

▶ Postmenopausal women, with the loss of endogenous estrogen, undergo serious bone loss and also have a heightened susceptibility to cardiovascular diseases. Although estrogen replacement ameliorates both of these processes, it also brings with it risks for tumors of the reproductive tissues. Can the effects of estrogen be "unbundled" (i.e., can the beneficial effects on bone and blood vessels be retained without gaining the cancer risks)? Some estrogen analogues are mixed antagonists/agonists; tamoxifen is the best known example. In experimental animals, some of these agents seem to prevent bone loss without much effect on reproductive tissues. In addition to the cancer risk, postmenopausal uterine bleeding is a major reason that women give up use of estrogens. Thus, success with these analogues would not only help the bone and cardiovascular diseases but markedly enhance compliance. Overall, this approach seems to be a promising lead in developing better agents with which to replace estrogens in postmenopausal women.

J. Roth, M.D.

Local Concentrations of Macrophage Colony-stimulating Factor Mediate Osteoclastic Differentiation

Perkins SL, Kling SJ (Univ of Utah, Salt Lake City)
Am J Physiol 269:E1024–E1030, 1995   5–38

Background.—The hematopoietic cytokine macrophage colony-stimulating factor (M-CSF) is required for the differentiation of osteoclasts and macrophages from bone marrow precursor cells. Stromal coculture techniques can be used to study osteoclast formation in vitro. These techniques were used to clarify the role of M-CSF in determining the differentiation of hematopoietic precursor cells into osteoclasts or monocytes and macrophages.

Methods and Results.—The study used ST-2 stromal cell/murine bone marrow cell culture to determine the effects of increasing levels of M-CSF on macrophage and osteoclast differentiation. When exogenous M-CSF was added to culture, tartrate-resistant acid phosphatase decreased by 98% in dose-dependent fashion. At the same time, there was a 2.5-fold increase in nonspecific esterase-staining macrophages. Significant decreases were also noted in indicators of osteoclast functional activity, such as ^{125}I-labeled calcitonin binding and calcitonin-stimulated adenosine 3',5'-cyclic monophosphate production. After 6 days in coculture, the ability of added M-CSF to inhibit osteoclast formation was substantially reduced. When neutralizing anti–M-CSF was added early in coculture, it also inhibited osteoclast formation. This effect decreased after day 9.

Conclusions.—The effects of M-CSF on osteoclast differentiation seem to occur early, during the proliferative phase of osteoclast formation. Whether hematopoietic precursor cells will ultimately differentiate into macrophages or osteoclasts may be influenced by local high M-CSF concentrations. As increasing concentrations of M-CSF were added to the in vitro system used, monocyte and macrophage formation increased and osteoclast-like cell formation was inhibited.

▶ Bone represents the sum of effects of bone-forming osteoblasts and bone-lysing osteoclasts. In earlier studies, a mouse model lacking M-CSF was found to have severe osteopetrosis that responded well to the injections of this hematopoietic cytokine. In the untreated mouse, macrophages are absent, as are osteoclasts. The injection of M-CSF was associated with the appearance of osteoclasts. In this study, using an in vitro cellular model, the researchers showed that antibodies against M-CSF prevented the conversion of macrophages to osteoclasts, providing a further boost to the evidence that the macrophages are the source of the osteoclasts and that specific cytokines induce this transformation. It is not difficult to envision that in the near future a direct mechanism for regulating bone density without having to involve other tissues of the body will be regulation of the number and the activity of the osteoclasts and osteoblasts. In this way, new therapies can be devised that will sustain the mineral density of the long bones without necessarily affecting other tissues.

J. Roth, M.D.

Bisphosphonates Induce Osteoblasts to Secrete an Inhibitor of Osteoclast-mediated Resorption

Vitté C, Fleisch H, Guenther HL (Univ of Berne, Switzerland; Institut Biomédical des Cordeliers, Paris)
Endocrinology 137:2324–2333, 1996   5–39

Background.—Bisphosphonates, which are analogues of pyrophosphate, strongly inhibit bone resorption. The inhibiting action of bisphosphonates is believed to be caused by the metabolic damage of actively resorbing osteoclasts after ingestion of these compounds bound to bone. Recent research has shown that a coculture of isolated osteoclasts with osteoblasts pretreated with bisphosphonate inhibits osteoclastic resorption. Whether the bisphosphonate-generated inhibition results from these compounds reducing the synthesis of the osteoclast-stimulating activity or from osteoblasts synthesizing an osteoclast resorption inhibitor was determined.

Methods and Findings.—The osteoblastic cell line CRP 10/30, which produces osteoclast-stimulating activity, and isolated rat osteoclasts cultured on ivory were used. The bisphosphonates ibandronate and alendronate, at a concentration of 10^{-7}, induced osteoblasts to synthesize an osteoclast inhibitor that decreased pit formation by more than half. The inhibitor was heat and proteinase labile, with a molecular mass of 1–10 kd. Resorption pit reduction was paralleled by a decline in tartrate-resis-

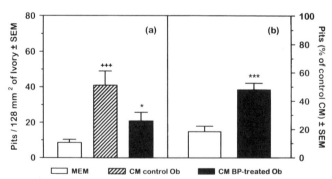

FIGURE 1.—Effects of minimal essential media (*MEM*) and conditioned media (*CM*) of untreated (*control*) and bisphosphonate (*BP*) (*ibandronate*)-treated osteoblastic CRP 10/30 cells on pit formation of isolated rat osteoclasts. A, average number of pits found on 128 mm² of ivory surface. B, data are presented as the number of pits expressed as a percentage of the number of pits formed by CM of control cells. Each *bar* represents the mean ± standard error of mean of 12 individual experiments. Each experiment was performed with different CM and osteoclast preparations of different animal pools. *Asterisk*, $P < 0.005$; *3 asterisks*, $P < 0.001$ (vs. control CM). *3 plus signs*, $P < 0.001$ (vs. MEM). (Courtesy of Vitté C, Fleisch H, Guenther HL: Bisphosphonates induce osteoblasts to secrete an inhibitor of osteoclast-mediated resorption. *Endocrinology* 137(6):2324–2333, 1996. Copyright The Endocrine Study.)

tant acid phosphatase–positive mononucleated and multinucleated cells. The mean area resorbed per pit was unchanged. The inhibitor apparently affected osteoclast formation and/or survival and not the osteoclast resorption activity. Rat preosteoblastic cells and rat dermal fibroblasts did not produce the inhibitor (Fig 1).

Conclusions.—Osteoblasts in vitro appear to mediate the action of bisphosphonates on bone resorption by synthesizing an inhibitor of osteoclast recruitment and/or survival. This finding emphasizes the important role that osteoblasts play in regulating resorption of osteoclastic bone.

▶ Tremendous interest has been generated by the recent introduction of alendronate, a third generation bisphosphonate, for the treatment of osteoporosis and Paget's disease. Moreover, several other highly effective bisphosphonates (ibandronate, residronate, and tuludronate) are currently being studied in clinical trials. One problem with the earlier bisphosphonates, such as etidronate, was that, depending on the dose, these agents had depressing effects on both formation and resorption of bone. As a group, the newer agents have been mainly designed to depress osteoclastic bone resorption, which presumably occurred because of absorption of the drug onto hydroxyapatite crystals, followed by direct effects of the agent on the resorbing osteoclast. Recent studies, however, point to the osteoblast as the mediator in this process. Not unexpectedly, the osteoblast, under hormonal stimulation, promotes osteoclastic resorption. This finding has previously been shown to be the mechanism by which parathyroid hormone, 1,25(OH) vitamin D_3, interleukin-1, and the tumor necrosis factors turn on osteoclastic bone resorption. Inhibition of the synthesis of an osteoclast-stimulating factor, or synthesis of a direct inhibitor of osteoclastic function, might be involved. The results point to a protein inhibitor of the osteoclast between 1 and 10 kd. Both ibandronate and alendronate had similar effects on depressing osteoclast number and on the formation of resorption pits.

The increase in bone mass in patients treated with bisphosphonate appears to plateau after 4–5 years. Although the reasons for this are not certain, the completion of previous bone remodeling units (remodeling transients) has been suggested as 1 possibility. These results also suggest that osteoblastic failure after long exposure to bisphosphonate could, in turn, result in a decrease in osteoclastic inhibition and a subsequent increase in bone resorption.

J.R. Shapiro, M.D.

Overexpression of the Granulocyte Colony-stimulating Factor Gene Leads to Osteoporosis in Mice

Takahashi T, Wada T, Mori M, et al (Sapporo Med Univ, Japan)
Lab Invest 74:827–834, 1996

5–40

Background.—The survival, proliferation, differentiation, and function of mature neutrophil granulocytes and their precursors are influenced by

TABLE 1.—Measurements of the Femoral Shaft in Transgenic Mice and Their Littermate Controls*

	Littermate controls (*n* = 7)	Transgenic Mice (*n* = 7)
Periosteal perimeter†	4.176 ± 0.181	4.565 ± 0.267§
Endcortical perimeter†	2.826 ± 0.142	3.722 ± 0.213§
Cortical area‡	0.7232 ± 0.0586	0.658 ± 0.043‖
Marrow area‡	0.554 ± 0.064	0.9683 ± 0.1267§
Average cortical width‡	0.221 ± 0.009	0.162 ± 0.017§

*Values are means ± standard deviation.
†Expressed as millimeters.
‡Expressed as square millimeters.
§Significant difference between transgenic mice and littermate controls, *P* < 0.01.
‖Significant difference between transgenic mice and littermate controls, *P* < 0.05.
(Courtesy of Takahashi T, Wada T, Mori M, et al: Overexpression of the granulocyte colony-stimulating factor gene leads to osteoporosis in mice. *Lab Invest* 74(4):827–834, 1996.)

the glycoprotein granulocyte colony-stimulating factor (G-CSF). Although G-CSF was originally isolated as a hematopoietic growth factor, evidence has suggested that it functions on a wide variety of cells. The function of G-CSF on bone cells in vivo was investigated.

Methods.—The bone tissue of transgenic mice that overexpress G-CSF was examined. Human G-CSF is increased under the direction of SRα promoter in these mice. Radiographic, routine histologic, and histomorphometric analyses of bone tissue were performed, as was serum biochemical assay. Nontransgenic littermates were also studied.

Findings.—In vertebral bodies and long bones, cortical thinning, accompanied by enlarged bone marrow cavities, was demonstrated radiographically. Histologic analysis revealed a reduced number and thickness of trabecular bones and cortical thinning in lumbar vertebrae and femur specimens. The number of mature neutrophilic granulocytes was increased in the enlarged bone marrow cavities, with no apparent changes in other cell types. The transgenic mice showed significantly increased static and dynamic parameters, which reflected bone resorption. There were no significant differences, however, in the parameters that reflected bone formation. Although transgenic and control mice had similar serum levels of calcium, phosphorus, and alkaline phosphatase, the transgenic mice had significantly greater serum levels of serum osteocalcin (Table 1).

Conclusions.—Osteoporosis developed in transgenic mice that expressed G-CSF because of increased osteoclastic activity. Collectively, G-CSF may negatively affect bone homeostasis in vivo.

▶ This article provides in vivo evidence that excessive production of a cytokine, in this case G-CSF, can lead to bone loss and osteoporosis. The list of cytokines that produce a similar end point includes interleukin-1 (IL-1) and IL-6, both of which have been implicated in the development of osteoporosis in postmenopausal women. Similarly, transgenic overproduction of IL-4 has recently been reported to induce osteoporosis, perhaps by a mechanism that includes an osteoblastic product that activates osteoclastic differentiation from monocytic precursors.[1] The mechanism that leads to increased osteoclastic differentiation and bone loss, however, may be more complex: Alterations in hormonal status (menopause) or the presence of tumors, such as multiple myeloma, may stimulate the production of several cytokines that act in concert to increase resorption of bone. Equally intriguing are the variations that occur in osteoblast and osteoclast cell receptors, which are another level of potential complexity. It is certain that the more we learn about the complex interactions at the level of the osteoblast–osteoclast multicellular unit, the better will be our ability to counter those processes that lead to osteoporotic fractures.

J.R. Shapiro, M.D.

Reference

1. Lewis DB, Liggitt HD, Effmann EL, et al: Osteoporosis induced in mice by overproduction of interleukin 4. *Proc Natl Acad Sci U S A* 90:11618–11622, 1994.

Role of Calcium Intake in Modulating Age-related Increases in Parathyroid Function and Bone Resorption
McKane WR, Khosla S, Egan KS, et al (Mayo Clinic and Found, Rochester, Minn; Rowett Research Inst, Aberdeen, Scotland)
J Clin Endocrinol Metab 81:1699–1703, 1996   5–41

Background.—The increased serum parathyroid hormone (PTH) and bone resorption occurring in elderly women make a significant contribution to age-related bone loss. Secretory patterns of PTH also are abnormal in elderly women. Previous studies of the effects of increased calcium level on PTH levels have not allowed sufficient time for complete adaptation to the change in calcium intake and have not looked at the effects on circadian patterns of PTH secretion. The effects of 3 years of controlled calcium intake—at either usual or high levels—on serum PTH, parathyroid gland secretory reserve capacity, and bone resorption were evaluated.

Methods.—Twenty-eight healthy elderly women with normal bone density for their age were studied. The patients were assigned to 3 years at their usual calcium intake level (mean, 20 mmol/day) or at a high-calcium intake level (mean, 60 mmol/day). Measurements of serum PTH and urinary excretion of deoxypyridinoline (Dpd)—a new marker of bone resorption—were made in these 2 groups of women and in a control group of normal young adult women. In addition, parathyroid gland secretory capacity was measured after induction of hypocalcemia by EDTA infusion.

Results.—Twenty-four-hour serum PTH values were 36% lower and mean urinary Dpd values 25% lower for elderly women in the high-calcium intake group compared with those in the usual-calcium intake group. The values measured in the high-calcium group were similar to

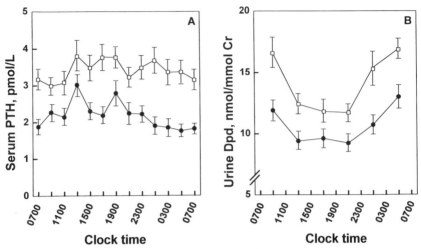

FIGURE 1.—**A,** serum parathyroid hormone (*PTH*) as a function of time in the usual calcium group (*open squares*) and the high calcium group (·) of elderly women. There was a significant time effect in both groups (*P* < 0.001) and also a significant group effect (*P* < 0.005), with the low calcium intake group having consistently higher PTH levels. **B,** urinary deoxypyridinoline (*Dpd*) as a function of time in the usual calcium group (*open squares*) and the high calcium group (·) of elderly women. There was a significant time effect in both groups (*P* < 0.001) and also a significant group effect (*P* < 0.005) with the low calcium intake group having consistently higher urinary Dpd values. (Courtesy of McKane WR, Khosla S, Egan KS, et al: Role of calcium intake in modulating age-related increases in parathyroid function and bone resorption. *J Clin Endocrinol Metab* 81(5):1699–1703, 1996. Copyright The Endocrine Society.)

those of young, premenopausal women, whereas the usual-calcium intake group had significantly higher values than the young women. A circadian pattern was apparent for both mean serum PTH and urinary Dpd, with consistently elevated levels over 24 hours for the high-calcium intake group (Fig 1). There was evidence that the high- and usual-calcium intake groups had differing circadian rhythms. Both groups showed an increase in urinary Dpd at night, but this increase was not as high in the high-calcium group. The high-calcium group also had significantly lower parathyroid gland secretory capacity than the usual-calcium group.

Conclusions.—Elderly women have an increased need for calcium, and failure to increase their calcium intake contributes to the development of increased PTH activity and bone resorption. Both of these abnormalities can be reversed by a high calcium intake. The nocturnal increase in bone resorption is not completely abolished by a high calcium intake, adding to the evidence that only a portion of bone resorption is PTH dependent. Long-term clinical trials will be needed to prove that calcium supplementation can prevent age-related bone loss.

▶ There is mounting evidence that increasing dietary calcium intake is useful for limiting bone loss in elderly (late postmenopausal) women.[1] Calcium supplementation is not effective in decreasing bone loss resulting from estrogen deficiency during the decade after the menopause. This article supports a role for increased dietary calcium intake in elderly women and suggests that suppression of PTH secretion is important in limiting bone resorption. However, note that calcium intake was relatively high, 2,000 mg/day, and that the low-calcium group ingested 900 mg/day, more than the 800 mg/day established as the recommended daily allowance for calcium. Is the currently recommended 1,500 mg/day supplement effective in suppressing nocturnal PTH secretion? More information is needed.

A question frequently asked is, When during the day should the calcium supplement be taken? Earlier studies advised taking calcium at bedtime to suppress nocturnal increases in PTH. In this study, high calcium intake blunted but did not abolish the nocturnal increase in bone resorption, which is consistent with the recent observation that bone-resorbing activity at night was not fully abolished by anti-PTH antibodies.[2] Calcium absorption is improved by taking it at mealtimes. Taking part of the calcium supplement at bedtime also may improve its effectiveness.

J.R. Shapiro, M.D.

References

1. Reid IR, Ames RW, Evans MC, et al: Effect of calcium supplementation on bone loss in postmenopausal women. *N Engl J Med* 328:460–464, 1993.
2. Latakos P, Blumshon A, Eastell R, et al: Circadian rhythm of in vitro bone resorbing activity in human serum. *J Clin Endocrinol Metab* 80:3185–3190, 1995.

Stable Expression of the Nuclear Vitamin D Receptor in the Human Prostatic Carcinoma Cell Line JCA-1: Evidence That the Antiproliferative Effects of 1α,25-Dihydroxyvitamin D3 Are Mediated Exclusively Through the Genomic Signaling Pathway
Hedlund TE, Moffatt KA, Miller GJ (Univ of Colorado, Denver)
Endocrinology 137:1554–1561, 1996

5–42

Background.—The secosteroid hormone 1α,25-dihydroxyvitamin D_3 [1,25-$(OH)_2D_3$] regulates the growth and differentiation of human prostate cancer cells. However, the exact mechanisms underlying these effects are unclear. This hormone can act through nongenomic signaling pathways involving a membrane-associated receptor as well as genomic pathways involving the nuclear vitamin-D receptor (VDR). The ability of the stereoisomer 1β,25-$(OH)_2D_3$, which acts as a potent antagonist of the membrane-associated receptor but a weak agonist of the nuclear receptor, to ablate the effects of 1,2-$(OH)_2D_3$ was assessed.

Methods and Findings.—The human prostate cell line JCA-1 was used. This cell line does not express detectable numbers of VDRs and is apparently not affected by 1,25-$(OH)_2D_3$ in growth studies. The cells were transfected stably with a wild-type VDR complementary DNA construct. Transfection resulted in the expression of high-affinity nuclear VDRs, a dose-dependent inhibition of growth by 1,25-$(OH)_2D_3$, and a significant

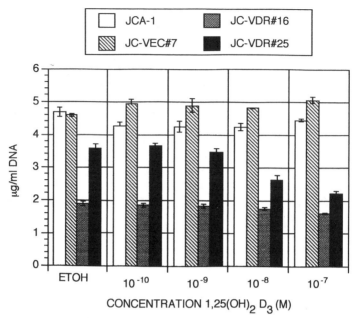

FIGURE 4.—Dose-dependent inhibition of growth by 1,25-(OH)$_2$D$_3$ in parental cells (*JCA-1*), vector-transfected cells (*JC-VEC 7*), and vitamin-D receptor (VDR)–transfected cells (*JC-VDR 16* and *25*). Cultures were treated with the designated concentration of 1,25-(OH)$_2$D$_3$ or ethanol vehicle control for 6 days. Monolayers were harvested for DNA quantitation to measure changes in growth. Each value represents the mean of triplicate samples ± SE. (Courtesy of Hedlund TE, Moffatt KA, Miller GJ: Stable expression of the nuclear vitamin D receptor in the human prostatic carcinoma cell line JCA-1: Evidence that the antiproliferative effects of 1α,25-dihydroxyvitamin D3 are mediated exclusively through the genomic signaling pathway. *Endocrinology* 137(5):1554–1561, 1996. Copyright The Endocrine Society.)

increase in 24-hydroxylase upregulation by 1,25-(OH)$_2$D$_3$ compared with controls (Fig 4).

Conclusions.—The expression of nuclear VDR is sufficient to mediate the antiproliferative effects of 1,25-(OH)$_2$D$_3$ on prostate cancer cells. The stereoisomer 1β,25-dihydroxyvitamin D$_3$ did not block these antiproliferative effects. Thus, nongenomic mechanisms of action apparently are not required for growth inhibition by 1,25-(OH)$_2$D$_3$.

▶ 1α,25-dihydroxyvitamin D$_3$, the active metabolite of vitamin D$_3$, is the principal mediator of the vitamin-D endocrine system. This article is of considerable interest for 2 reasons: (1) it illustrates the differential role of membrane receptors acting through nongenomic pathways, and that of nuclear receptors binding to DNA (genomic) in determining hormone action; and (2) it presents data indicating mechanisms through which 1α,25-dihydroxyvitamin D$_3$ diminishes the proliferation of prostatic carcinoma cells.

Membrane-bound VDRs mediate several nongenomic effects of 1α,25-dihydroxyvitamin D$_3$.[1] These include the hormone action to increase calcium transport, alter phospholipase C activity, and increase alkaline phosphatase levels. The genomic receptor controls cellular growth and differentiation by binding to hormone-responsive elements in DNA. The nongenomic pathway may influence the genomic response to the hormone, an issue this paper seeks to define. The antiproliferative effect of 1α,25-dihydroxyvitamin D$_3$ appears to be mediated by the genomic pathway. Not only is this action of vitamin D of potential therapeutic importance, the study presents data that may be useful in the design of vitamin-D analogues that may be even more potent in suppressing the growth of prostatic cancer. This question was addressed by Skowronski et al., who observed that synthetic analogues of vitamin D$_3$ having reduced calcemic activity retained antiproliferative effects on prostatic cancer cells.[2] Interestingly, significant antiproliferative activity was retained by analogues with tenfold less affinity for the VDR than the native hormone.

J.R. Shapiro, M.D.

References

1. Baran DT: Nongenomic actions of the steroid hormone 1 alpha, 25-dihydroxyvitamin D3. *J Cell Biochem* 56:303–306, 1994.
2. Skowronski RJ, Peehl DM, Feldman D: Actions of vitamin D3 analogs on human prostatic cancer cell lines: Comparison with 1,25-dihydroxyvitamin D3. *Endocrinology* 136:20–26, 1995.

Effects of Reciprocal Treatment With Estrogen and Estrogen Plus Parathyroid Hormone on Bone Structure and Strength in Ovariectomized Rats

Shen V, Birchman R, Xu R, et al (Helen Hayes Hosp, New York; Columbia Univ, New York)
J Clin Invest 96:2331–2338, 1995

5–43

Introduction.—Although antiresorptive agents have been able to prevent bone loss associated with postmenopausal osteoporosis, these agents have not been able to restore lost bone mass. Cancellous bone loss has been halted and some lost bone mass and structure has been restored with a treatment regimen combining antiresorptive and anabolic agents, such as parathyroid hormone (PTH). To maintain newly gained bone mass, the use of an antiresorptive agent has been proposed. An examination was conducted to determine if estrogen therapy alone could preserve newly gained bone. After prolonged use of estrogen, the beneficial effects of parathyroid hormone were studied in an animal model of postmenopausal osteoporosis.

Methods.—Six-month-old rats were ovariectomized and treated for 8 weeks with an intermittent injection of 30 μg/kg per day of rat PTH plus 15 μg/kg per day of 17β-estradiol, 17β-estradiol-alone, or vehicle. After a group from each treatment regimen was killed, during the next 8 weeks, the rest of the rats were either crossed over to their reciprocal treatment, maintained on their previous treatment, or administered vehicle only.

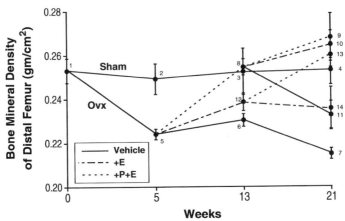

FIGURE 4.—Effects of combined parathyroid hormone plus estradiol and crossover treatments on bone mineral density at the distal femur. Numbered points represent group numbers. (Reproduced from *The Journal of Clinical Investigation*, 1995, vol 96, pp 2331–2338, by copyright permission of The American Society for Clinical Investigation.)

All of the rats were killed at the end of the second 8-week treatment period.

Results.—Estrogen alone can maintain gains in bone mass, trabecular connectivity, and mechanical strength induced by PTH. Bone mineral density of the distal femur was measured because it is a cancellous-rich region of the femur and indicated that the combined parathyroid and estrogen treatment increased the parameters of connectivity (Fig 4). However, when both agents are withdrawn, the effects are reversed. In the rats with established osteopenia who had estrogen therapy alone, full beneficial effects were observed with the addition of PTH at a later date. There was little change in cancellous bone volume during the second 8-week period of treatment with PTH plus estrogen, supporting the idea that there is a plateau in the action of PTH on cancellous bone.

Conclusions.—A promising approach to the treatment of osteoporosis may be the combined and/or sequential use of antiresorptive and anabolic agents. Because of its ability to increase connectivity parameters and thicken trabecular plates, treatment with combined estrogen and PTH can be effective in preventing and treating estrogen deficiency–induced bone loss. The plateau effect of PTH on cancellous bone may be a result of more anabolic action in the cancellous bone, indicating that the maximum benefit was achieved earlier.

▶ The topic of osteoporosis treatment has received considerable exposure because of the recent availability of an effective third generation bisphosphonate, alendronate. Clinically, the relevant issues are the site specific effectiveness of antiresorptive agents (spine vs. hip) and a plateau effect seen with both estrogen and the first-generation bisphosphonate, etidronate, after 3–5 years of treatment. This has been ascribed to the well-known coupled activity of osteoblasts and osteoclasts: decreasing resorption eventually decreases bone formation. Combining an antiresorptive agent with one that increases bone formation (PTH) would seem optimal.

In this study, one objective was to see if PTH would maintain the estrogen-induced gain in bone mass in the ovariectomized rat. Although the anabolic effects of PTH occur even after estrogen replacement, there seemed to be little increase in cancellous bone volume during the second 8-week period of treatment with PTH plus estrogen. Although the authors attribute this plateau to early rapid bone formation, I suggest that if seen in human trials, it would decrease the long-term effectiveness of PTH therapy. Cyclic therapy may be a solution.

For an informative review on the subject of the clinical applications of measuring bone turnover, refer to the article by Marcus.[1]

J.R. Shapiro, M.D.

Reference

1. Marcus R: Biochemical assessment of bone resorption and formation. *Bone* 18: 15S–16S, 1996.

Age-Dependent Reduction in Insulin Secretion and Insulin mRNA in Isolated Islets From Rats

Perfetti R, Rafizadeh CM, Liotta AS, et al (NIH, Baltimore, Md)
Am J Physiol 269:E983–E990, 1995   5–44

Purpose.—Aging and the age-related decrease in glucose tolerance are major risk factors for the development of non–insulin-dependent diabetes mellitus (NIDDM). In approximately 70% of elderly patients with diabetes, the disease onset is thought to occur when the β-cells stop producing enough insulin to overcome insulin resistance. The age-related changes in β-cell physiology were studied in detail in rats.

Methods.—Isolated islets from male Wistar rats of various ages were studied. The analysis included insulin release from single cells, total pancreatic insulin content, and insulin mRNA concentrations for islet-specific genes.

Results.—With 10 minutes of glucose stimulation, islets from 6-month-old rats had 40% more insulin-secreting cells than islets from 24-month-old rats. At 1 hour, 67% of islets from the young rats vs. 51% of those from the old rats were secreting insulin. Islets from the older rats also had a lower amount of insulin secreted by each β-cell. Islet size and the number of β-cells increased with age, but whole pancreas insulin content was significantly less in organs from 24-month-old rats than in those from 6-month-old rats. Islets from 24-month-old rats had insulin mRNA concentrations of half the newborn value, although there was only a modest decrease in glucagon mRNA concentrations.

Conclusions.—Wistar rats show a progressive, age-related decline in β-cell activity. The changes in β-cell physiology noted in this study may play an important role in the increasing risk of diabetes with age. Further research is needed to determine the biochemical and molecular mechanisms causing the physiologic age adaptation of β-cell secretion and replication.

► These authors, colleagues of mine in Baltimore, have shown that islets from 24-month-old rats are less sensitive to glucose than islets of 6-month-old rats. When exposed to glucose, a smaller percentage of the islets from the older rats secrete insulin than do those of younger rats. Similarly, the total insulin output per secreting islet is less from the older rats than from the younger ones. Even at the highest glucose concentrations, more of the young cells secreted insulin than did the old cells, and the young cells each secreted more than the insulin secreting cells from the old. The mRNA content of the islet cells decreased progressively with age. On the other hand, mRNA for glucagon and somatostatin changed little or not at all. This age-dependent diminution in sensitivity to glucose in vitro is an important first step in trying to understand the changes in the islet cells that occur in vivo with aging. Further studies will be needed to delineate the mechanisms and how relevant these findings in the rat are to human populations.

J. Roth, M.D.

Effects of Aging on Glucose Regulation During Wakefulness and Sleep
Frank SA, Roland DC, Sturis J, et al (Univ of Chicago)
Am J Physiol 269:E1006–E1016, 1995   5–45

Background.—Aging is associated with glucose intolerance, less efficient sleep, and disturbances of circadian rhythm. Studies of normal adults have shown that sleep and circadian rhythm have important effects on glucose regulation. The effects of time of day, sleep, and growth hormone (GH) secretion on glucose tolerance and insulin secretion were studied in older men.

Methods.—The study included 8 modestly overweight older men (mean age, 65 years; mean body mass index, 29) and 8 weight-matched young men. Data from lean young men participating in a previous study were also analyzed. All men were studied during 53 hours of constant glucose infusion, including 8 hours of nocturnal sleep, 28 hours of continuous wakefulness, and 8 hours of daytime sleep. This study design permitted assessment of the effects of time of day in the absence of sleep and of the effects of sleep at an abnormal time. The subjects' glucose, insulin, C-peptide, and GH concentrations were assessed every 20 minutes, and their insulin and GH secretion rates were calculated by deconvolution.

Results.—Sleep was shallower and more fragmented in the older men than in the younger men. Although all groups showed significant glucose increases in association with sleep, the increases in insulin secretion occurring after sleep were significantly reduced in the older men. The older men had a normal increase in glucose from morning to evening while they were awake, but no proportional increase in insulin secretion.

Conclusions.—The decreased glucose tolerance observed in older adults is associated not only with insulin resistance but also with reduced β-cell sensitivity to the effects of sleep and circadian rhythm on glucose regulation. The reduced sleep-associated increase in elderly individuals probably reflects age-related changes in a number of different factors. The reduction in β-cell responsivity could play a role in the age-related development of impaired glucose tolerance.

▶ Aging in humans is often associated with the deterioration of glucose tolerance, which is ascribed largely to peripheral insulin resistance, although investigators have also shown abnormalities in insulin secretion. When the authors infused glucose continuously for a 2-day period, they detected a decrement in glucose tolerance with aging, which was associated with insulin resistance and also a relative insensitivity of the β-cell to glucose. Variables such as sleep, weight, and other features of the aging human are discussed in the article.

J. Roth, M.D.

Decline of Plasma Growth Hormone Binding Protein in Old Age
Maheshwari H, Sharma L, Baumann G (Northwestern Univ, Chicago)
J Clin Endocrinol Metab 81:995–997, 1996   5–46

Background.—As individuals age, their growth hormone (GH) secretion and plasma insulin-like growth factor (I) levels decline. These changes may contribute to the age-related changes in body composition, including decreased lean body mass and increased adipose tissue mass. Growth hormone secretion begins to decline during the third decade of life, but changes in muscle mass and strength are not apparent until later. It could be that the action of GH in older adults is affected by age-related changes in GH receptor function. Plasma levels of GH binding protein (GHBP) are believed to indicate the level of GH receptor in tissues and thus an individual's responsiveness to GH. Patterns in GHBP level were investigated in 50 women and men.

Methods.—The study included normal adults—37 women and 13 men—ranging in age from 60 to 98 years. A standard GH-binding assay was performed to measure GHBP activity in plasma of all subjects.

Results.—Plasma GHBP activity declined progressively from age 60 years onward (Fig 1). The level of GHBP for study participants aged 60–65 years was about twice as high as that of participants in their 90s. This was in contrast to the previously reported stability of GHBP activity in adults aged 20–60 years (Fig 2). Plasma insulin-like growth factor-I was negatively correlated with age and positively correlated with GHBP (Fig 3).

Conclusions.—Beginning at age 60 years, plasma GHBP activity, and presumably GH receptor activity, declines progressively with age. Older adults may have GH resistance in addition to reduced GH secretion, which may add to their changes in body composition and frailty. For the oldest

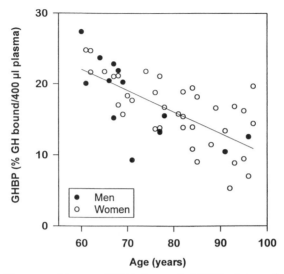

FIGURE 1.—Plasma growth hormone (*GH*) binding protein (*GHBP*) activity as a function of aging in individuals older than 60 years. The GH binding protein activity is defined as the percentage of GH bound to 400 μL plasma under standardized conditions. *Line* represents the regression line. There is a significant negative correlation between age and GHBP ($r = -0.688$; $P < 10^{-6}$). (Courtesy of Maheshwari H, Sharma L, Baumann G: Decline of plasma growth hormone binding protein in old age. *J Clin Endocrinol Metab* 81(3):995–997, 1996. Copyright The Endocrine Society.)

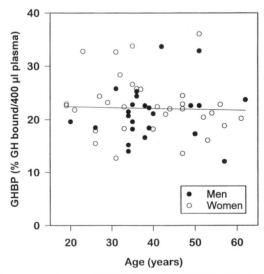

FIGURE 2.—Plasma growth hormone (*GH*) binding protein (*GHBP*) activity in younger adults, using the same assay method and symbols as in Figure 1. No significant correlation is present. This figure was redrawn using data reported in Mercado M, Carlsson L, Vitangcol R, et al: Growth hormone-binding protein determination in human plasma: A comparison of immunofunctional and growth hormone-binding assays: *J Clin Endocrinol Metab* 76:1291–1294, 1993. (Courtesy of Maheshwari H, Sharma L, Baumann G: Decline of plasma growth hormone binding protein in old age. *J Clin Endocrinol Metab* 81(3):995–997, 1996. Copyright The Endocrine Society.)

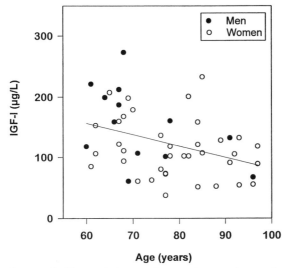

FIGURE 3.—Plasma insulin-like growth factor-I (*IGF-I*) as a function of aging in humans. Symbols as in Figure 1. The correlation is statistically significant ($r = -0.424$; $P < 0.001$). (Courtesy of Maheshwari H, Sharma L, Baumann G: Decline of plasma growth hormone binding protein in old age. *J Clin Endocrinol Metab* 81(3):995–997, 1996. Copyright The Endocrine Society.)

individuals, the combination of decreased GH production and GH resistance amounts to a particularly severe functional GH deficiency.

▶ Growth hormone binds to its receptors and thereby activates them, generating in the target cell the characteristic program we associate with GH. In addition to activating the receptors, binding of GH to its receptors stimulates the release of a portion of the receptor into the circulation. These pieces of the receptor found in the circulation are referred to as the plasma GHBP. Plasma levels of GHBP correlate positively with the level of GH action in a wide range of conditions. In essence, the level of GHBP reflects some end result of GH interactions with GH receptors. Thus, under conditions of known low GH, the GH binding protein levels are low, whereas in acromegaly the binding hormone levels are elevated.

The authors of this article have applied this approach to the problem of GH secretion and action in old age. With old age, the levels of insulin-like growth factor-I, thought to reflect in some cases GH action, are depressed. Similarly, the area under the curve of GH secretion, especially at night, is reduced as a function of increasing age. Is there a somatopause, that is, a physiologic GH deficiency similar to the estrogen deficiency of the menopause? Many studies are focused on trying to answer just this question through the administration of insulin-like growth factor-I, GH, or GH-releasing hormones. The finding in this study that the levels of GHBP in plasma decline in old age would suggest that GH interaction with its receptors in a physiologically meaningful way is reduced. Because the GHBP in plasma is relatively stable and not subject to the rapid fluctuations such as in GH and less subject to the physiologic decline as in insulin-like growth factor-1 raises this as an excellent marker worthy of exploration. Indeed, the decline in GHBP from ages 60 to 100 years appears to show a more straightforward relationship to age than does the decline in insulin-like growth factor-1. It also contrasts with the steady levels of GHBP found from ages 20 to 60 years. It will be interesting to see whether longitudinal measurements provide more information than the cross-section measurements described here. The authors interpret this as an example of GH resistance. I would see it more like the decreased levels of GHBP in GH deficiency.

The GH receptor belongs to a very large family of receptors including prolactin receptors as well as a wide range of cytokine and chemokine receptors. It may be that measuring the soluble forms of these receptors will turn out to be a very useful device for learning about actions of these and other related intercellular communication molecules in vivo; the levels of the cytokines in plasma may be very low and the major actions may be at the local level. Thus, the serum level of "binding protein" in some situations may be the best integrated measure of the biologically relevant interaction of hormone (or hormone-like molecule) with its receptor.

J. Roth, M.D.

Age-Related Changes in Amylin Secretion
Edwards BJ, Perry HM, Kaiser FE, et al (St Louis Univ, Mo; Ripley Med Clinic, Miss; Pfizer Inc, Groton, Conn)
Mech Ageing Dev 86:39–51, 1996   5–47

Background.—The pancreatic peptide amylin (islet amyloid polypeptide) has been shown in in vitro and in vivo studies to affect glucose metabolism. Glucose intolerance and diabetes mellitus become more frequent with aging. The amylin response to a glucose challenge was assessed in adult subjects of various ages.

Methods.—The cross-sectional study included 30 healthy, lean adults in 3 age groups: 20–40 years, 41–60 years, and 61–90 years. All underwent a standard 75-g oral glucose tolerance test, after which glucose, insulin, and amylin concentrations were measured.

Results.—The 3 groups were similar in terms of body mass index and body composition. The 2 younger groups were comparable in their glucose concentrations and insulin secretion values, whereas the older subjects had a slower increase in insulin secretion. There was no significant difference in amylin secretion by sex. Amylin secretion was greater in the young and old subjects compared with the middle-aged subjects, although the amylin concentration was slower to increase among the older subjects than among the young subjects. In each age group, the insulin to amylin ratio was variable, indicating that insulin and amylin were not cosecreted in a fixed ratio. Maximum amylin and increase in amylin were significantly associated with a glucose concentration of more than 120 mg/dL at 2 hours after glucose challenge.

Conclusions.—Amylin secretion in response to glucose challenge is greater in younger and older adults than in middle-aged adults. There is a correlation between glucose and amylin, which may indicate that amylin plays a counterregulatory role. Alternatively, amylin may simply reflect the age-related impairment of glucose metabolism. Further studies are needed to determine the role played by amylin in the hyperglycemia of aging.

▶ This article explores age-related aspects of the physiology of pancreatic islet amyloid polypeptide, an interesting protein in search of physiologic significance. Amylin, a 37–amino-acid peptide produced by the islet β cell shares 50% homology with the calcitonin gene-related peptide (CGRP), a non–β-cell peptide.[1] Amylin is deposited in pancreatic islets in patients with non–insulin-dependent diabetes mellitus, but apparently has little effect on islet function.[2] What is interesting are the multiple activities ascribed to this protein related to carbohydrate metabolism. In muscle, amylin opposes glycogen synthesis, activates glycogenolysis and glycolysis, and increases lactate output. However, in keeping with its relationship to calcitonin/CGRP, amylin has also been found to reduce serum calcium and increase renal excretion of calcium.[3] In this study, the secretion of amylin is followed after a standard glucose tolerance test in young, middle-aged, and older subjects. An effect of amylin on glucose homeostasis is suggested by relationship of both maximum amylin and increase in amylin and a glucose concentration of more than 120 mg/dL at 2 hours. Some questions are: Why do middle-aged subjects have lower amylin secretory response compared with younger and older individuals, and how this could relate to abnormal glucose metabolism? Could this be related to muscle mass? It remains to be decided whether amylin secretion regulates glucose metabolism or merely reflects impaired glucose metabolism with age. This requires additional study.

J.R. Shapiro, M.D.

References

1. Castillo MJ, Scheen AJ, Lefebvre PJ: Amylin/islet amyloid polypeptide: Biochemistry, physiology, patho-physiology. *Diabete et Metabolisme* 21:3–25, 1995.
2. Bennett WM, Smith DM, Bloom SR: Islet amyloid polypeptide: Does it play a pathophysiological role in the development of diabetes? *Diabetic Medicine* 11:825–829, 1994.
3. Miles PD, Deftos LJ, Moosa AR, et al: Islet amyloid polypeptide (amylin) increases the renal excretion of calcium in the conscious dog. *Calcif Tissue Int* 55:269–273, 1994.

Neurobiology of Aging

Circadian Locomotor Rhythms in Aged Hamsters Following Suprachiasmatic Transplant

Hurd MW, Zimmer KA, Lehman MN, et al (Univ of Toronto; Univ of Cincinnati, Ohio)
Am J Physiol 269:R958–R968, 1995   5–48

Objective.—Changes in sleep and activity are a common source of problems for older patients. In rodents, ablation of the suprachiasmatic nucleus (SCN), which is the location of a circadian pacemaker in mammals, will disrupt circadian rhythms. These rhythms can then be restored by fetal SCN grafts. In animals with only partial lesions of the SCN, simultaneous expression of the host and transplant donor rhythms can be observed. The changes that occur with partial SCN ablation are comparable to the age-related changes in activity rhythms occurring in humans, with shortened period, reduced amplitude, and fragmentation. The ability of fetal SCN grafts to restore rhythmicity in animals without experimental lesions was examined.

Methods and Results.—Cross-genotype fetal SCN tissue block grafts were placed in aged hamsters with intact SCNs. The transplanted fetal "clock" was shown to express itself in an aged animal with reduced amplitude or fragmented pattern of activity. In contrast, no such expression was noted in young animals receiving fetal SCN grafts or in aged animals receiving cortical tissue grafts. Three different patterns of expression were noted in aged animals receiving fetal SCN grafts: complete donor dominance of locomotor rhythms, relative coordination between the donor and host rhythms, and spontaneous switching between the 2 rhythms. In some cases, either of the 2 rhythms was expressed for a prolonged period.

Conclusions.—Fetal SCN grafts can restore circadian rhythmicity in aged rodents with intact SCNs. The pattern of rhythmicity expressed after grafting may vary with the relative amplitude or strength of signals produced by the native and transplanted SCNs. The donor SCN's influence on the host's behavior may occur through neural or humoral interactions at the postsynaptic target of the host SCN in the midline thalamus.

▶ For decades, brain transplants were so far-fetched that they became the subject of several genres of jokes. Now it is clear that brain tissue can be transplanted and may well substitute for the missing parts. Moreover, it is likely that residual host cells at the transplant site may give instructions to the transplant as to how to behave and what to do.

In this study, the authors turn to a long-standing problem of the elderly relating to changes in sleep and activity patterns associated with daily rhythms. Disruption of these daily rhythms is a common problem in elderly individuals. Experimentally, disruptions of the rhythms can be produced in rodents by ablation of the SCN, the site of a pacemaker in mammals. The authors show how the transplanted pacemaker may completely take over if there is no donor rhythm, but that when there is either an intact or a partially intact donor pacemaker, the graft interacts with the residual pacemaker to achieve some modus vivendi. Earlier studies showed that transplants would restore rhythms to animals with hypothalamic lesions that had lost their rhythms. When the lesion in the host animal is incomplete, it is possible to discern 2 distinct activity rhythms driven by 2 different pacemakers. Factors that determine whether the donor or the transplant rhythm will dominate are being studied further by the authors.

J. Roth, M.D.

For the Cortex, Neuron Loss May Be Less Than Thought
Wickelgren I (Brooklyn, NY)
Science 273:48–50, 1996   5–49

Introduction.—Although aging is associated with cognitive changes, these changes are selective and do not preclude normal functioning in healthy older individuals. It has long been assumed that these cognitive changes are caused by widespread cell death in the brain. However, recent studies have indicated that biological changes in healthy aging brains are more subtle.

Neuron Loss.—It was assumed that cortical neuron loss was an inevitable and irreversible process of aging. However, the discovery that a common method of preparing histologic specimens of brain tissue causes shrinkage of cortical tissue, particularly of young cortical tissue, raised the possibility that reduced cell density measures simply reflected this tissue shrinkage. In addition, the advanced methods recently developed for screening for brain pathologies have raised the possibility that brains with dementias may have inadvertently been included with normal brains, thus skewing the findings regarding cell death.

Age-Related Changes.—Animal studies and some human studies have revealed no correlations between cortical cell counts and age or between cortical cell counts and cognitive function in diverse areas, although patients with dementia do appear to have significant brain cell death. Imaging studies have provided evidence that myelin breakdown may be related to most changes associated with normal aging. In addition, an age-related decrease has been observed in the density of the N-methyl-D-aspartate receptor for the neurotransmitter glutamate, essential for learning and memory. The concentrations of both the receptor and the neurotransmitter may decline with age.

Conclusion.—The finding that cortical neurons may not be lost in normal aging opens the door for potential interventions to prevent subtle memory deficits, including drug therapy to compensate for deficiencies of neurotransmitters or of receptors or to prevent demyelinization.

▶ In this article, Ingrid Wickelgren reviews changing ideas about cell loss and the aging brain. Based on studies done in 1955, it was suggested that aging was associated with up to a 40% loss of neurons. Loss of mental capacity with aging was attributed to these losses in neurons.

In the past decade, several challenges to this concept have arisen. One is a methodological challenge suggesting that young brains shrink on fixation more than aged ones and, thereby, artifactually show a higher density of neurons than do the older ones. Another criticism was raised by Robert Terry at the University of California, San Diego, who suggested that the early studies did not distinguish elderly patients who had Alzheimer's disease or other serious degenerative diseases of the brain known to be associated with nerve cell loss; he suggested that when one eliminates the brains of those patients who are known to have degenerative disorders, nerve cell losses were not noted in brains from the aged. Another challenge is based on a study that showed that large neurons may become smaller with age rather than being lost, but give the appearance of a loss of cellularity.

Recent results from a collaborative study from several centers have shown that the entorhinal cortex and the superior temporal sulcus, 2 areas that have important roles in cognitive function, remain intact with aging yet undergo severe devastation with dementia.

Another recent challenge suggests that the loss in brain size with aging may be the result of a loss of white matter, i.e., of myelin. The loss of myelin could slow brain function as well as impair the health of the nerve cells without destroying them. A change in the density of the N-methyl-D-aspartate receptor for glutamate has also been noted. This receptor is thought to play an important role in establishing memory.

In summary, the idea that there is a massive loss of neurons with normal aging has been undermined by multiple findings including those that suggest that the nerve cells may undergo shrinkage without death and that this shrinkage may be associated with a decreased number of receptors or of neurotransmitters, and possibly even alterations in function. Restoring neurons that are below par to normal function is quite a different task than trying to replace neurons that have died. This provides new targets and optimism for both preventive and therapeutic approaches to the problem.

J. Roth, M.D.

Schwann Cell Apoptosis at Developing Neuromuscular Junctions Is Regulated by Glial Growth Factor
Trachtenberg JT, Thompson WJ (Univ of Texas, Austin)
Nature 379:174–177, 1996   5–50

Objective.—Reinnervation of denervated muscle fibers in adults occurs through axonal regeneration, whereas reinnervation of partially denervated muscle occurs through sprouts from intact axons. Recent studies suggest that the induction and guidance of axonal outgrowth in muscle reinnervation is regulated by Schwann cells (SCs). Compared with adult muscle, neonatal muscle shows deficient reinnervation of muscle after denervation. The responses of SCs to denervation in neonatal muscles were examined in rats.

Findings.—The terminal SCs of hind limb rat muscles were observed using polyclonal antibodies against the glial antigen S100. When the muscles were denervated in the early postnatal period, SCs rapidly disappeared from the developing neuromuscular junction. Further studies suggested that apoptosis, programed cell death, was responsible for the disappearance of the SCs. Apoptosis of SCs in response to denervation decreased with increasing age. When glial growth factor (a neuregulin trophic factor found in developing sensory and motor neurons) was injected in vivo, SC apoptosis was prevented.

Conclusions.—Schwann cells seem to play a key role in regulating nerve growth. Denervation of neonatal muscle results in apoptosis of SCs, which may explain the deficient reinnervation and axonal sprouting in newborns; a glial growth factor can prevent this apoptosis. Trophic interactions between the axon and SCs seem to influence the normal development of the neuromuscular system.

▶ It is becoming increasingly clear that cells have 2 sets of choices that partially overlap: to divide or not to divide, and to die an apoptotic death or to live. These decisions seem to be highly influenced by humoral factors, released by the cell itself or by its neighbors, interacting with specific receptors on the target cell. In this study, the SCs played a key role in helping nerves regrow. In neonates, the SCs undergo apoptotic death, which can be overcome by providing a glial growth factor. Increasingly, physiology and pathophysiology will be defined in terms of these autocrine and paracrine kinds of systems.

J. Roth, M.D.

Cellular and Molecular Biology

The Transmembrane Form of Tumor Necrosis Factor Is the Prime Activating Ligand of the 80 kDa Tumor Necrosis Factor Receptor

Grell M, Douni E, Wajant H, et al (Univ of Stuttgart, Federal Republic of Germany; Hellenic Pasteur Inst, Athens, Greece; Hoffmann–La Roche Limited, Basel, Switzerland; et al)

Cell 83:793–802, 1995   5–51

Introduction.—Tumor necrosis factor (TNF) is an important mediator of inflammatory, immunologic, and pathophysiologic reactions. There are 2 separate species of TNF, a 26-kd membrane-expressed form (mTNF) and a soluble 17-kd cytokine (sTNF). There also are 2 distinct membrane receptors ($TNFR_{60}$, with a molecular weight of 60 kd; and $TNFR_{80}$, with a molecular weight of 80 kd). Tumor necrosis factor receptor$_{60}$ appears to be the main signal transducer of TNF-induced cellular responses, but the signal capacity and functional role of $TNFR_{80}$ are unknown. New findings regarding the functional significance of $TNFR_{80}$ were reported.

Findings.—Experiments in several different systems, including T-cell activation, thymocyte proliferation, and granulocyte/macrophage colony-stimulating factor production, showed that mTNF is superior to sTNF in activating the $TNFR_{80}$ receptor. The $TNFR_{60}$ receptor also is signaled by mTNF, and the cooperativity between these receptors brings much stronger cellular responses than possible with sTNF alone. There also was evidence that mTNF activation of $TNFR_{80}$ led to completely different TNF responses, for example, making tumor cells that had been resistant to the cytotoxic activity of sTNF sensitive to mTNF-mediated toxicity.

Conclusions.—Tumor necrosis factor receptor$_{80}$ responds differently to the 2 forms of TNF. The major physiologic activator of $TNFR_{80}$ appears to be mTNF, not sTNF. The local response of tissues reactive to external stimuli appears to be controlled by $TNFR_{80}$, which may therefore play a key physiologic role in local inflammatory responses.

▶ Typically, when we think of signaling agents, we think of a soluble signal molecule released from a cell traveling to another cell and there interacting with cell surface receptors as the initiating event in the cellular response. In this article, the authors show that a form of TNF, instead of being soluble in the medium, is actually held in the membrane by a transmembrane segment; the activation of the receptor occurs as a cell membrane–cell membrane interaction. As noted in Abstract 5–35, we are increasingly recognizing these complementary molecules on the surface of 2 different cells that participate in an active cellular communication process.

J. Roth, M.D.

YY1 and Sp1 Transcription Factors Bind the Human Transferrin Gene in an Age-Related Manner
Adrian GS, Seto E, Fischbach KS, et al (Univ of Texas, San Antonio)
J Gerontol 51A:B66–B75, 1996   5–52

Introduction.—Transferrin (TF) is an iron-binding protein that plays many important roles in managing the body's iron supply. Serum TF concentrations decrease with age, which probably has adverse effects for elderly individuals. The aging regulation of human TF in transgenic mice carrying chimeric human TF-chloramphenicol acetyltransferase (TF-CAT) transgenes were studied. These animals show decreased liver expression of TF transgenes with age, the result of decreased gene transcription. The expression of the human TF-CAT transgene and its regulation during aging were described.

Findings.—Electrophoretic mobility shift assays and antibody-recognition studies were done in transgenic mice. The results showed that the 5' regulatory elements of the human TF gene were bound by 3 YY1 proteins (Y1, YY1-a, and YY1-b) and an Sp1-like transcription factor. As the mice aged, their YY1-a and YY1-b activities increased and their Sp1-like binding activity decreased. No age-related change in the binding activity of YY1 was apparent.

Conclusions.—The human TF gene has previously unrecognized binding sites for YY1 and Sp1 transcription factors, which show age-related differences in their binding activities. Sp1 is a positive transcription factor, and YY1 can act as a negative one. Thus, the age-related changes in their activities could be responsible for decreased transcription of the human TF transgene, and for the age-related decline in serum TF concentrations.

▶ Iron plays a vital role not only in erythropoiesis, but also in growth of all cells. Transferrin is important for in vivo management of iron. It has an antioxidant role because it has a high affinity for ferric ions, which, when free, promote oxidative damage of proteins and other macromolecules. Iron bound to transferrin is used for red blood cell formation. Elderly individuals commonly have a reduced serum concentration of transferrin. The authors try to define what nuclear factors may be leading to this diminished level of transferrin.

The expression of any given gene is highly regulated in both positive and negative ways by proteins that bind upstream of the DNA that codes for the protein. To study these proteins, it is common to create a chimeric gene; the region immediately upstream of the gene of interest (all by itself, without the portion that codes for the protein) is linked instead to a reporter gene, whose product is easy to measure. In this study, the authors chose the gene for the bacterial enzyme CAT, which ordinarily is absent in mammals, and used CAT expression as a first approximation of what the normal gene does when it is linked to its upstream regulatory region. This artificial gene (the immediate upstream region of the human transferrin gene linked to the coding region of the CAT gene), when placed permanently into the genome of mice, is expressed and its expression changes in an age-related fashion. With aging, the binding of negative response factors increases and the binding of positive stimulatory factors diminishes, which provides a clue to what may be driving the age-related decrement in expression of this gene in humans. This model in the mouse now provides an opportunity to go back to the humans to determine if indeed these mechanisms, discovered in mice, contribute substantially to the age-related change in humans.

J. Roth, M.D.

Requirement of an ICE-Like Protease for Induction of Apoptosis and Ceramide Generation by REAPER
Pronk GJ, Ramer K, Amiri P, et al (Chiron Corp, Emeryville, Calif; Univ of California, San Francisco)
Science 271:808–810, 1996 5–53

Purpose.—Previous genetic studies of *Drosophila melanogaster* embryos suggest that the 65–amino-acid REAPER (RPR) protein governs apoptosis during embryonic development. Although the mechanisms underlying cell death caused by RPR are unknown, it has some homology to the death domains of Fas and tumor necrosis factor-α (TNF-α), which are involved in apoptosis in mammals. Cell lines in which RPR expression and RPR-mediated cell death could be induced were studied to determine whether RPR uses cellular components similar to those used by the transmembrane receptors for Fas ligand and TNF-α.

Findings.—When RPR expression was induced in *Drosophila* Schneider cells, apoptosis followed rapidly. This apoptotic effect was blocked by the peptide N-benzyloxycarbonyl-Val-Ala-Asp-fluoromethylketone (Z-VAD-fmk). Thus, some interleukin-1β converting enzyme (ICE)-like protein seemed to be needed for RPR to function. As RPR-induced apoptosis occurred, ceramide production increased. This effect was also blocked by Z-VAD-fmk, suggesting that an ICE-like protease was also required for ceramide generation.

Conclusions.—The apoptotic signaling pathways used by RPR, an intracellular protein in *Drosophila*, are similar to those used by the transmembrane receptors Fas and tumor necrosis factor receptor type 1 in vertebrates. The induction of apoptosis by RPR and the accompanying increase in ceramide both appear to depend on ICE-like proteases. The findings suggest that, from an evolutionary standpoint, the biochemical pathways leading to apoptosis are highly conserved among species and among the different factors initiating apoptosis.

▶ Genetic studies have implicated RPR protein as having an important role in carrying out programmed cell death (apoptosis). An ICE-like protease is required for RPR to function and for the generation of ceramide, which is believed to be a second messenger in the pathway by which 2 vertebrate transmembrane receptors, *Fas* and TNFR-I, carry out their apoptosis. The remarkable similarity between the fruit fly (*Drosophila*) and worm (*Caenorhabditis*) pathways for apoptosis with those of humans have made them extraordinarily powerful tools in uncovering the human system by genetic techniques.

J. Roth, M.D.

6 Geriatric Nursing

Introduction

The research base that underlies the practice of geriatric nursing continues to grow. The articles in this chapter have been chosen to address issues that nurses face regardless of practice setting, as well as those specific to the long-term care setting. For example, research on triggers of myocardial ischemia (Abstract 6–1), a meta-analysis of the effectiveness of weight-loss strategies for type II diabetes (Abstract 6–2), and a qualitative study of Parkinson's disease (Abstract 6–3), provide information that geriatric nurses can use in developing interventions with the subpopulations with these conditions regardless of setting.

Also included are research articles in which the relationship between nursing interventions and patient outcomes are explored. Much of this work is new and will require further monitoring. One example is the report of an interdisciplinary home hospitalization program for older adults (Abstract 6–9).

Geriatric nurses, regardless of setting, work closely with caregivers as well as patients. Qualitative research provides insight into the caregiving experience. Nurses often have a central role in helping patients and caregivers make treatment decisions for themselves and their relatives. Research articles that can assist nurses to more effectively work with patients and family members who find themselves confronted with difficult treatment decisions are included.

Articles in the final section of this chapter provide promising insights and potential interventions for those who provide nursing care to the frail elderly population in long-term care settings. These articles address issues such as pressure ulcers (Abstract 6–14), restraints and falls (Abstract 6–15), and disruptive behaviors (Abstracts 6–16 and 6–18). The pilot work about the use of behavioral interventions to promote functional feeding (Abstract 6–17) and bathing (Abstract 6–18) in patients with behavioral disturbances looks especially promising. The long-term care staff's job morale and functioning are discussed in the final article in this section (Abstract 6–19). It is important to note that it was the system stressors and work climate, not the patient care demands, that had a negative impact on staff.

Sharon K. Ostwald, Ph.D., R.N., C.S.

Diseases With New Interventions for Nursing

Triggers of Myocardial Ischemia During Daily Life in Patients With Coronary Artery Disease: Physical and Mental Activities, Anger and Smoking
Gabbay FH, Krantz DS, Kop WJ, et al (Univ of the Health Sciences, Bethesda, Md; Cedars-Sinai Med Ctr, Los Angeles; Georgetown Univ, Washington, DC; et al)
J Am Coll Cardiol 27:585–592, 1996   6–1

Introduction.—In patients with coronary artery disease, transient myocardial ischemia occurs during many activities, not just during strenuous exercise. Studies have shown that cold, mental stress, anger, and cigarette smoking can trigger myocardial ischemia. Few studies have investigated the effect of emotional states or mental stress on ischemia during daily life. To determine the potency of physical activity, mental activity, emotional states, and cigarette smoking as triggers of ischemia, a study was done in patients with coronary artery disease.

Methods.—Sixty-three patients with coronary artery disease who were between 43 and 77 years of age kept a validated structured diary of physical and mental activities and moods. All patients underwent ECG monitoring. Physical and mental activities were evaluated and classified according to 5 levels of intensity.

Results.—Ischemia occurred most often during physical and mental activities that were moderately intense. Most of the patients' time was spent doing physical and mental activities of low intensity, but the risk of ischemia was the highest during intense physical activities and stressful mental activities. The amount of time in ischemia was higher for physical and mental activities of high intensity. The amount of time in ischemia was 5% for high-intensity activities and 0.2% for low-intensity activities. Strenuous physical activity and intense anger were strong ischemia triggers. At the onset of ischemia, heart rates increased with the intensity of the activity or mental state. Among patients who smoked, the risk of ischemia was more than 5 times higher when the patients were actually smoking. Coffee and alcohol consumption also were associated with ischemia, but after controlling for concurrent cigarette smoking, this relation disappeared.

Conclusions.—During daily life, ischemia can be triggered in patients with coronary artery disease by activities of high and low intensity. Anger and smoking are strong triggers of ischemia. Mental activities are as strong as physical activities in triggering ischemia. Coffee and alcohol consumption are associated with ischemia only when associated with smoking. The diary system used in this investigation was previously validated in a series of studies. However, this method still relies on patient self-report.

▶ These authors contribute to our understanding of the triggers of myocardial ischemia in the daily life of individuals with coronary artery disease. Of particular interest is the extent to which anger triggers ischemia. Although laboratory studies have shown a relation between mental and emotional stress and myocardial ischemia, the extent to which this occurs in daily life has not previously been well characterized. This study shows that mental distress, such as intense anger, is as potent an ischemic trigger as strenuous exercise. Other studies have implied that stress-induced ischemia may be associated with poor prognosis,[1] suggesting the importance of identifying those individuals who are particularly reactive and instituting interventions. Nonpharmacologic behavioral interventions, such as biofeedback and relaxation, may prove to be important adjunctive therapy to pharmacologic treatments.

S.K. Ostwald, Ph.D., R.N.

Reference

1. Jain D, Burg M, Souter R, et al: Prognostic implication of mental stress-induced silent left ventricular dysfunction in patients with stable angina pectoris. *Am J Cardiol* 76:31–35, 1995.

Promoting Weight Loss in Type II Diabetes
Brown SA, Winter M, Upchurch S, et al (Univ of Texas, Austin; Univ of Texas, Houston; Audie L Murphy Mem Veterans Hosp, San Antonio, Tex)
Diabetes Care 19:613–624, 1996   6–2

Background.—Obesity is common among people with type II diabetes, and weight loss is among the most important and challenging management goals. To determine the relative efficacy of different strategies to promote weight loss in individuals with type II diabetes, a meta-analysis of the applicable research was performed.

Methods.—A literature search was conducted to identify both published and unpublished data related to weight loss promotion in patients with type II diabetes. Bibliographies; MEDLINE and other databases; theses created by persons seeking master degrees in nursing, public health, and nutrition; and the Center for Disease Control were among those resources searched. Specific inclusion criteria included the participation of the patients in various weight loss strategies and that outcomes of the studies were measured by weight loss. The search yielded 89 studies involving 1,800 patients that met the inclusion criteria. Based on data distribution, the ages of these patients were divided into those younger than 55 years and those older than 55 years. The features from each of these studies, including methodology, sample size, and research quality, were then coded on forms created for this purpose. There were 80 variables and 23 outcomes that were defined in a detailed coding book. Effect sizes were calculated for each weight loss strategy and each outcome variable.

Results.—With the exception of surgery, dietary strategies alone, which resulted in an average reduction of 20 lb, produced the greatest changes in body weight. However, statistically significant weight reduction occurred

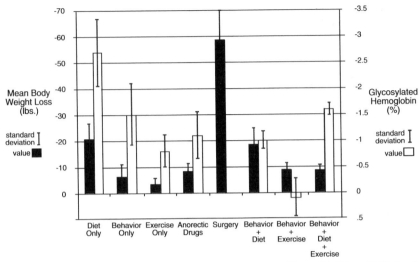

FIGURE 1.—Major outcomes of intervention strategies. (Courtesy of Brown SA, Winter M, Upchurch S, et al: Promoting weight loss in type II diabetes. *Diabetes Care* 19:613–624, 1996.)

with all interventions (Fig 1). Either diet alone or the combination of behavioral therapies, diet, and exercise resulted in the largest decreases in glycosylated hemoglobin. Surgery and diet alone produced the greatest decreases in fasting blood sugar levels. Dietary interventions also had the greatest effect on total cholesterol and triglyceride levels. The effects of dietary intervention alone remained stable for at least 6 months, whereas the effects of behavioral therapy diminished over time and other strategies had little short-term effects. With regard to age, effects of weight loss–promoting interventions were higher for those patients who were younger than 55 years of age, except for the effects of behavioral therapy on mean body weight and glycosylated hemoglobin levels. The effects of diet alone were twice as high in the younger patient group than in the older patient group. A large improvement in body mass index was noted in patients older than 55 years of age.

Conclusions.—The most effective strategies other than surgery to promote weight loss in patients with type II diabetes were diet interventions, although all interventions had some impact. Diet interventions also had the most prolonged effect.

▶ The treatment of type II diabetes remains a major challenge for health care professionals. Because at least 80% of patients with type II diabetes are obese, weight loss strategies constitute an important approach to long-term management. This article offers an excellent, comprehensive meta-analysis of the literature in this area. The authors' findings that dietary strategies alone are the most effective for promoting weight loss and that the effects are 2-fold higher in patients younger than age 55 than in those 55 years and older are very interesting. The article raises many questions regarding the role of current therapeutic approaches, such as American Dietetic Association dietary restrictions, behavioral therapy, surgery, and anorectic drugs.

S.K. Ostwald, Ph.D., R.N.

Day-to-Day Demands of Parkinson's Disease
Habermann B (Univ of San Francisco)
West J Nurs Res 18(4):397–413, 1996   6–3

Introduction.—Most studies on Parkinson's disease have concentrated on depression, psychological adjustment to the disease in the elderly, and variables that predict psychological adaptation. There is little information on this disease from the perspective of the individual. To describe the demands of daily living experienced by middle-aged individuals with Parkinson's disease, interviews were conducted and research was done.

Procedure.—Three interviews were conducted during a 3-month period with 16 individuals with Parkinson's disease. The patients were between 42 and 59 years of age; 9 were men. The severity of disease ranged from stage 1 to stage 3 using the Hoehn and Yahr modified staging. The transcribed interviews were interpreted using thematic analysis, analysis of exemplars, and search for paradigm cases. Various strategies were used to ensure the credibility of the research. The demands of Parkinson's disease mentioned by participants included acknowledging symptoms, seeking medical help, dealing with emotional responses and a changing body, gaining formal and practical knowledge, and dealing with unpredictability.

Acknowledging Initial Symptoms and Seeking Help.—Initial symptoms mentioned by participants varied from handwriting cramping, toes curling, difficulty getting toothpaste out of the tube, and changes in stride while running. Many individuals encountered physicians who negated these experiences and suggested that they were insignificant. Many did not get the attention of their physicians until their symptoms had worsened, and by this time the patients were concerned about brain tumors or strokes.

Dealing With Emotional Responses and a Changing Body.—Although some participants expressed relief that they had Parkinson's disease, they still felt anger and denial, especially because they had a disease that normally affected much older people. They spoke of having to think about movements that were once automatic and prereflective. They had to remind themselves how to do the simplest things, like waving goodbye or scrambling an egg. Many began to think of their bodies as uncooperative.

Gaining Knowledge.—These individuals wanted to know more about Parkinson's disease, but their physicians gave them little information, spent little time with them, and ignored issues of self-care and day-to-day coping. Although the participants read as much information as they could about Parkinson's disease, they also realized that their own experiences could tell them what was best for themselves. Learning about medication dosing, their responses to medication, and the effects of diet and activities on medication and daily functioning was a process common to all.

Dealing With Unpredictability.—The unpredictability of how they would function at any given moment became a day-to-day and a long-term demand for these individuals. They used various strategies to compensate for this unpredictability, but the control they had was limited. Because of the uncertainty of their futures, these participants focused on the present and planned minimally for the future.

Discussion.—To improve our understanding and management of Parkinson's disease and other chronic illnesses, we must understand the range of demands that individuals face every day and what it is like to experience the illness. These participants reported a lack of caring and nurturing practices and a glaring lack of acknowledgment of their concerns by health care professionals. There has been limited chronic illness research specific to Parkinson's disease.

▶ This qualitative study, which explores the meaning of having Parkinson's disease from the perspective of the individual, broadens our understanding of what it is like to have a chronic, degenerative, and progressive illness. Habermann skillfully illustrates, through the words of individuals with Parkinson's disease, the complexity and range of demands that persons with the disease face on a daily basis. These demands include acknowledging symptoms and seeking help; balancing emotional responses; dealing with a changing body; gaining formal and practical knowledge; and dealing with unpredictability, changing roles, sense of identity, and relationships. Understanding these demands is the basis on which interventions are built, and this can truly assist individuals with Parkinson's disease, or any other chronic disease, in coping with their chronic illness on a daily basis.

S.K. Ostwald, Ph.D., R.N.

The Relationship of Hospital Process Variables to Patient Outcome Post-Myocardial Infarction
Proctor TF, Yarcheski A, Oriscello RG (Elizabeth Gen Med Ctr, New Jersey; State Univ of New Jersey, Newark)
Int J Nurs Stud 33(2):121–130, 1996 6–4

Introduction.—One recent outcomes study found that age was the only significant predictor of patient outcome after myocardial infarction (MI), not stage of illness, comorbidity, complications, or intensity of treatment. More research is needed to identify other predictors of patient outcome after MI. The conceptual model of Donabedian provides a rationale for linking hospital process variables to patient outcome variables. Previous meta-analyses have found that nursing and medical care and the information provided to patients have significant effects on patient outcomes, particularly nursing care. The effects of hospital environment on outcomes have been less well investigated, although this environment has been found to affect certain physiologic and psychologic outcomes. The impact of these hospital process variables, as rated by patients, on patient outcomes after MI were evaluated.

Methods.—Sixty-eight adult patients with MI (49 men and 19 women; mean age, 62 years; 60% Caucasian) were studied at the time of hospital discharge. The 4 hospital process variables were assessed using the Patient Judgment of Hospital Quality Questionnaire. The patients' knowledge and their clinical, psychologic, and functional status at discharge were assessed with the Revised Haussman and Hegyvary Outcome Criteria Instrument for Acute Myocardial Infarction. This outcome measure provided information about the subscales of general health status; rest and sleep; activities of daily living; knowledge of general health, medication, activity, and nutrition; and anxiety.

Results.—Pearson correlations between the hospital process variables and the patient outcome measure found that patient outcomes were significantly and positively correlated with nursing care and hospital environment. Medical care and information provided during hospitalization had no significant effect on outcome. On stepwise multiple regression analysis, nursing care was the only significant predictor of patient outcome at discharge; it explained 16% of the variance. Nursing care was significantly correlated with all 3 of the other hospital process variables. On further analysis, patient outcome was significantly related to education and occupation but not to age, sex, stage of MI, or comorbidity.

Conclusions.—Nursing care is the only hospital process variable that is a significant predictor of patient outcome after MI. Both nursing care and hospital environment are positively correlated with patient outcome, which is consistent with Donabedian's conceptual model that suggests a link between process and outcome variables. At a time when patient outcomes research is increasingly important, there is a need for more explanatory theory regarding those outcomes.

▶ Much of the literature about patient outcomes has focused almost exclusively on medical interventions and patient satisfaction with their health status. This article is of interest because it explores the relationship among patients' outcomes after myocardial infarction and their evaluation of 4 hospital process variables: nursing care, medical care, information, and hospital environment. The finding that patient perception of nursing care was the only process variable that was a predictor of patient outcome at the time of discharge suggests that more attention needs to be given to the effect of nurses' skill, competence, and caring on patient outcomes.

S.K. Ostwald, Ph.D., R.N.

The Effects of a Discharge Information Intervention on Recovery Outcomes Following Coronary Artery Bypass Surgery

Moore SM (Case Western Reserve Univ, Cleveland, Ohio)
Int J Nurs Stud 33:181–189, 1996   6–5

Background.—The small amount of research done on the effectiveness of discharge information on recovery after coronary artery bypass surgery (CABG) has focused on compliance with coronary risk-reduction behaviors. However, the postoperative physical and psychological functioning of the patient are also important, but unstudied, aspects of CABG recovery, particularly with the increasing number of patients who are discharged early. The efficacy of an audiotaped discharge intervention with respect to physical function and psychological distress was evaluated in patients recovering from CABG.

Methods.—Eighty-two patients undergoing their first CABG surgery were assigned to either the experimental group, which received the intervention plus standard discharge information, or the comparison group, which received only standard discharge information. The intervention consisted of a 15-minute audiotape that described typical recovery experiences in sensory terms, the duration and sequence of such events, and coping strategies. One month after surgery, the patients were interviewed to assess psychological distress with the Profile of Mood States and physical function with the Sickness Impact Profile.

Results.—The 2 groups were similar in age, the number of grafts, preoperative cardiac functional status, and employment status, but had significant differences in sex, length of hospital stay, and education. The patients in the intervention group reported that the information was accurate in describing their experiences and helpful. This group had significantly better physical functioning than the comparison group at 1 month postoperatively, but did not differ from the comparison group in psychological functioning. Physical functioning correlated significantly with age and the length of hospital stay. However, the intervention effect remained significant after controlling for these factors.

Conclusions.—The addition of specific sensory information and coping instructions to discharge information can enhance physical functioning in patients recovering from CABG. The lack of psychological effect raises questions about the timing of the assessment and the processes through which information reduces stress.

▶ This article presents an innovative, inexpensive way to provide discharge information to patients after CABG. The author used the theory of self-regulation as the basis for the development of a 15-minute audiotape that included information about expected experiences during recovery from CABG and instructions for coping with those experiences. The audiotape intervention produced positive effects on physical function at 1 month compared to results in patients who received the usual cardiac discharge information. This type of intervention may be especially helpful for elderly patients who are discharged from the hospital or undergo special treatments for a wide variety of problems. Hagopian reports success with audiotapes that increase self-care behaviors among individuals who are undergoing radiation therapy.[1] These audiotapes, like those of Moore, cover side effects that patients may experience and suggested self-care activities to relieve them. This low-cost intervention may provide more accurate information in a timely way because it allows patients to pace themselves and repeat topics of particular interest to them. Audiotaped information also has a special benefit for patients who have difficulties with literacy or vision, not uncommon problems among the elderly population.

S.K. Ostwald, Ph.D., R.N.

Reference

1. Hagopian GA: The effects of informational audiotapes on knowledge and self-care behaviors of patients undergoing radiation therapy. *Oncol Nurs Forum* 25:697–700, 1996.

Caregiving and Dementia: The Impact of Telephone Helpline Services
Coyne AC, Potenza M, Nose MAB (COPSA Inst for Alzheimer's Disease and Related Disorders, Piscataway, NJ; Univ of Medicine and Dentistry of New Jersey, Piscataway)
Am J Alzheimer's Dis July/Aug:27–32, 1995   6–6

Background.—Dementia substantially affects the functioning of patients and family caregivers. Although social and psychological interventions have been shown to have a significant potential for benefit for both patients and caregivers, these resources are underutilized. The single largest determinant of service underutilization is knowledge and awareness of programs. The relationship between contact with a telephone helpline and utilization rates and caregiver burden and depression was assessed.

Methods.—Ninety-eight caregivers for patients with dementia who called a helpline were mailed a questionnaire measuring resource use, burden, and depression. The subjects were randomly assigned to 2 groups: a control group that received standard helpline services during the single initial call, and an experimental group that received biweekly follow-up calls from the staff during a period of 8 weeks. After the 8-week study period, the subjects were mailed another questionnaire.

Results.—Fifty-one caregivers completed and returned both questionnaires, including 23 in the experimental group and 28 in the control group. Resource use increased over time in both groups, but increased more dramatically in the experimental group. The burden score decreased during the study period in the experimental group and increased in the control group (Fig 2). There were no significant changes in depression scores over time in either group.

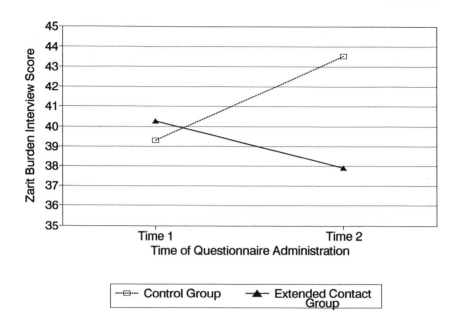

FIGURE 2.—Mean Zarit Burden Interview score as a function of group (control vs. extended contact) and time of questionnaire administration. (Courtesy of Coyne AC, Potenza M, Nose MAB: Caregiving and dementia: The impact of telephone helpline services. *Am J Alzheimer's Dis* July/Aug:27–32, 1995.)

Conclusion.—Sustained contact with a telephone helpline specializing in dementia can increase resource utilization and reduce psychological burden for family caregivers of patients with dementia.

▶ It is somewhat surprising that a biweekly telephone call during an 8-week period could have such a favorable impact on caregiver burden. This article reports the effectiveness of a telephone helpline providing information, referral, education, and counseling to caregivers of persons with dementia. Caregivers who received biweekly telephone calls from helpline personnel demonstrated greater use of community resources and less burden than caregivers who had only one contact with the helpline. This intervention has the potential for wide implementation by chapters of the Alzheimer's Association who have helplines in place or as a low-cost service that is offered as an important part of a network of services provided by HMOs to families of enrollees with dementia.

S.K. Ostwald, Ph.D., R.N.

From Research to Practice: The Effects of the Jointly Sponsored Dissemination of an Arthritis Self-Care Nursing Intervention

Goeppinger J, Macnee C, Anderson MK, et al (Univ of North Carolina, Chapel Hill; East Tennessee State Univ, Johnson City; Univ of Zimbabwe, Harare; et al)

Appl Nurs Res 8(3):106–113, 1995   6–7

Objective.—For patients with arthritis and other chronic diseases, self-care is both supplementary and complementary to the care delivered by health care professionals. Community-based nursing interventions that are of proven effectiveness in enhancing self-care among diverse groups of people with arthritis are needed. Previous reports have described the "Bone Up On Arthritis" (BUOA) program, a community-based, self-care nursing intervention for arthritis, including a randomized study documenting its effectiveness. However, the costs of finding community leaders to perform the intervention were prohibitively high. Also, the good results were obtained in a relatively homogeneous sample of older, rural white women with osteoarthritis. This study sought to determine whether the program could be effectively delivered by volunteers in a sample that differed in demographic and disease characteristics.

Methods.—The sample included 154 patients with various kinds of arthritis identified at 4 different chapters of the Arthritis Foundation. Compared with previous studies, the sample included more variety in types of arthritis, more ethnic groups, a broader age range, and men as well as women. Volunteer resource people were trained to implement the BUOA program in its home study format. The content of the self-care lessons, presented in audiotapes and booklets, included exercise, joint protection, depression, medications, nutrition, and more. The patient outcome measures, which included self-care behavior, helplessness, pain, dysfunction, and depression, were assessed by questionnaire before and after the BUOA intervention.

Results.—All of the measured outcomes improved significantly after the intervention. Clinically significant improvements were noted in helpless-

TABLE 3.—Participant Changes in The 4-Sites Study (*n* = 154)

Variable/Measure	Pretest M	Posttest M	Difference	Paired *t* (P)
Self-care behavior (Self-Care Behaviors Inventory)	49.97	57.17	7.20	3.02 (2)*
Helplessness (Arthritis Helplessness Index)	35.50	34.13	−1.37	−3.99 (2)†
Pain (Pain Index)	22.56	20.88	−1.68	−3.93 (2)*
Dysfunction (Disability Scale, Health Assessment Questionnaire)	1.34	1.27	−0.08	−2.41 (2)*
Depression (Center for Epidemiologic Studies Depression Scale)	18.31	15.19	−3.12	−4.64 (2)†

*P ≤ .03.
†P = .000.

(Courtesy of Goeppinger J, Macnee C, Anderson MK, et al: From research to practice: The effects of the jointly sponsored dissemination of an arthritis self-care nursing intervention. *Appl Nurs Res* 8(3):106–113, 1995.)

ness, pain, and especially depression (Table 3). The improvements were similar to those achieved in the original sample, after statistical control for differences in age and initial level of depression.

Conclusion.—The BUOA arthritis self-care intervention is effective even when delivered by community volunteers and in groups different from those for which it was originally intended. With this flexible program, volunteers can effectively complement professional resources in a cost-effective manner. The program is acceptable to people with arthritis, although more work is needed to improve its acceptability in rural populations, particularly those of native American and Hispanic-American backgrounds.

▶ This article is important because it demonstrates that an educational nursing intervention to improve self-care in persons with arthritis can be disseminated in other locations through local volunteer organizations, while maintaining the positive results demonstrated by researchers in a randomized trial of the intervention. The cost of using health care professionals to deliver community-based interventions that have been shown to be effective can be prohibitive and hinder the dissemination of important interventions that promote healthy living among elderly populations and those with chronic diseases. This study demonstrates that self-care nursing interventions were effective when offered by community volunteers and suggests that trained and motivated volunteers from agencies such as the Arthritis Foundation can extend and complement professional nursing resources in a cost-effective manner.

S.K. Ostwald, Ph.D., R.N.

Multidisciplinary Team Intervention

Controlled Trial of a Geriatric Case-Finding and Liaison Service in an Emergency Department

Miller DK, Lewis LM, Nork MJ, et al (St Louis Univ, Mo)

J Am Geriatr Soc 44:513–520, 1996   6–8

Background.—A visit to the emergency department (ED) may be considered a sentinel event in a geriatric patient. Previous studies have demonstrated the positive impact of comprehensive geriatric assessment programs in other settings. Therefore, a comprehensive geriatric assessment program was developed for the ED and its effects were evaluated, particularly with regard to the frequency of geriatric problems in older patients visiting the ED, the cost-effectiveness of the program, and the effects of the intervention on outcomes.

Methods.—For an 11-month period, geriatric assessments were offered to elderly patients on alternate days. Using a structured schedule, the nurse assessed patients for functional status, severity of illness, delirium, dementia, depression, nutritional status, visual and hearing deficits, incontinence, and the patient's perceived need for dental care and social services. The evaluation was summarized for consultation with the ED staff, after which suggestions were made for resources, and assistance in arranging appointments was offered. Each evaluated patient was matched by sex and age to a control patient seen within the same week. Experimental and control patients were called 3 months later to determine health status and utilization of suggested services. The cost of identifying particular geriatric problems was determined.

Results.—Geriatric assessments were complete for 385 patients and revealed a high prevalence of daily living dependency, poor nutrition, visual and hearing deficits, incontinence, and the need for dental or social services, with a moderate prevalence of affective disorders, a 6% to 21% prevalence of delirium, and a 10% prevalence of dementia. Dementia was the most difficult and, therefore, most expensive problem to identify, followed by delirium and affective disorders. Dental and social problems were most prevalent (77%) and least expensive to identify, requiring only approximately $1 to $5 per problem to identify (Table 2). Compliance

TABLE 2.—Prevalence of Identified Geriatric Problems and Efficiency of Case Identification Among 385 Evaluated Intervention Subjects

Problem	Estimated Minutes Per Evaluation	Identified/Total (%)	Cost per Problem Identified
Geriatric medical needs			
Functional status			
≥1 Basic ADL dependency	1.5	94/385 (24.4)	$ 2.54
≥3 Intermediate ADL dependencies	1.5	208/385 (54.0)	1.15
Delirium			
Definite		2/374 (5.6)	44.13
Probable		17/374 (4.5)	24.39*
Possible		42/374 (11.2)	11.58*
Dementia (given no delirium)	9	23/260 (8.5)	42.02
Depression	5		
Major (GDS ≥ 15)		20/268 (7.5)	27.67
Minor or other affective problem (GDS 1–14)		18/268 (6.7)	14.56*
Undernutrition/Nutritional risk			
Body mass index ≤21	1	72/384 (18.8)	2.20
Mid-arm circumferences < norm	1	83/384 (21.6)	1.91
≥5% weight loss in previous 3 mo.	0.5	83/385 (21.6)	0.96
Any positive undernutrition factor	2.5	155/384 (40.4)	2.56
Visual deficit (<20/100 with lenses)	2	91/283 (32.2)	2.57
Hearing deficit by Whisper Test	1	90/317 (28.4)	1.45
Urinary or bowel incontinence	0.5	125/382 (32.7)	0.63
All medical problems combined†	26.2‡	839/385 (82.1)§	4.96
Dental and social problems			
No access to dentist		205/385 (53.2)	0.23
Unmet Social Service Needs		410/385 (51.9)§	1.32
All dental and social problems combined	3.7	615/385 (77.0)§	0.96
Medical, dental and social combined†	29.9‡	1454/385 (91.3)§	3.27

*Number of problems identified includes all previous categories in same section. In essence, this evaluates the effect of different cutpoint criteria for follow-up or referral.

†Includes all categories of positivity in medical problems, except "possible" delirium, which was excluded.

‡Actual time per evaluated subject. Not a simple sum of other times in column because not all measures were obtainable on all subjects.

§Percent of subjects who had at least 1 of the indicated problems.

Abbreviations: ADL, activities of daily living; *GDS,* Geriatric Depression Scale.

(Courtesy of Miller DK, Lewis LM, Nork MJ, et al: Controlled trial of a geriatric case-finding and liaison service in an emergency department. *J Am Geriatr Soc* 44(5):513–520, 1996.)

with the suggestions was 61.6% among the primary care physicians but only 36.6% among patients and families. There were few differences in outcomes at 3 months between the intervention and control patients. The intervention patients tended to have fewer visits to the ED and to have more new advance directives during follow-up than the control patients, but these differences were not statistically significant. In particular, the number of newly initiated dental and social services were similar in the 2 groups.

Conclusion.—The geriatric assessments identified a high number of geriatric problems in older patients visiting the ED. These problems, except possibly for dementia, could be identified at a reasonable cost. However, outcomes were not significantly affected by the intervention, largely because of the poor compliance of patients and families with the recommendations and the lack of control over care delivery after the ED visit.

▶ This study demonstrates the ability of an advanced practice nurse to identify functional, geriatric, dental, and social service needs of geriatric patients being seen in an inner city ED while they are waiting to be treated. To the degree that the purpose of the program was cost-effective case finding, the program was effective. However, the randomized intervention group who received information and referral for their unmet needs did not have significantly better outcomes on the measures tested. It is unrealistic to expect that providing patients with information and referrals for newly identified needs, unrelated to the reason for the ED visit, will produce outcomes such as decreased mortality or less frequent ED use or nursing home institutionalization 3 months later.

This study does, however, identify the importance of the ED as a site for identifying needs of underserved elderly without a primary care provider. A more intensive intervention that could move underserved elderly into a community-based system of primary care might, indeed, have positive outcomes, such as decreased use of the emergency room and better utilization of appropriate services.

S.K. Ostwald, Ph.D., R.N.

Decreased Hospital Utilization by Older Adults Attributable to a Home Hospitalization Program
Stessman J, Ginsberg G, Hammerman-Rozenberg R, et al (Hadassah Univ, Mount Scopus, Jerusalem; Inst of Geriatric Medicine, Jerusalem)
J Am Geriatr Soc 44:591–598, 1996   6–9

Background.—It is generally agreed that long-term home care for the elderly has many social and medical benefits. However, there is disagreement about the cost-effectiveness of home care vs. hospital care. There is little information about the comparative costs of short-term home care and acute and geriatric hospital care. To compare the cost-effectiveness of a short-term home health care program for the elderly and a regular ambulatory care program with hospitalization as needed, 2 programs were compared over a 26-month period.

Methods.—The Home Hospitalization program was initiated in 1991 with the goal of shortening or preventing hospitalizations. Patients older than 65 years were referred to this program (study group) or to routine medical care (control group), and the costs of the 2-programs were compared.

Results.—Costs were analyzed and compared for the first 26 months the Home Hospitalization program was in operation. During this time, 741 elderly patients received care for 37,290 days at an average daily cost of $30.06 in 1992 and $23.64 in 1993. In the study group, the average hospital stay per person decreased from 2.80 days in 1991 to 2.65 days in 1992, to 2.54 days in 1993. In the control group, the average hospital stay increased from 2.62 days in 1991 to 2.70 days in 1992, to 2.71 days in 1993. In the study group, the average geriatric hospital stay decreased from 1.49 days in 1991 to 1.34 days in 1992, to 1.33 days in 1993. In the control group, the average geriatric hospital stay decreased from 1.64 days in 1991 to 1.58 days in 1992, and then increased to 1.68 days in 1993. The estimated savings of $5.54 million for 20,773 general hospital days and $0.98 million for 8,486 geriatric hospital days was greater than the $0.97 million cost of the program. The cost-benefit ratio was 5.7:1. Patient satisfaction was high.

Conclusions.—Patients who were carefully selected and supported received cost-effective, technically advanced, short-term care in their home. A short-term program such as the Home Hospitalization program can reduce total health care costs associated with hospitalization in the elderly and may be suitable in other developed countries.

▶ Patients and families have consistently expressed the desire for health care delivery models that will increase the patient's ability to receive care at home. Although considerable discussion has occurred in the United States about the cost-effectiveness of community-based long-term care and its ability to substitute for nursing home care, little discussion has occurred about the use of short-term home care as a substitute for acute and subacute hospitalization.

These authors present a home hospital model in which patients older than 65 years with acute or subacute illnesses, who would otherwise be hospitalized, are cared for at home by a cadre of physicians, nurses, therapists, and ancillary personnel, and supported by the patients' family. During a 2-year period, they showed not only a high degree of patient satisfaction but also a decrease in hospitalization rates and a 5.7:1 cost-benefit ratio.

S.K. Ostwald, Ph.D., R.N.

Strategies for Educating Patients and Caregivers

Caregiving as Women's Work: Women's Experiences of Powerfulness and Powerlessness as Caregivers
Rutman D (Univ of Victoria, Canada)
Qual Health Res 6:90–111, 1996   6–10

Background.—Family caregiving is most frequently provided by women. To create public policy that supports these caregivers in social and material ways, an understanding of the caregiving experience and of what is needed to support caregiving is needed. Two groups of caregivers were brought together to describe factors that contribute to their feelings of powerlessness and powerfulness.

Methods.—Five unpaid family caregivers and 8 women who were professional caregivers in addition to their unpaid family caregiving responsibilities participated in workshops. During the workshops, the participants described an ideal caregiving situation and recounted situations in which they felt powerless and in which they felt powerful. The workshops were audiotaped, and the audiotapes were transcribed. The transcripts were coded and analyzed to identify themes and concepts related to powerfulness and powerlessness.

Results.—Caregiver powerlessness was related to 4 major themes: a lack of recognition of the caregiver's competence, a lack of control, clashes between the values and preferences of the caregiver and the care receiver, and the lack of responsiveness of the health care system. In addition, the family caregivers identified the need to suppress their own emotions as another cause of powerlessness. The caregivers reported feelings of powerfulness in response to the knowledge that their expertise was valued, the ability to make beneficial changes for the care receiver, the opportunity to share their knowledge and skills, and opportunities to take care of their own needs.

Conclusions.—Public policy that supports family caregiving should foster the full participation of these caregivers in personal and health care planning for the patient through recognition of the unique value of the knowledge the caregivers have of the patient's preferences, values, needs, and life history. The power differentials between family and professional caregivers must be eliminated. This may be partially accomplished by a redefinition of "care" to include and legitimate the nonmaterial, relational features of caregiving that can have real benefits for the patients. In addition, policies should be developed to promote caregiver self-care.

▶ This qualitative study of women's experiences as formal and informal caregivers expands our understanding of the concept of power as experienced by women who provide care to others. Themes of powerlessness and powerfulness cut across paid and unpaid caregivers. The critical incidents shared by caregivers make it clear that respect and recognition for their knowledge and competencies are central to their sense of power and/or

Chapter 6–Geriatric Nursing / **357**

fulfillment as caregivers. The message is clear that health care providers must recognize caregivers as partners and bridge the communication gulf between professional and family caregivers.

S.K. Ostwald, Ph.D., R.N.

Information Needs, Sources of Information, and Decisional Roles in Women With Breast Cancer
Bilodeau BA, Degner LF (Manitoba Cancer Treatment and Research Found, Winnipeg, Canada; Univ of Manitoba, Winnipeg, Canada)
Oncol Nurs Forum 23:691–696, 1996   6–11

Background.—To participate effectively in treatment decisions patients with cancer need information on treatment options and side effects, prognosis, and how to cope with the effects of their disease and its treatment. The preferred and actual roles of women with recently diagnosed breast cancer in treatment decisions, determined sources of information, and identified information needs were studied.

Methods.—Seventy-four women were included in the cross-sectional survey study. The patients performed control preferences card sorting, completed the Thurston scaling of information needs, and ranked information sources.

Findings.—Forty-three percent of women preferred and 57% assumed passive roles in the decision-making process. Older women especially preferred and assumed passive roles. Thirty-seven percent of the women preferred to have a collaborative role, although only 19% were able to take such roles (Table 2). Personal sources of information—physicians, nurses, friends, and relatives—were preferred to written sources. Women with higher levels of education found medical journals more relevant than those with less education. Most women's information needs included disease stage, the likelihood of being cured, and treatment options. Self-care and sexuality issues were ranked as least important. However, older women ranked self-care issues as more important (Fig 3).

Conclusions.—Personal sources of information were preferred to written sources among women with newly diagnosed breast cancer. Women who wish to take a collaborative role in treatment decisions may find it difficult to assume such a role.

TABLE 2.—Distribution of Preferred and Actual Roles in Treatment Decision Making

	Active Role	Collaborative Role	Passive Role
Preferred role	20%	37%	43%
Actual role	24%	19%	57%

Note: n = 74
(Bilodeau BA, Degner LF: Information needs, sources of information, and decisional roles in women with breast cancer. *Oncol Nurs Forum* 23:691–696, 1996.)

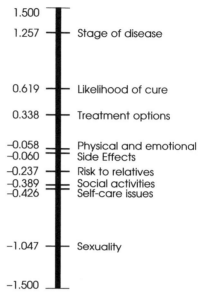

1.500
1.257 — Stage of disease

0.619 — Likelihood of cure
0.338 — Treatment options

−0.058 — Physical and emotional
−0.060 — Side Effects
−0.237 — Risk to relatives
−0.389 — Social activities
−0.426 — Self-care issues

−1.047 — Sexuality

−1.500

Scale Value for perceived relevance for each information
need (1.5 greatest relevance, −1.5 least relevance)

FIGURE 3.—Hierarchical profile of information needs of women recently diagnosed with breast cancer ($n = 74$). (Bilodeau BA, Degner LF: Information needs, sources of information, and decisional roles in women with breast cancer. *Oncol Nurs Forum* 23:691–696, 1996.)

▶ Although nurses and physicians believe they provide patients with adequate information about diagnoses and options, patients often disagree. This article presents an intriguing way to describe preferred and actual treatment decision roles and information needs of women newly diagnosed with breast cancer. Women newly diagnosed with breast cancer reported information about their disease as their most important need and information about sexuality as least important, in spite of articles to the contrary in the popular press. More women (43%), especially older women, preferred a passive role in treatment decisions. That same preference for a passive role (52%) was reported in a similar study of women newly diagnosed with breast cancer in the United Kingdom.[1] It is dangerous, however, to assume that all women prefer a passive role and not remain open to those who wish a collaborative or active role. Similar studies are under way in other countries that use the same card sort procedure to examine cultural differences in decision-making preferences.

Reference

S.K. Ostwald, Ph.D., R.N.

1. Beaver K, Luker KA, Owens RG, et al: Treatment decision making in women newly diagnosed with breast cancer. *Cancer Nursing* 19:8–19, 1996.

▶↓ Alzheimer's disease affects approximately 4 million individuals in the United States, devastating families as well as the individuals with the disease. Eventually most families will be forced to make decisions regarding life-sustaining treatments for their relatives. These 2 articles (Abstracts 6–12 and 6–13) illustrate a qualitative and a quantitative approach to this ethical dilemma. Hurley et al. present a 4-phase model for achieving consenses about treatment decisions for Alzheimer's patients, based on a qualitative analysis of observational and interview data obtained from nurse and family caregivers. This model supports the integration of clinical and ethical judgments and clarifies the importance of ongoing interactions between family members and health care providers.

S.K. Ostwald, Ph.D., R.N.

Reaching Consensus: The Process of Recommending Treatment Decisions for Alzheimer's Patients
Hurley AC, Volicer L, Rempusheski VF, et al (Edith Nourse Rogers Mem Veterans Hosp, Bedford, Mass; Northeastern Univ, Boston; Boston Univ; et al)
Adv Nurs Sci 18(2):33–43, 1995   6–12

Background.—When a patient with a terminal illness loses the capability to make decisions, family members and caregivers may experience uncertainty in treatment planning. Decision making in such circumstances is ethically guided by either the patient's self-determination (via an advance directive) or an effort to decide what options are in the patient's best interest. The nature of dementia of the Alzheimer's type (DAT) is such that decisions tend to be made by the latter method, by a designated surrogate decision maker and the health care team. This process of decision making was studied in a 25-bed dementia special care unit that offers a hospice approach to patients with DAT.

Methods.—At a family conference, the surrogate decision maker makes decisions about the level of care that the patient will be provided. This is termed the advance proxy plan. Nurses provide recommendations for the surrogate decision maker to consider and incorporate the advance proxy plan into the treatment plan. Data regarding this process were obtained through observation and interview of nurse caregivers and family surrogate decision makers at 15 consensus meetings, on the unit, and/or privately or through medical records.

Findings.—A model was developed for achieving consensus in decision making (Fig 1). The patient decline construct comprises the concepts of dignity, need for protection, quality of life, and regression. The degree to which the staff feels the surrogate decision maker is capable of carrying out his or her specific responsibilities is termed family coping; the staff must assess the surrogate decision maker's coping and attempt to enhance it. Staff professional development includes the abilities of the staff to help

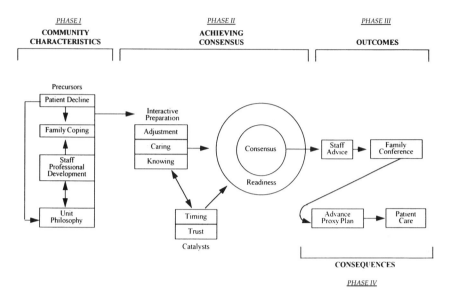

FIGURE 1.—Achieving consensus: The process of recommending treatment decisions for patients with Alzheimer's disease. (Courtesy of Hurley AC, Volicer L, Rempusheski VF: Reaching consensus: The process of recommending treatment decisions for Alzheimer's patients. *Adv Nurs Sci* 18(2):33–43, 1995. Copyright 1995 Aspen Publishers, Inc.)

build the surrogate decision maker's self-esteem and provide preparation, assurance of care, and reinforcement of the surrogate decision maker's power to change his or her mind. Unit philosophy refers to the ethical and clinical principles that undergird hospice care. Achieving consensus requires interactive preparation (adjustment, caring, and knowing) and the catalysts of timing and trust. Timing of decision making must reflect the most psychologically correct moment. Mutual respect and honesty between the staff and patient's family are crucial. After readiness of the family and staff is achieved, a dynamic group decision making mechanism results in staff consensus regarding the recommendation to be presented at the family conference. The SDM then makes decisions about provision of care.

Conclusions.—The concepts and constructs in this model met the criteria for judging the merits of a grounded theory study; they were empirically grounded and linked systematically in the data. Nurses cannot realistically separate assessment of the family from assessment of the patient. The integration of clinical and ethical judgments in designing patient care is supported by the model; practicing nurses need the opportunity to make such judgments appropriate to an advance proxy plan. Staff would also benefit from the opportunity to develop skills to facilitate consensus among family members and staff.

►↓ When presented with hypothetical situations, most of us indicate that, if we experienced severe cognitive decline, we would choose to forgo life-sustaining treatments. However, empirical studies such as this one raise questions about those hypothetical decisions. Although it is preliminary and hypothesis-generating, this study raises interesting questions about the factors that influence decisions and the role of health care providers in providing information and support, especially for those who choose to forgo life-sustaining treatments in the face of critical illness or coma in their spouses.

S.K. Ostwald, Ph.D., R.N.

Life-Sustaining Treatment Decisions by Spouses of Patients With Alzheimer's Disease
Mezey M, Kluger M, Maislin G, et al (New York Univ; Univ of Pennsylvania, Philadelphia)
J Am Geriatr Soc 44:144–150, 1996   6–13

Background.—The family members of many patients with Alzheimer's disease (AD) must make difficult decisions about life-sustaining treatment. However, no one to date has reported on how patient or proxy characteristics affect proxy decisions to consent to or forgo life-sustaining treatment.

Methods.—Fifty spouse caregivers of patients with AD were studied prospectively. Spouses were presented with 2 scenarios—critical illness and irreversible coma—and rated their agreement with, certainty of, and comfort with 4 treatments: resuscitation, breathing machine, feeding tube, and antibiotics. Eighteen patients had a durable power of attorney for health care, and 20 had a living will. Twenty-six had neither.

Findings.—Approximately half the spouses said they would forgo resuscitation for the patient with a critical illness; 28 would forgo a breathing machine; 21, a feeding tube; and 5, antibiotics. Five spouses said they

---

TABLE 2.—Spouses' Anticipated Decisions to Forgo Life-Sustaining Treatment in the Face of Critical Illness (*n* = 50) and Irreversible Coma (*n* = 50)

	Forgo Treatment				
	Critical Illness		Coma		
	n	%	*n*	%	*P* Value
Cardiopulmonary resuscitation	24	48	44	88	< 0.0001
Breathing machine	28	56	44	88	< 0.0001
Feeding Tube	21	42	42	86	< 0.0001
Antibiotics	5	10	34	68	< 0.0001
All four treatments	5	10	33	66	< 0.0001
All but antibiotics	17	34	42	84	< 0.0001

Note: McNemar's test for correlated proportions.
(Courtesy of Mezey M, Kluger M, Maislin G, et al: Life-sustaining treatment decisions by spouses of patients with Alzheimer's disease. *J Am Geriatr Soc* 44(2):144–150, 1996.)

TABLE 3.—Spouse Comfort With Anticipated Decision to Consent to or Forgo Treatment in the Face of Critical Illness (n = 50)

| | Comfort with Decision | | | | |
| | Consent to Tx | | Forgo Tx | | |
	n	%	n	%	P Value
Cardiopulmonary resuscitation	40	80	26	52	< 0.001
Breathing machine	37	74	28	56	< 0.001
Feeding tube	39	79	26	52	< 0.001
Antibiotics	47	93	20	40	< 0.001

Note: Chi-square test for independent samples.
(Courtesy of Mezey M, Kluger M, Maislin G, et al: Life-sustaining treatment decisions by spouses of patients with Alzheimer's disease. *J Am Geriatr Soc* 44(2):144–150, 1996.)

would forgo all treatments. Twelve said they would forgo all but antibiotics (Table 2). Spouses were significantly more likely to forgo treatment if the patient were in a coma than if he or she were critically ill. Spouses were also more certain about decisions related to coma. Certainty and comfort were significantly, positively correlated (Table 3). Spouses who said they would consent to treatment were more comfortable with their decisions than those who said they would forgo it. The spouses of patients with stage 7 disease were more likely to forgo resuscitation than the spouses of those with stages 4–6 disease. For the critical illness scenario, poorer quality of life (as rated by the spouses) was associated with a greater likelihood that spouses would forgo feeding tubes. Highly burdened spouses tended to consent to treatment.

Conclusions.—The spouses of patients with AD are likely to forgo life-sustaining treatment if the patient is in a coma. Spouses are less certain of their decisions in the event of critical illness. Health care professionals need to provide additional support to spouses who forgo treatment compared with those who consent to treatment. Spouses should be asked which factors are important to them when they make decisions about treatment.

Miscellaneous Long-term Care Issues

Multi-Site Study of Incidence of Pressure Ulcers and the Relationship Between Risk Level, Demographic Characteristics, Diagnoses, and Prescription of Preventive Interventions
Bergstrom N, Braden B, Kemp M, et al (Univ of Nebraska, Omaha; Creighton Univ, Omaha, Neb; Rush Univ, Chicago; et al)
J Am Geriatr Soc 44:22–30, 1996
6–14

Background.—Differences in past studies have made it difficult to compile consistent data on the incidence and etiology of pressure ulcers. The incidence of pressure ulcers in varied populations, demographic characteristics, and the impact of primary diagnosis on the development of pressure ulcers were determined in a cohort study.

Methods.—A total of 843 patients were randomly selected from 2 skilled nursing homes, 2 university tertiary care hospitals, and 2 Veterans'

TABLE 1.—Demographic Characteristics of Randomly Selected Subjects According to Pressure Ulcer Outcome (0,1,2) and Clinical Setting

Pressure Ulcer Outcome	Tertiary Care (n = 306)			Veteran Administration Medical Centers (n = 282)			Nursing Home (n = 255)			Total (n = 843)		
	0*	1†	2‡	0*	1†	2‡	0*	1†	2‡	0*	1†	2‡
Age												
n	280	9	17	261	8	13	194	18	43	735	35	73
X	53.8	61.7	61.2	62.4	65.6	65.9	73.0	73.6	79.7	61.9	68.7	72.9
SD	17.9	20.8	15.5	11.5	6.9	15.6	12.0	8.6	9.3	16.2	13.3	14.6
Range	19–99	28–84	36–86	25–91	54–73	42–102	29–92	56–91	55–95	19–99	38–91	36–102
F, df, P	(2.17, [2,303], P = NS)			(0.85, [2,279], P = NS)			(6.29, [2,252], P = .002)			(18.1, [2,840], P = .0001)		
Braden Scale Score												
n	280	9	17	261	8	13	194	18	43	735	35	73
X	19.4	19.8	17.4	20.5	17.9	15.4	19.3	17.4	16.1	19.8	18.1	16.3
SD	2.7	5.1	4.0	2.4	4.1	3.5	2.4	2.5	2.6	2.5	3.7	3.2
Range	11–23	8–23	9–23	11–23	12–23	9–22	9–23	12–21	10–22	8–23	8–23	9–23
F, df, P	(0.01, [2,303], P = NS)			(9.24, [2,279], P = .0001)			(13.19, [2,252], P = .0001)			(59.92, [2,840], P = .0001)		
Sex												
% Male	90	3	7	92	3	5	79	8	13	89	4	7
% Female	93	3	4	100	0	0	74	6	20	84	4	12
	(NS)			(NS)			(NS)			(χ^2 = 6.175, [2], P = .05)		
Race												
% White	89	4	7	92	4	4	74	8	18	85	5	10
% Black	100	0	0	93	0	7	91	3	6	95	<1	4
% Other	100	0	0	100	0	0	100	0	0	100	0	0
	(NS)			(NS)			(NS)			(P = <.003)		

*0 = No pressure ulcer.
†1 = Stage I pressure ulcer present on 2 consecutive observations.
‡2 = Stage II pressure ulcer present on at least 1 observation.
(Courtesy of Bergstrom N, Braden B, Kemp M, et al: Multi-site study of incidence of pressure ulcers and the relationship between risk level, demographic characteristics, diagnoses, and prescription of preventive interventions. J Am Geriatr Soc 44(1):22–30, 1996.)

TABLE 3.—Logistic Regression Predicting Pressure Ulcer Development Using Demographic Characteristics, Braden Scale Score, and Preventive Measures

	OR	95% CI	χ^2	P
Variables in Model				
Turning Prescription	.68	0.37–1.22	1.68	.195
Pressure Reduction	.80	0.49–1.30	0.81	.368
Braden Scale	1.30	1.19–1.41	36.05	< .001
Age	.97	0.95–0.98	15.56	< .001
Race	2.73	1.25–5.98	6.29	.012
Sex	0.93		0.08	.773
Intercept			1.60	.206
Model χ^2			121.80	< .001
Degrees of Freedom			6	

(Courtesy of Bergstrom N, Braden B, Kemp M, et al: Multi-site study of incidence of pressure ulcers and the relationship between risk level, demographic characteristics, diagnoses, and prescription of preventive interventions. *J Am Geriatr Soc* 44(1):22–30, 1996.)

Administration Medical Centers (VAMCs). The patients had no pressure ulcers on admission. Sixty-three percent of the patients were male, and 79% were white. The mean age was 63 years (Table 1).

Findings.—Pressure ulcers developed in 12.8% of the patients. The incidence was 8.5% in tertiary care centers, 7.4% in VAMCs, and 23.9% in nursing homes. In a logistic regression analysis, factors that predicted pressure ulcers were lower Braden Scale scores, older age, and white race. When the Braden Scale score was included in the regression, primary diagnosis did not significantly predict the development of pressure ulcers. Braden Scale scores and white race predicted use of turning, whereas Braden Scale scores, white race, and female sex predicted use of pressure reduction (Tables 3, 4, and 6).

Conclusions.—The basis of prescriptive decisions for the prevention of pressure ulcers should be risk assessment rather than primary diagnosis or demographic factors. Risk assessment should enable health care providers to make better use of turning and support surfaces.

TABLE 4.—Logistic Regression Models Predicting Pressure Ulcer Development Using the Braden Score or Mobility and Activity Subscale Scores and Selected Primary Diagnoses

	Braden Scale not in Model				Braden Scale in Model			
	OR	95% CI	χ^2	P	OR	95% CI	χ^2	P
Variables in Model								
Braden Scale					1.37	1.28, 1.48	75.76	< .001
Mobility	1.72	1.27–2.33	12.21	< .001				
Activity	1.46	1.13–1.88	8.20	.004				
Cardiovascular Diagnosis	2.49	1.14–5.48	5.18	.023				
Intercept			5.5	.018			36.31	< .001
Model χ^2			48.04	< .001			85.36	< .001
Degrees of Freedom			2				1	

(Courtesy of Bergstrom N, Braden B, Kemp M, et al: Multi-site study of incidence of pressure ulcers and the relationship between risk level, demographic characteristics, diagnoses, and prescription of preventive interventions. *J Am Geriatr Soc* 44(1):22–30, 1996.)

TABLE 6.—Logistic Regression Predicting Prescriptive Practices in Pressure Ulcer Prevention Based on Level of Risk (Braden Scale Score), Age, Race, and Sex

	Turning				Pressure Reduction			
	OR	95% CI	χ^2	P	OR	95% CI	χ^2	P
Variables in models								
Braden Scale	1.6	1.45–1.73	103.83	< .001	1.29	1.22–1.37	73.80	< .001
Age	.99	0.98–1.01	.02	.893	1.00	0.99–1.01	0.21	.645
Race	2.66	1.21–5.81	6.02	.014	1.90	1.26–2.86	9.39	.002
Sex	.94	0.58–1.53	.06	.806	.32	0.23–0.43	50.64	< .001
Intercept			38.61	< .001			22.75	< .001
Model χ^2			161.66	< .001			168.57	< .001
Degrees of Freedom			4				4	

(Courtesy of Bergstrom N, Braden B, Kemp M, et al: Multi-site study of incidence of pressure ulcers and the relationship between risk level, demographic characteristics, diagnoses, and prescription of preventive interventions. *J Am Geriatr Soc* 44(1):22–30, 1996.)

▶ Pressure ulcers are a persistent and costly threat to institutionalized frail elderly, and the annual cost of pressure ulcer treatment in the United States is as high as $7 million. The 1992 publication of the Agency for Health Care Policy and Research Clinical Practice Guidelines, *Pressure Ulcers in Adults: Prediction and Prevention*, established the standard for assessment and prevention in all settings.[1] The nurse researchers in this article found an average incidence rate of 12.8% in a sample of 843 residents followed up for up to 4 weeks in 6 long-term care settings in 3 geographical regions. These findings, together with those of Olson, Langemo, Burd, et al., who found an incidence rate of 13.4% over 2 weeks for patients admitted to an acute care setting,[2] emphasize the importance of implementing a formal system of need assessment and aggressive prevention protocols for all institutionalized elderly on admission to the facility.

S.K. Ostwald, Ph.D., R.N.

References

1. Panel for the Prediction and Prevention of Pressure Ulcers in Adults: *Pressure Ulcers in Adults: Prediction and Prevention.* Clinical Practice Guideline, number 3. Rockville, MD, Agency for Health Care Policy and Research, 1992 Public Health Service, US Dept of Health and Human Services, AHCPR publication 92-0047.
2. Olson B, Langemo D, Burd C, et al: Pressure ulcer incidence in an acute care setting. *J Wound Ostomy Continence Nurs* 23:15–22, 1996.

Physical Restraint Use and Falls in Nursing Home Residents
Capezuti E, Evans L, Strumpf N, et al (Univ of Pennsylvania, Philadelphia)
J Am Geriatr Soc 44:627–633, 1996   6–15

Objective.—Although elderly nursing home residents are sometimes restrained to prevent falls, studies indicate that restraints not only do not lower the risk of falls but may increase the risk of restraint-related death or injury. The association between restraint use and falls was examined in a longitudinal clinical trial of nursing home residents comparing fall rates among residents consistently restrained and never restrained.

Methods.—Restraint status was determined by nurse interviewers at 3 time points approximately 1 month apart. Each determination was made twice a day during a 72-hour period. The number of times a resident was restrained was recorded. Restraint scores of 1–27 were classified as "low," whereas scores of 28–54 were classified as "high." Falls, injuries, cognitive status, and psychoactive drug use were recorded. The results were analyzed statistically using chi-square tests and multivariate analysis.

Results.—The 322 residents were 84% female, 95% white, and had an average age of 84 years. Of these, 119 were restrained. There were 149 residents who had at least 1 fall and 85 who fell 2 or more times. There were no injuries in 63 falls, minor injuries in 68, and serious injuries in 18. Ambulatory residents accounted for 55.2% of falls and nonambulatory residents for 34.8%; nonconfused residents accounted for 48.1%, confused residents for 45%, nonrestrained residents for 49.3%, and restrained residents for 41.2%. The risks of falls (1.65) and recurrent falls (2.46) were highest in the restrained confused ambulatory subgroup. The risks of falls and recurrent falls for the rest of the residents were 0.49 and 0.42. The injury rate from falls was highest in the high-intensity restraint group (39%) as compared with the low-intensity restraint group (25.6%). Nonconfused nonambulatory restrained patients had a fall risk of 0.28, a recurrent fall risk of 0.48, and an injury risk of 0.42 (Table 4). Residents

TABLE 4.—Effect of Restraint Use on Fall/Injury Risk in 3 Subgroups of Nursing Home Residents

	Adjusted Odds Ratio and 95% CI			
Outcome	Confused Ambulatory ($n = 89$)	Confused Nonambulatory ($n = 102$)	Nonconfused Nonambulatory ($n = 39$)	Tests for Significance* Chi-square/P
Falls	1.24 (0.49, 3.14)	0.81 (0.32, 2.01)	0.28 (0.05, 1.58)	2.41, $P=.30$
Recurrent falls	2.11 (0.84, 5.33)	0.32 (0.11, 0.97)	0.48 (0.05, 4.72)	6.79, $P=.03$
Fall with any injury	1.58 (0.62, 4.04)	2.50 (0.75, 8.35)	0.42 (0.04, 4.01)	2.25, $P=.33$

*Interaction chi-square derived from multiple logistic regression ($df = 2$) controlling for psychoactive drug use.
Abbreviation: CI, confidence interval.
(Courtesy of Capezuti E, Evans L, Strumpf N, et al: Physical restraint use and falls in nursing home residents. *J Am Geriatr Soc* 44(6):627–633, 1996.)

who received psychoactive drugs had a fall risk of 1.78 when compared with residents who did not receive such drugs.

Clinical Significance.—The use of restraints does not significantly lower the risk of falls or injuries from falls in nursing home residents, regardless of cognitive status. Restraint use and psychotropic drug use may actually increase the risk of falls. These findings suggest that interventions to promote mobility may be beneficial in reducing the risk of falls.

Conclusions.—Restraints do not lower the risk of falls or injuries from falls in nursing home residents. The use of psychoactive drugs increases the risk of falls.

▶ Physical restraints continue to be used in nursing homes in spite of the accumulating data suggesting that restraints do not prevent falls and may cause serious problems such as pressure ulcers, contractures, incontinence, muscle weakness, and increased confusion. This article adds to the increasing evidence that restraints are not associated with a significantly lower risk of falls or injuries, especially among those residents of concern to nursing staff because of their wandering and poor judgment. For this group of confused ambulatory residents, who are most likely to be restrained, restraint use in this study was actually associated with increased falls, as well as recurrent falls. Despite the methodologic limitations of the studies in this area, it is clear that the current direction of developing restraint-free environments is appropriate and that the outdated practice of routinely applying restraints to residents to prevent falls should be abolished.

S.K. Ostwald, Ph.D., R.N.

Nurses' Acceptance of Behavioral Treatments and Pharmacotherapy for Behavioral Disturbances in Older Adults
Burgio LD, Hardin JM, Sinnott J, et al (Univ of Alabama, Birmingham; Towson State Univ, Md; Univ of Pittsburgh, Pa; et al)
Appl Nurs Res 8(4):174–181, 1995   6–16

Background.—Elderly patients often demonstrate behavioral disturbances. These have traditionally been managed with pharmacotherapy, usually neuroleptic medication. However, this practice has recently been questioned with the development of behavioral interventions. The clinical recommendation of behavioral interventions is largely dependent on their acceptability. Therefore, the acceptability of 2 behavioral treatments and haloperidol was investigated in a group of nurses with a special interest in geriatric patients.

Methods.—A random sample of nurses who were members of the Gerontological Society of America were sent 1 of 12 vignette conditions that varied the patient's cognitive capacity, living situation, and medical problem. The respondents were asked to evaluate the appropriateness of treatment with differential reinforcement of incompatible behavior (DRI), time-out from positive reinforcement (time-out), and haloperidol. Also included was a demographic survey form and the Treatment Evaluation Inventories to measure the effects of the patient's cognitive capacity, living situation, and medical problem on treatment acceptability.

Results.—Acceptability differed significantly, with the DRI procedure receiving the highest acceptability ratings, followed by time-out and finally haloperidol. Acceptability of the treatments was significantly related to the patient's living situation and cognitive capacity. In addition, the nurse's education, age, and experience with geriatric patients were significantly related to acceptability ratings.

Conclusions.—To nurses with a special interest in geriatric issues, it is more acceptable to treat behavioral disturbances in elderly patients with behavioral treatments than with pharmacotherapy. Their acceptance is mediated by both personal and patient factors.

▶ Behavioral interventions, long used by psychologists, are gaining acceptance among other health professionals. In previous research, Burgio et al. demonstrated that physicians assigned higher acceptability ratings to behavioral treatments for behavioral disturbances in older adults and the lowest ratings to haloperidol.[1] In this article, Burgio and colleagues explore nurses' acceptance of behavioral treatments and haloperidol for patients with behavioral disturbances who reside in nursing homes and community settings. Like physicians, nurses rated the acceptability of behavioral treatments higher than haloperidol, with nurses with the most contact with geriatric patients and specialty training in geriatrics or gerontology showing the greatest acceptance of behavioral treatments. This acceptability among nurses is especially important because in nursing homes and home health care settings, nurses play the dominant role in both choosing and supervising the use of behavioral interventions.

S.K. Ostwald, Ph.D., R.N.

Reference

1. Burgio LD, Sinnott J, Janosky JE, et al: Physician's acceptance of behavioral treatments and pharmacotherapy for behavioral disturbances in older adults. *Gerontologist* 32:546–551, 1992.

Nursing Interventions to Promote Functional Feeding
van Ort S, Phillips LR (Univ of Arizona, Tucson)
J Gerontol Nurs Oct:6–14, 1995   6–17

Background.—Patients with dementia typically demonstrate a decline in self-feeding abilities as their cognitive ability declines, which puts them at increased risk for malnutrition and weight loss. Staff feeding activities typically do not encourage or maintain patient autonomy and become increasingly time-consuming and difficult. Contextual and behavioral nursing interventions were designed to encourage functional feeding in demented patients in long-term care. The efficacy of these interventions were evaluated.

Methods.—Eight demented residents who required feeding assistance, but were able to sit in a chair, interact with the caregiver, and were not typically combative, were studied. The residents were weighed and videotaped during 2 lunches and 2 dinners at baseline. The contextual intervention was then implemented for 2 weeks, after which the subjects were videotaped and weighed again. In the contextual intervention, all noise and distractions were minimized, all subjects were seated at the table next to self-feeding residents with the food and their name card directly in front of them, finger food was placed in the subjects' hands, and feeder interruptions were avoided until the meal was over. The behavioral intervention was then used with 4 subjects, after which they were again videotaped and weighed. This intervention included the use of individualized verbal and tactile prompts, role modeling, cue synchronization, and reinforcement to elicit and sustain feeding behaviors. The videotapes were coded to determine changes in feeding behaviors.

Results.—Both interventions produced more sustained feeding-related behaviors, improved the match between the resident's functional abilities and the level of assistance offered by the feeder, and maintained the residents' weights. No more time was required for feeding with the contextual intervention, even though the residents ate and drank more, refused less, and demonstrated more self-feeding, food touching, and interaction with the feeder. The behavioral intervention did require more time, but increased independent self-feeding.

Conclusions.—Nursing interventions to modify the feeding environment can promote self-feeding without an increase in the time and resources needed for meals. A behavioral intervention that used systematic prompting, cuing, and behavioral guidance also promoted self-feeding, although it did require more time. Both interventions promoted self-feeding and maintained the weight of the residents. Nursing interventions can be implemented for demented older adults in a long-term care setting to promote functional feeding and improve the mealtime interaction.

▶ As dementia increases, caregivers report less self-feeding, which results in weight loss and increased time devoted to feeding activities. Family caregivers and nursing home staff often find feeding activities to be frustrating, as well as time consuming. Researchers have shown that aggressive behaviors are increased around mealtimes for patients with dementia. As described in this article, nursing interventions that modify the environment (contextual) and match the caregiver's level of assistance with the resident's ability (behavioral) resulted in the consumption of more food, more self-feeding, and no decrease in weight. Nurses who work in long-term care settings may find the Feeding Behaviors Inventory developed by Durnbaugh, Haley and Roberts to be helpful in the assessment of problem feeding behaviors.[1] In addition, specific menus and strategies to increase self-feeding among patients with dementia are discussed by Ford.[2]

S.K. Ostwald, Ph.D., R.N.

References

1. Durnbaugh T, Haley B, Roberts S: Assessing problem feeding behaviors in mid-stage Alzheimer's disease. *Geriatr Nurs* 17:63–67, 1996.
2. Ford G: Putting feeding back into the hands of patients. *J Psychosoc Nurs* 34:35–39, 1996.

Behavioral Analysis and Nursing Interventions for Reducing Disruptive Behaviors of Patients With Dementia
Boehm S, Whall AL, Cosgrove KL, et al (Univ of Michigan, Ann Arbor, Gerontology Metro Medical Group, Allen Park, Mich)
Appl Nurs Res 8(3):118–122, 1995   6–18

Background.—Psychological research has developed several effective behavioral interventions for use with elderly patients. Behavioral interventions are based on behavioral analysis, and focus on antecedent events, the small steps of the behavior that require intervention, and the consequences of the behavior. These observations then inform behavioral modeling. The feasibility of using behavioral analysis and behavioral modeling in designing a nursing intervention to decrease disruptive and abusive behaviors in elderly, institutionalized patients was studied.

Methods.—Selected staff members in 2 nursing homes were trained in the principles of behavioral analysis and observed and recorded the disruptive behaviors of 1 selected patient with dementia in each institution, along with the antecedents and consequences of these behaviors. These observations were used to develop a behavioral plan for each of the 2 patients, which was implemented by trained staff. Disruptive behaviors during bathing with 1 patient and during shaving with the other patient were observed while the individualized behavioral plan was being implemented, when the plan was withdrawn, and again during a second intervention phase.

Results.—The baseline observation sessions included 6–9 disruptive and abusive behaviors by the 2 patients. These behaviors were reduced to 0–1 when the behavior plan was implemented during both intervention phases. When the intervention was withdrawn, the disruptive behaviors returned with similar frequencies. The implementation of the behavioral plan resulted in a reduced need for nursing staff resources, with only 1 (compared with 4) staff members needed for bathing and shaving.

Conclusions.—The use of behavioral analysis to design nursing interventions, including systematic cues and consequences, is a feasible approach for the reduction of disruptive and abusive behavior in patients with dementia.

▶ This small feasibility study addresses a problem frequently encountered in nursing homes: disruptive and aggressive behaviors exhibited by persons with dementia during personal cares, such as bathing. The authors use modeling to teach nurses how to use behavioral analysis to design nursing interventions. Although most of the literature in behavioral gerontology is found in the field of psychology, behavioral interventions clearly have implications for nursing practice. These findings suggest that nurses who use behavioral analysis can recognize cues and consequences that support disruptive behaviors and alter their approach to provide systematic cues and consequences that support cooperative behavior in patients.

S.K. Ostwald, Ph.D., R.N.

Effects of Work Stressors and Work Climate on Long-term Care Staff's Morale and Functioning
Schaefer JA, Moos RH (Ctr for Health Care Evaluation, Palo Alto, Calif; Stanford Univ, Calif)
Res Nurs Health 19:63–73, 1996   6–19

Background.—There is increasing evidence of associations between work stressors and a negative work climate and distress, low job satisfaction, decreased job performance, and physical and mental health problems among health care staff members. Most of this research has been cross-sectional, which limits understanding of the effects of these factors over time. Therefore the relationships between work stressors and climate and job morale and functioning were analyzed in long-term health care staff members surveyed twice at an interval of 8 months.

Methods.—A total of 405 long-term staff members from 14 nursing facilities completed the Work Stressors Inventory, which assesses supervisor/physician relationships, general job tasks, patient care tasks, and workload and scheduling, and the Work Environment Scale, which assesses coworker cohesion, autonomy, and clarity. The respondents also completed a questionnaire measuring job satisfaction, intent to stay, and job-related distress. These questionnaires were completed again 8 months later. The contributions of work stressors and work climate to job morale and functioning were analyzed in multivariate analyses controlling for age, race, and job position.

Results.—There was little change over time in work stressors, work climate, job morale, or job functioning. Problems in the supervisor/physician relationships were associated with decreased job satisfaction and intent to stay and increased job-related distress. Increased job task stressors correlated with job-related distress, depressed mood, and physical symptoms, whereas increased patient care task stressors correlated with greater job satisfaction. Workload and scheduling stressors were the strongest predictors of poor job morale and functioning. These work stressor indices explained 5% to 21% of the morale and functioning variance.

Work climate plus work stressor variables explained 13% to 33% of the variance in staff morale and functioning. Greater co-worker cohesion was associated with increased job satisfaction and intent to stay. Job satisfaction was also positively related to job clarity. More autonomy was associated with more intent to stay and less distress.

Work stressors were more predictive of staff morale and functioning at follow-up than were work climate variables, which were nevertheless still significant. As predictors of staff outcome at follow-up, the initial assessments of work stressors were only significant in relation to job-related distress, depressed mood, and physical symptoms, but not job morale. Initial assessments of the work climate did not significantly predict follow-up staff outcomes.

Conclusions.—Both work stressors and work climate significantly and independently affect job morale and functioning in long-term health care staff members. The importance of good working relationships to staff morale indicates that system-level interventions to change the work environment should be designed as well as education and in-service interventions.

▶ Documentaries about the horrors of nursing homes contribute to the general public's perspective that long-term care facilities are stressful and undesirable places to work. Furthermore, high rates of turnover among staff, especially unlicensed staff members, support the perception that the work is unrewarding. On the contrary, Schaefer and Moos found that it is the system stressors and work climate, not the patient care demands, that have the broadest negative impact on staff. Stresses related to caring for chronically ill and dying patients with complex needs enhanced the staff's sense of self-confidence and were linked to more job satisfaction and less job-related distress, depression, and physical symptoms. As is true with other types of caregivers, long-term care staff members are able to provide a better quality of care over time when they are supported, respected, and empowered to cope within a cohesive work group.

S.K. Ostwald, Ph.D., R.N.

Subject Index*

A

Abdominal
cramping after radiation therapy for
prostate cancer localized to pelvis,
96: 68
pain
myocardial infarction and,
unrecognized, *96:* 89
after radiation therapy for prostate
cancer localized to pelvis, *96:* 68
Abuse, *95:* 163–164
alcohol
delirium after elective noncardiac
surgery and, *95:* 92
in general practice, use of brief
screening instruments for, *96:* 228
risk factors for, *95:* 163
Accident
motor vehicle, and Alzheimer's disease,
95: 278
ACE (*see* Angiotensin, -converting enzyme
inhibitors)
Acetaminophen
protective effect in Alzheimer's disease,
96: 278
Acetohexamide
hypoglycemia and, serious, *97:* 70
2-Acetylaminofluorene
-induced DNA repair in hepatocytes (in
rat), *95:* 317
Acetylcholine
endothelium-dependent
hyperpolarization in mesenteric
artery to (in rat), *95:* 337
Activity(ies)
associated with successful aging, *97:* 2
of daily living
hierarchical structure, *95:* 62
limitations in, and cognitive
functioning, *96:* 208
tests in detecting, staging, and
tracking Alzheimer's disease,
97: 166
limitation in hospitalized patients, and
pressure ulcer risk factors, *96:* 107
physical (*see* Physical, activity)
Acupuncture
after stroke, effect on functional
outcome, *95:* 301
Acute care
Acute Care for Elders, randomized trial
of, *96:* 51

issues in long-term care, *96:* 169–177
settings, inaccessibility of advance
directives on transfer from
ambulatory setting to, *97:* 117
Acutely ill
functional outcomes of, randomized
trial of care in hospital medical
unit especially designed to improve,
96: 51
ADDTC
diagnostic criteria for vascular
dementia, comparison with other
diagnostic criteria, *97:* 244
Adenohypophysis
prolactin release from, basal and
dopamine-inhibited (in rat),
95: 327
Adenosine
adenylyl cyclase sensitivity to, effect of
increased concentrations of proteins
G_i1 and G_i2 on, *96:* 350
triphosphatase activities in atrophic,
angulated skeletal muscle fibers (in
rat), *95:* 351
Adenylyl cyclase
activation in adipocytes, age-dependent
changes in (in rat), *96:* 360
sensitivity to inhibitory and stimulatory
agonists, effect of increased
proteins G_i1 and G_i2 on (in rat),
96: 349
Adhesion
molecules, recombinant, chemokines
regulate T cell adherence to,
97: 283
Adipocytes
beta-adrenergic subtypes and adenylyl
cyclase activation in, age-dependent
changes in (in rat), *96:* 360
differentiation promoted by
prostaglandin J_2 metabolite,
97: 313
gene expression in, impaired
β-adrenergic receptor-mediated
regulation of (in rat), *96:* 352
proteins G_i1 and G_i2 concentration
increase in, and sensitivity of
adenylyl cyclase to inhibitory and
stimulatory agonists (in rat),
96: 349
Adipose
tissue, components of renin-angiotensin
system in (in rat), *97:* 314

---

* *All entries refer to the year and page number(s) for data appearing in this and previous
editions of the* YEAR BOOK.

373

Author Index